Speech Audiometry

UK   Taylor & Francis Ltd, 4 John St, London WC1N 2ET

USA   Taylor & Francis Inc., 242 Cherry St, Philadelphia, PA
19106–1906

Copyright © Taylor & Francis Ltd 1987

British Library Cataloguing in Publication Data

Speech audiometry.
   1. Audiometry   2. Hearing disorders—Diagnosis
   I. Martin, Michael, *1933–*
   617.8'8607544   RF294

   ISBN 0-85066-641-4
   ISBN 0-85066-638-4 (pbk)

Library of Congress Cataloging-in-Publication Data

Speech audiometry.
   Bibliography: p.
   Includes index.
   1. Audiometry, Speech.   I. Martin, Michael, OBE.
[DNLM: 1. Audiometry, Speech.   2. Hearing Disorders—
diagnosis.   3. Speech Perception.   WV 272 S7417]
RF294.5.S6S625   1987   617.8'075   87–10074

Typeset by
Katerprint Typesetting Services, Oxford
Printed in Great Britain by
Redwood Burn Ltd, Trowbridge, Wiltshire.

CONTENTS

List of Contributors   vii

Preface   ix
M. Martin

1   **Basic Properties of Speech**   1
    R. Wright

2   **Towards a Theory of Speech Audiometry Tests**   33
    P. Lyregaard

3   **Speech Tests in Quiet and Noise as a Measure of Auditory Processing**   63
    M.E. Lutman

4   **Equipment for Speech Audiometry and its Calibration**   75
    H. Fuller

5   **The German Path to Standardization in Speech Audiometry**   89
    K. Brinkmann

6   **Speech Audiometry for Differential Diagnosis**   109
    P.I.P. Evans

7   **The Uses and Misuses of Speech Audiometry in Rehabilitation**   129
    R. Green

8   **Speech Tests of Hearing for Children**   155
    A. Markides

9   **Speech Perception Tests for the Profoundly Deaf**   171
    A.B. King

10   **Testing Visual and Auditory Visual Speech Perception**   179
    G. Plant and J. Macrae

11   **Speech Audiometry in the USA**   207
    B. Kruger and R.M. Mazor

12   **The Scandinavian Approach to Speech Audiometry**   237
    S. Arlinger

13   **Speech Audiometry in Australia**   247
    J. Bench

14   **Speech Tests in Audiological Assessment at the National Acoustic Laboratories**   255
    P. Dermody and K. Mackie

15   **Some Aspects of Speech Tests in Non-European Languages**   279
    J.J. Knight

Appendix: Equipment for Speech Audiometry: A Draft Standard   287

References   295

Index   319

ACKNOWLEDGMENTS

I am grateful to Mark Lutman of the MRC Institute of Hearing Research for encouraging me to proceed with editing this book when he was unable to join me in the venture.

The advice and encouragement of Mary Plackett, Chief Librarian of the RNID, is much appreciated as is the help of the library staff.

Finally, the support of Margaret, my wife, in putting up with the editing that occupied so much time at home is greatly appreciated.

CONTRIBUTORS

S. Arlinger
Department of Audiology
Regionsjukhuset (RiL)
581 85 Linkoping
Sweden

J. Bench
Lincoln Institute of Health Sciences
School of Communication Disorders
625 Swanston Street
Carlton, Vic. 3053
Australia

K. Brinkmann
Physikalisch-Technische
Bundesanstalt
Postfach 3345
D–3300 Braunschweig
FR Germany

P. Dermody
National Acoustic Laboratories
126 Greville Street
Chatswood, NSW 2067
Australia

P.I.P. Evans
Audiology and Human Effects
Group
Institute of Sound and Vibration
Research
The University
Southampton
Hampshire SO9 5NH
UK

H. Fuller
National Physical Laboratory
Teddington
Middlesex TW11 0LW
UK

R. Green
Audiology Unit
Royal Berkshire Hospital
London Road
Reading
Berkshire RG1 5AN
UK

A.B. King
The Royal National Institute for the
Deaf
105 Gower Street
London WC1E 6AH

J.J. Knight (Retd.)
Institute of Laryngology and Otology
Grays Inn Road
London WC1
UK

B. Kruger
Kruger Associates
37 Somerset Drive
Commack
NY 11725
USA

M.E. Lutman
MRC Institute of Hearing Research
University of Nottingham
University Park
Nottingham NG7 2RD
UK

P. Lyregaard
Oticon Research Unit
Eriksholm
243 Kongevejen
DK-3070 Denmark

K. Mackie
Speech Communication Research
Section
National Acoustic Laboratories
126 Greville Street
Chatswood, NSW 2067
Australia

J. Macrae
National Acoustic Laboratories
126 Greville Street
Chatswood, NSW 2067
Australia

A. Markides
Department of Audiology and
Education of the Deaf
Manchester University
Manchester
UK

R.M. Mazor
Audiology & Speech Language
Pathology
Department of Otorhinolaryngology
Albert Einstein College of Medicine
1300 Morris Park Avenue
Bronx, NY 10461
USA

G. Plant
National Acoustic Laboratories
126 Greville Street
Chatswood NSW 2067
Australia

R. Wright
The Royal National Institute for the
Deaf
105 Gower Street
London WC1E 6AH

Preface

The idea for this book originated from the first of a series of one day courses entitled Updates in Audiology put on by the British Society of Audiology (BSA) in 1983. The Education Committee of the BSA originated the idea of a series of one day courses which would be aimed at experienced workers in the broad field of audiology who it was felt would appreciate short courses that would not teach basics but would refresh and update their knowledge on current practice in areas that they were not particularly expert in. It was not intended that these courses should be reviews of research activities, but of course would take note of the relevance of research to current practice.

The first course, which was organised by Mark Lutman from the MRC Institute of Hearing Research and myself, was greatly oversubscribed and it became apparent that not only was there a great interest in the subject but there was a clear gap in the perception of what speech audiometry was thought to be able to do and what its advantages and disadvantages really were. Furthermore, although the subject is often written about in learned journals there was limited information available suitable for the average practitioner dealing with the day to day handling of patients. This book however is not a textbook but aims to draw attention to what is important in the many varied aspects of speech audiometry.

While the BSA course was intended to reflect practice in the UK it was apparent that much could be learned from practices elsewhere, Consequently a number of colleagues around the world were asked if they would contribute on the practices from their own countries or areas. I am very grateful to them for broadening the scope of this book to give it an international dimension that is so important today; no one can now afford to work in a multidisciplinary field such as audiology without being aware of developments in other countries.

The first two chapters of the book deal with the basics of speech production and perception and an approach to a theoretical basis for speech audiometry. In the UK, many practitioners of speech audiometry, because of their training, have little appreciation of the complexities of speech perception, and Richard Wright's Chapter sets out a hierarchical approach that poses the question as to what needs to be considered in undertaking speech audiometry, but leaves us to answer the question! Paul Lyregaard states that 'our knowledge of the factors mediating speech intelligibility is rudimentary', which in itself is a sobering thought for those undertaking speech audiometry, but sets out a theoretical framework which gives an understanding of the problems involved and indicates the wide variance that can occur with different tests, a point that other contributors refer to and which many practitioners largely ignore.

Mark Lutman then looks at the effect of noise on speech perception as this is probably the most difficult problem that faces hearing aid users and which is often not taken into account, as speech audiometry is normally undertaken in quiet.

There is overwhelming support from all contributors that the use of recorded material is essential in order to obtain reliability in all but a few circumstances. This therefore requires that the equipment used for this purpose is calibrated and capable of producing speech of reasonable quality. Hilary Fuller draws attention to equipment and calibration needs and appended to her chapter is the outline of a draft proposal on the technical requirements for speech audiometers produced by the working group, WG19, of IEC Technical Committee 29. It will remain to be seen whether or not this, in some form, is acceptable in the future as an international standard. Very few countries have progressed very far in standardizing speech audiometry due to the difficulties involved. West Germany is an exception to this and Klaus Brinkmann describes the background and current state of the relatively advanced level of standardization that now exists in Germany. Of note in this and other chapters is the start of the use of Compact Audio Discs for recording and replaying speech test material.

The audio disc under microprocessor control has very considerable advantages for speech audiometry in that it can store very large amounts of speech material with very high quality on one side of a disc. The disc is also almost indestructable and with microprocessor control can be made to reproduce very precisely and rapidly any item recorded in any order. However, great care has to be taken in the preparation of the material before it is recorded owing to the very high cost of producing the initial masters.

Chapters 6, 7 and 8 then deal with the areas which are usually associated most closely with speech audiometry, i.e., differential diagnosis, rehabilitation and the testing of children.

Phillip Evans points out the small range of material used in the UK and in particular the use of monosyllabic words rather than spondees which are widely used in the USA. He draws attention to methods of scoring and recording speech audiometric results for diagnostic purposes as well as describing test procedures. Methods for differentiating sensory and peripheral disorders are discussed.

One of the widest uses of speech audiometry is in rehabilitation and Roger Green's chapter may well cause concern to some readers as he questions many of its uses. In particular, he reinforces Paul Lyregaard's material on minimal differences for significantly different scores and shows the differences required for some current materials.

Andreas Markides describes speech tests of hearing for children setting out the criteria and material used in the UK, particularly that which originates from Manchester University.

Speech audiometry has tended to make an unwritten assumption that the person being tested can understand at least some of the material being presented. Profoundly deaf people in most cases will achieve a zero score on conventional speech material, but this is not to say that they do not discriminate some parts of speech. Angela King describes techniques that begin to determine what abilities profoundly deaf people have for understanding speech, even if that understanding is far from complete.

Geoff Plant and John Macrae then describe ways in which the ability to lipread, or speechread, can be assessed. As is well known, the visual and audiovisual path is important for people with even small degrees of hearing loss but becomes crucial for those with severe, profound and total losses. This aspect is of course not covered by tests which use only an auditory test signal and therefore may well not give a true picture of the communication abilities of the deaf person. The authors stress the importance of the tests in attempting to provide a comprehensive aural rehabilitation programme for hearing impaired people.

The remaining chapters in the book deal with the practice of speech audiometry in the USA, Scandinavia and Australia. Barbara Kruger and Rosemarie Mazor comprehensively review the status of speech audiometry in the USA; they also remind us of the terminology used there. Stig Arlinger describes the practices in Scandinavia which vary more than might at first be assumed in a group of countries that are noted for their work in the fields of speech and hearing. An overview of speech audiometry in Australia is then given by John Bench which is followed by a detailed account of the practices in the National Acoustic Laboratories in Australia, which provide audiological services throughout the country to children, war veterans and pensioners. John Knight takes the opportunity to remind us that not all the world by any means speaks English or even Western European languages and that special consideration has to be given to the construction of non-European speech audiometric tests. The value of knowing about practices in other countries is that it highlights both the common elements and the differences that may well cause us to consider our own practices.

In conclusion it is as well to consider how far speech audiometry has progressed to date. The following Editorial for the November 1967 edition of *Sound*, written by the late T. S. Littler, gives us a viewpoint of twenty years ago.

About 40 years ago the Acoustical Society of America was founded and the first number of its journal was published in October 1929. In looking through its first volume it is a sobering experience to find that, by that time, practically all we know about the essentials of speech testing was completed, although it was not until during the Second World War that articulation testing had a new stimulus in its application to the supra-threshold testing of the speech interpreting potentials of deaf patients: this became known as speech audiometry. Speech audiometry had previously been introduced as a crude form of threshold detectability in the 1930s and was known as a screening test for sifting out children whose hearing was sub-normal from an ordinary school population and it was in regular use by many educational authorities until about 1950. . . Speech sounds contain so many clues regarding their identity that we can recognise them from only a part of this information and no matter how we choose our speech material, we can never expect to get the same information regarding hearing disability as that obtainable from specially designed tests using pure tones or critically defined spectra of pure tones where there is not the same redundancy inherent in speech information. The difficulty appears to be in designing non-redundant test signals that can be used for testing hearing ability and interpretation at levels above threshold, and so one still goes on experimenting with varieties of speech signals for this purpose when it is considered that tests using pure tones are unsatisfactory. . . The design of word lists needs to be clearly understood before one can fully appreciate their application to an assessment of hearing ability and the limits of their sensitivity: apart from individual intrinsic intelligibility of different words and phonemes, one must be careful to examine whether one is giving appropriate weighting to the value of consonants as compared with vowels in the contribution to the intelligibility of speech. A list of speech testing material will give an articulation curve which reflects the inherent design of the experimenter. Thus the designing of speech testing methods will be expected to be the subject of continuous experiment as well as open to criticism of its aim.

The readers of this book will have to decide how far we have come in twenty years of experimentation and, hopefully, from the material assembled here, be able to judge for themselves as to whether the aims of speech audiometry are being met.

Michael Martin

Chapter 1

Basic Properties of Speech

R. Wright

Many areas of research and clinical practice involve some aspect of speech, and many people are thus expected to have some knowledge of the subject. But what kind of knowledge? Linguistics, phonetics, psychology, acoustics, signal processing, physiology, communication engineering: there is no end to it. It is tempting to assume that one's own innate knowledge will suffice, at least for clinical subjects like audiology. After all, most of us are (given normal hearing and a few other favours) expert in the use of speech; is that not sufficient?

It is not enough when dealing clinically with hearing loss, because we are then intervening in a process which has gone wrong. No mechanical knowledge may be required to drive a car, but we should like rather more when faced with a breakdown. One useful aspect of the multidisciplinary nature of speech studies is that quite a lot of information is available at the introductory level. There are excellent texts to introduce linguistics, phonetics, the physics of sound and of speech, and the basics of psychoacoustics and speech perception.

This chapter will refer to all the above areas at an introductory level, but the reader is referred to Denes and Pinson (1963), Fry (1979), Gimson (1980), Ladefoged (1962, 1982) and Moore (1982) for a more complete introduction. None requires a degree in maths or other prerequisites. They all take the time and space to provide a proper foundation, whereas this chapter is only a summary, a list of findings.

Given a basic understanding at the introductory level, this chapter will try to emphasize two particular aspects of speech:

1. the importance of viewing speech as something very different from a sequence of sounds. It is usual to introduce phonetics with a description of 'the sounds'; this approach leads to many problems. It encourages a view that speech can be adequately described at a single level of analysis. This in turn makes it awkward to introduce linguistics and a heirarchy of descriptive levels. It is then equally awkward to describe prosodic aspects

1

such as stress and intonation. They tend to be introduced as something added to speech more or less as an optional extra or afterthought. This chapter will go very much to the opposite extreme, and will try to cover almost all of speech perception without recourse to a segmental description.

2. the importance of decision making. Speaking and hearing are often treated as opposite ends of a 'speech chain'; articulatory phonetics is often viewed as opposed to acoustic phonetics; but the speaker and hearer are joined in the task of making a set of decisions concerning units at various linguistic levels. Speech perception will therefore be presented in terms of a set of yes/no (or at worst three-way) decisions, and the acoustic characteristics which encode the speaker's decisions and provide the cues to the listener's decisions.

This approach is not meant to be idiosyncratic. Hearing impairment only becomes a problem for speech when decisions about the speech signal begin to be made incorrectly. By and large, many segmental decisions can be incomplete before communication begins to be affected (because they were not necessary for correct decisions at higher levels). This process can only begin to be adequately explained by consideration of a heirarchy of suprasegmental aspects of the decision making involved in speech perception. The point of speech audiometry is to provide a methodology which tests a person's ability to make these decisions.

The Speech Signal

Periodic and Aperiodic Waveforms

The physical description of speech usually begins with a consideration of waveforms (Figure 1). Speech at this level can be considered as simply a disturbance of the air pressure, a sound wave.

The first distinction to be made concerning waves is whether or not they repeat. A repetitive wave is termed *periodic*, as shown in Figure 1(a). A non-repetitive or *aperiodic* wave is shown in Figure 1(b).

Many interesting physical phenomena have a repetitive aspect, including the idealized vibration of the larynx when used for speech. The resultant periodic waves are essentially different from aperiodic waves, because they are completely described by one repetition (one period). Thus Figure 1(a) is a complete description whereas for the aperiodic wave, 1(b) the figure is only a portion, an incomplete description.

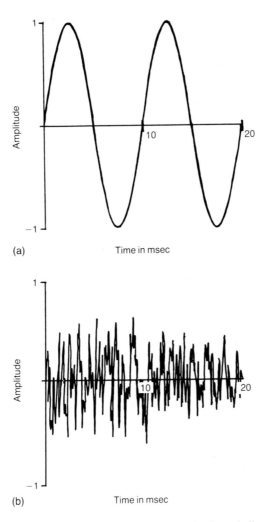

Figure 1. Periodic and Aperiodic Waveforms: (a) An example of a periodic wave, a 100 Hz pure tone; (b) An aperiodic waveform, random noise.

Properties of a Periodic Wave

A periodic wave is characterized by three properties:

(a) the period, which is the repetition interval.
(b) the amplitude, which is simply the height for the pure tone in Figure 1(a). (An exact definition of amplitude can be made for any periodic wave, however complicated the shape.)
(c) the wave shape (wave form).

3

The pure tone in Figure 2 has a period of 1 msec (0.001 second). Thus it repeats 1000 times per second and has a *fundamental frequency* of 1 kHz. The amplitude shown represents the quietest sound that the normal ear can hear at this frequency. In this case the amplitude has units of length, representing the actual amount of motion of notional small volumes of air. It should be noted that this motion is very small: it is of the order of the diameter of an air molecule!

It is more usual to give pressure rather than amplitude, because pressure can be directly measured. The equivalent pressure is also shown in Figure 2.

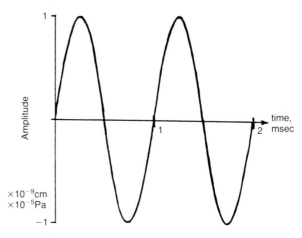

Figure 2.   A pure tone with a frequency of 1000 Hz, at a level corresponding to the detection threshold for normal hearing.

Wave Shape and Spectrum

The key to formally characterizing a wave form is presented in Figure 3, showing how a complicated shape is equivalent to a combination of pure tones, varying in period and amplitude. This principle was developed by the French mathematician (and Utopian socialist) Fourier, ca 1800, and is called *Fourier analysis*.

Fourier analysis shows that ANY periodic waveform can be represented as a combination of pure tones. Further, the frequencies of the pure tones to be used are specified: it is sufficient merely to use those tones whose frequencies are integer multiples of the fundamental frequency. These tones constitute a *Fourier series*. The wave shape can be exactly specified in terms of the amplitudes and phases of a set of pure tones. The lowest frequency tone (with period equal to that of the complicated waveform) is the *fundamental* of the Fourier series. The remaining tones are the *harmonics*, beginning with the second harmonic. This method of representation of waveforms is also called harmonic analysis.

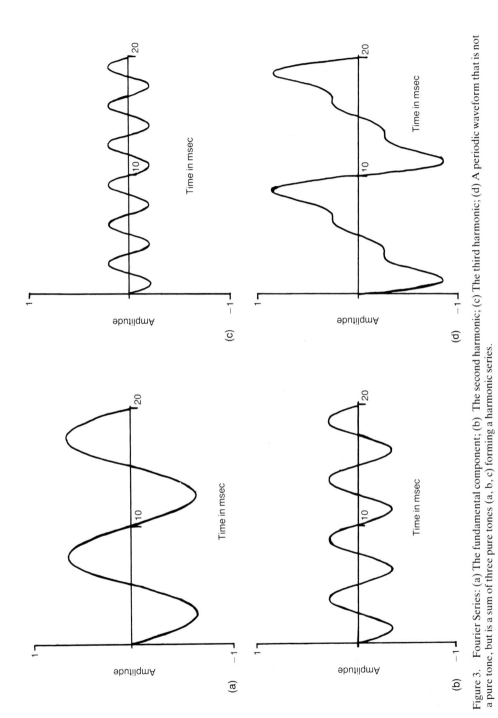

Figure 3.   Fourier Series: (a) The fundamental component; (b) The second harmonic; (c) The third harmonic; (d) A periodic waveform that is not a pure tone, but is a sum of three pure tones (a, b, c) forming a harmonic series.

A bar graph can be constructed showing the amplitude of each harmonic of the series, Figure 4. This shows the same information as in Figure 3, but in a compact way (especially if many more harmonics were to be used). This graph is a *line spectrum* or *discrete spectrum*.

Knowledge of the period, the overall amplitude, and the spectrum completely characterize a periodic signal. Further, the period is evident in the spectrum, and the overall amplitude is defined in terms of the individual amplitudes which constitute the spectrum. Thus the spectrum is a complete description of a periodic waveform.

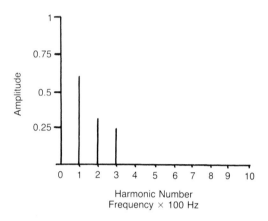

Figure 4.   The line spectrum for the waveform in Figure 3(d).

Aperiodic Waveforms

Fourier analysis can be extended to non-repetitive signals. A non-mathematical interpretation would be to consider such signals as actually having a period, but one of duration approaching infinity. Thus the fundamental frequency becomes very low (approaching zero), and the lines in the spectrum get very close together. The result is a *continuous spectrum*, a spectrum which has energy (or could have energy; some frequency regions may make no contribution) at all frequencies. Because it is impossible to draw an infinite number of vertical bars, it is conventional to just draw the tops of the bars. Figure 5 shows an aperiodic sound and its continuous spectrum.

It is worth emphasizing that sounds which occur at very low repetition rates can have very high frequency content. Thus although the normal ear is said to reach a lower frequency limit at about 20 Hz, this does not mean that one must slam a door at a frequency greater than 20 Hz in order to be heard. A person may slam a particular door once per day. This is not a very low frequency (one cycle/day) sound, because it is not a pure tone. It can be analysed as an aperiodic signal with a continuous spectrum, and with significant energy at audible frequencies.

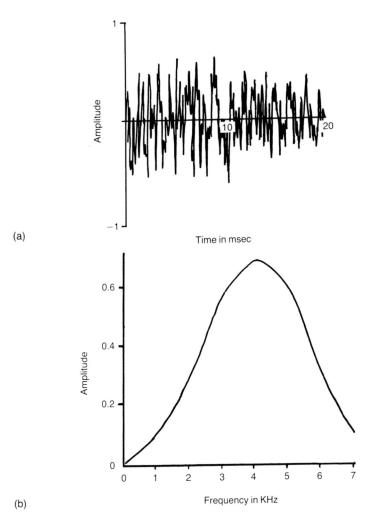

Figure 5.   Aperiodic signals: (a) A noise waveform; (b) The continuous spectrum of the noise waveform.

Duration

The fact that a waveform can be described in terms of amplitude, period, and spectrum has already been discussed. One more dimension is necessary: time. We wish to deal with speech signals, and so must describe signals which are of finite duration: they start and stop.

This involves a compromise with the definition of a periodic signal, and hence with the requirements of Fourier analysis. Speech signals will have a repetitive aspect, but will not be perfectly repetitive because of their finite

7

duration. Thus making a line spectrum from one period of a speech signal is an approximation: a very good approximation for a sustained sound with many similar periods; a poor approximation for a rapidly changing sound which is really not at all repetitive.

Given the above reservation concerning periodic signals, we can physically describe speech signals in terms of their amplitude, period, spectrum and duration. The duration is simply the time from the beginning to the end of the signal involved. If the signal changes over the course of its duration, then properly we need multiple values of amplitude, period and spectrum. A three-dimensional graph of spectrum vs time could be produced (amplitude vs frequency vs time) and this is exactly the information in a speech spectrogram, the basic tool of acoustic phonetics research (Figure 6).

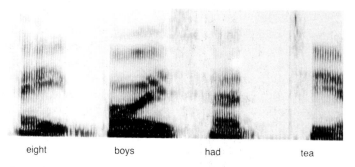

eight   boys   had   tea

Figure 6. A speech spectrogram, a three-dimensional representation of speech. Frequency is the vertical dimension, time is horizontal, and the signal level is represented by the amount of darkness.

Spectrogram courtesy IBM (UK) Science Centre, Winchester.

Psychoacoustics

The human observer is not just like a microphone and a Fourier analysis system. Human response on any physical dimension does not in general uniformly equate to the physical units which describe that dimension. This is the whole subject of psychophysical scaling, and deserves separate study in its own right. We can only summarize the most relevant results.

For each of the physical descriptions so far discussed (duration, amplitude, period and spectrum) we can present an equivalent perceptual description, Table I.

Perceptually speech sounds can thus be described in the following terms:

LOUDNESS. There is a proportionality effect to the perception of loudness (and pitch; and many other sensory phenomena): small changes to small signals are as significant as much larger changes to large signals. Thus a

Physical	*Perceptual*
Amplitude	Loudness
Period	Pitch
Spectrum	Quality
Duration	Length

Table I: Physical (Acoustic) and Perceptual (Auditory) Descriptions

change in sensation depends upon the *ratio* of the stimulus change to the size of the original stimulus. This is not at all the same as a *linear* response. In a linear system the sensation change (or measurement) depends only upon the stimulus change, and no ratio is involved. Most physical devices (like microphones) are built to have a linear response, and hence differ in a basic way from human auditory perception.

The decibel scale is a way of numerically coping with the wide range of sound levels. Human auditory processing is faced with the same problem, and also solves it by the use of a logarithmic relationship. Thus the decibel scale is an approximation to loudness, the auditory scaling of acoustic intensity.

So decibel steps should represent loudness steps. Indeed, one decibel is approximately the minimum detectable loudness change over a wide range of intensities and frequencies. Although decibels are still a physical measurement, a logarithmic conversion from linear physical measurements, the decibel uses a mathematical relation (the logarithm) which is a good approximation to the perceptual scaling for loudness.

A common problem in hearing impairment is the phenomenon of recruitment, in which a person is abnormally sensitive to changes in sound level. This can be viewed as an alteration to the proportionality constant in the logarithmic scaling such that loudness increases faster than for the normal ear.

PITCH. A periodic sound will produce a sensation of pitch. (So will other sounds; this is a complex subject and the reader is referred to Moore, 1982). Pitch is determined mainly by the repetition period.

It is a commonplace error to confuse fundamental frequency with the *amplitude* of the fundamental component in the line spectrum. This leads to the conclusion that if the amplitude of this component is reduced to zero, then the fundamental frequency is eliminated. People then marvel at the power of human perception in 'recovering' the 'missing' fundamental frequency (as in telephone bandwidth speech).

Simple inspection of the time waveforms can help clarify the issue. Figure 7(a) shows a signal and its spectrum; Figure 7(b) shows the same signal except the amplitude of the fundamental component is zero. As is evident from the figure, the obvious period is unaltered. Changing the amplitudes in the spectrum will change the quality, not the period. There is no missing

9

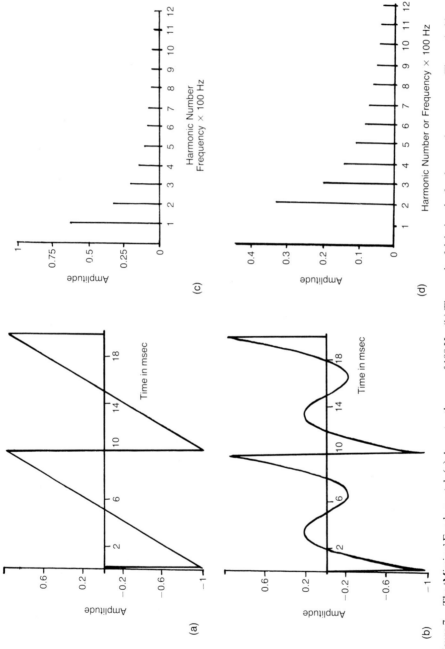

Figure 7. The 'Missing' Fundamental: (a) A sawtooth wave of 100 Hz; (b) The result of deleting the fundamental component. The period is unaffected; (c) The spectrum of (a), consisting of the fundamental and harmonics; (d) The spectrum of (b). The greatest common divisor of the harmonics is still the 'missing' fundamental.

fundamental as far as the eye (or the ear) is concerned: the period of Figure 7(b) is as evident as that of Figure 7(a). Further, even in the spectrum the fundamental frequency is still evident, as the harmonic spacing. In practice, as few as three higher harmonics (such as 17, 18 and 19 in Figure 8) are sufficient to produce a clearly evident periodicity (again, clear to the eye in the figure, and clear to the ear as an actual signal).

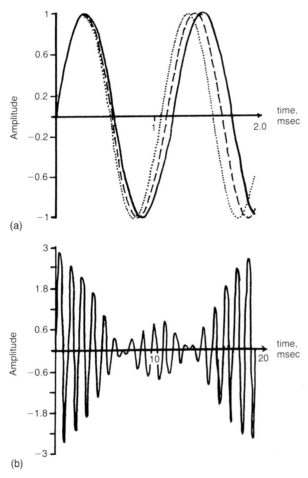

Figure 8. An extreme case of periodicity determined solely by higher harmonics: (a) The first cycles of pure tones at 850, 900 and 950 Hz, which are harmonics 17, 18 and 19 of a series beginning at 50 Hz; (b) The sum of the three very high harmonics, with obvious periocity at 20 msec corresponding to 50 Hz.

The basis of pitch in periodicity (NOT in strength of the fundamental of the spectrum) should be borne in mind in any consideration of pitch perception through either an impaired ear or a band-limiting device.

11

As with loudness, pitch relations are on approximately a log scale. Thus uniform intervals in pitch relate to uniform ratios in frequency. In music this leads to units such as semitones and octaves, which do not represent a fixed step size in physical terms, but rather represent a fixed ratio. Thus an octave is a doubling in frequency. And an octave rise in pitch can occupy a small (from 50 Hz to 100 Hz) or large (300 Hz to 600 Hz) frequency range. Both of these one-octave pitch rises would be perceived as being of approximately the same 'size'.

QUALITY. There is a difference between the sustained sounds produced by two different musical instruments playing the same note (i.e., same pitch, loudness and duration). In music this difference is called timbre but in speech it is called quality. The quality difference depends upon the spectrum, or equivalently the waveform.

For speech sounds, two vowels can be matched for pitch, loudness and duration, but their phonemic category (identity) will be determined by their quality.

LENGTH. Perception of length is not so regular as for pitch and loudness. There is not an accepted psychophysical scale in general use in audiology or phonetics, primarily because it is often unclear in speech just where any particular unit begin and ends (either perceptually or physically). Phoneticians use 'short' and 'long' to represent phonological contrasts (especially for vowels) which may or may not relate to perception of length, and may not be reducable to physical dimensions.

Linguistics

Speech is used for communication between persons. It is this role which is considered at the linguistic level.

Communication proceeds by the encoding (at the source) and the decoding (at the receiver) of information. The encoding and decoding consist of specific yes/no decisions operating upon various units which constitute a *linguistic hierarchy*. As with psychophysics and phonetics, linguistics is a major field of study in its own right.

Speech can be analysed for decision-making purposes according to the following (simplified!) linguistic hierarchy, summarized in Table II:

The UTTERANCE. An utterance constitutes the largest unit of *syntax*, which is the system of word-arrangement constraints.

The PHRASE (tone group). Within an utterance, divisions can be made into the major syntactic constituents. Acoustically the divisions may be marked with pauses or changes in fundamental frequency, or may be determined purely by syntactic structure. A defining characteristic of a tone group is that it has within it one main pitch change, called the *nucleus* of the *intonation*

Linguistic Unit	Decision System
Utterance	Syntax
Phrase	Intonation
Foot	Stress
Syllable	Vocalic vs Consonantal
Syllable-Part	Manner
Segment	Place

Table II: Hierarchy of linguistic units and their associated speech contrasts.

pattern. As soon as we attempt to divide an utterance into any smaller information-bearing units we must have pitch information, operating within an intonation system. The first decisions made about an utterance (first in terms of the size of the unit which the decision governs) are decisions based upon pitch perception.

The FOOT (stress group). The next level down requires the identification of stressed syllables, or at the very least the unit of 'stressed and following unstressed syllables', called the foot. Only a stressed syllable can carry an intonation marker (a pitch change), and thus only a stressed syllable can be the nucleus of a tone group. In English, an unstressed syllable MAY (not must; some do not) reduce, and a reduced syllable is shorter in length than an unreduced syllable. There is often also a difference in quality: the vowel in a reduced syllable 'reduces' to /I/ or /ə/.

Thus we see that just to divide an utterance into stress groups requires all of the perceptual dimensions except loudness, although the use of quality may not be necessary for the determination of stress. Rather it should be viewed as a correlate, with duration as the determiner. Similarly, loudness will also be affected (modulated) by stress and intonation patterns, as a secondary effect. Interestingly, when periodicity cues are removed (in whispered speech) intonation patterns can still be conveyed through the use of the secondary cue (correlate) of loudness; duration as a cue to stress is unaffected by presence or absence of periodicity.

The SYLLABLE. The foot is defined as a stressed syllable followed by any number of unstressed syllables. We have indicated that stress on a syllable is determined principally by duration. How is the syllable defined?

A syllable must have one and only one *syllable centre*, a sound with a vocalic role (a vocoid). Thus a foot divides into syllables, each of which has a centre (a vowel sound or another sound with a vowel role); then anything left over must attach to one or the other (preceeding or following in time) adjacent centres as a *syllable margin*. A part of the speech signal 'attached' to a following centre is thus *syllable initial*; otherwise it becomes *syllable final*.

13

The SYLLABLE-PART. Conventionally in English a syllable centre is a vowel, and an initial or final syllable margin is a consonant or consonant cluster. Additionally certain consonants may extend their roles to also serve as syllable centres. Thus 'syllabic' nasals or /r/ or /l/ are consonantal segments with a role (one level up) as syllable centres.

In English a syllable centre is either a single vowel, diphthong or syllabic consonant. A syllable margin, however, can consist of from zero to three consonants (and very rarely four as in 'twelfths').

It is possible to describe syllable parts without reference to vowels and consonants. From the decision making point of view a syllable centre requires a certain set of decisions about quality, and the margins require different decisions about 'manner'. Only one yes/no decision about each manner type may be 'loaded' onto a given syllable margin. This fact can be used to divide margins and thus divide syllables. This approach will be discussed in detail in the acoustic phonetics section.

The SEGMENT. The lowest-level unit is the individual speech sound. Decisions about speech at this level are *phonemic*; thus a phoneme is the minimum information bearing unit of the speech signal. It is only at this very lowest level that we encounter the units naïvely thought of as constituting speech. A wealth of interpretation must be accomplished before decisions at the segmental level are reached.

Of course, if only the stylized enunciation of isolated monosyllabic words is considered (as in some types of speech audiometry) then most of the higher levels are completely eliminated. We should at least be aware of what is being thrown away.

Acoustic Phonetics

This section will cover the description of speech (in particular, spoken English) in terms of the acoustic consequences of speech production, and the acoustic cues to speech perception. A complete description of speech would cover the many overall characteristics (voice quality, pitch range, rate; speaker sex, class, dialect, nationality) which must be present but do not encode a message. Thus there are overall features and contrastive features. The contrastive features carry the information, and require the decisions which form production and perception. The contrastive features will be the main concern of this discussion. This section will attempt to cover every speech decision (from top to bottom) and the associated acoustic cues.

As mentioned earlier, it is usual in introductory phonetics to concentrate on speech sound contrasts. Such an approach undervalues the linguistic complexity of speech, and leaves out decisions about syllable structure, stress and intonation. These higher linguistic levels also have contrasts, and are referred to collectively as prosodics or suprasegmentals. To give these aspects their due, this discussion will begin with prosodics and only arrive at segmentals after all the higher levels of decision making have been described.

Prosodic Aspects: Pitch, Length, Loudness

The last section endeavored to show how (at least for English) the whole shape of an utterance and all the perceptual decisions down to the level of the syllable are prosodic, meaning based on pitch and length and perhaps loudness, and not based on spectral quality or anything to do with individual speech sounds.

The first decision about an utterance is the division into tone groups, each with its major pitch change on the nucleus. For simple utterances there will be just one tone group, and one nucleus. The role of the pitch change to mark the nucleus is especially significant, as this will be the most important word in the utterance.

Pitch is primarily determined by the periodicity of the speech signal. In normal speech, median values for fundamental frequency range from about 120 Hz for adult male voices to 180 Hz for adult females and roughly up to 250 Hz for children. Variation about this median in ordinary speech does not usually span much more than an octave, and variation tends to be toward higher pitches. Thus the median is usually near the low end of a person's range. Most people are actually capable of producing nearly a two octave range of fundamental frequencies, but for speech they tend to use about an octave located (again) at the low end of their range of possibilities. Within a single utterance a range of half an octave is quite usual, though the variation can be anything from nearly zero (a dull monotone) to an octave or more (extreme emphasis).

The next decision concerns stressed and unstressed syllables. This is an area which has considerable variation from language to language. In English the stress system is rather complex, because two factors are principally involved: pitch and length.

The nucleus is not the only syllable in an utterance which may have a pitch change; other stressed syllables may have a pitch marker (pitch motion). The important distinction is that unstressed syllables can never have a pitch marker.

Furthermore, in English an unstressed syllable may reduce. The vowel duration may be shortened by 50% or more, and the vowel quality may also reduce to /I/ or /ə/.

Thus there are four sorts of syllable:

    1 — stressed plus pitch motion
    2 — stressed
    3 — unstressed but not reduced
    4 — reduced

The clearest distinction is the three-way division between 1, 2 and 3 together, and 4. Type 1 has a pitch motion, type 4 has shortened length, and types 2 and 3 are both of full length but without pitch motion.

Many discussions of this subject founder on treating stress as a question of separating type 2 vs 3. It is much clearer (and more important for speech perception) to begin with the very much easier separation of 1 vs 2 + 3 vs 4. Then type 2 vs type 3 can be put in proper perspective. It is not the first decision to be made regarding stress; rather it is the last. The physical basis of this decision is not well established. According to Ladefoged (1982) it relates to 'effort', but effort can manifest itself in any (or any combination) of the prosodic dimensions.

Typical conversational speech proceeds at 100 to 150 words per minute, or two to three words per second. Thus the syllabic rate is approximately five syllables per second. A stressed syllable marked with a pitch change can typically have a duration of 100 to 200 msec, and could extend to 500 msec or more. A reduced syllable can easily have a duration of less than 50 msec, and in the extreme can reduce to nothing.

Segmental Aspects: Vowel and Consonant Contrasts

At the segmental level information in the speech spectrum (and hence the sound quality) becomes important for the first time. Of particular interest is the change of quality with time, as quality on its own provides limited information.

Vowel Contrasts

A uniform tube (such as an organ pipe) has the property of resonance. Certain frequencies are favoured, others are subject to cancellation. For speech the resonant frequencies (or modes) of the vocal tract are called *formants*. Vowel perception is based mainly on the position in frequency of the first two formants, F1 and F2.

These two formants determine a two-dimensional space, as shown in Figure 9(a), which shows the F1 and F2 values for the vowels of American English. Perceptual studies have shown a close agreement between physical formant measurements and perceptual scaling of vowel similarities, as shown in Figure 9(b). Furthermore, the physical and perceptual data bear a striking similarity to the 'vowel quadrilateral' used in the traditional teaching of phonetics, Figure 9(c). Thus the vowel quadrilateral closely represents speech perception, although it is conventionally labelled in terms of speech production. Further, the perception is closely linked to the acoustic description of the vowels, not the articulatory description. Thus the real success of the vowel quadrilateral (and the cardinal vowels) in phonetics can be explained: it is a good description of perception, and phonetics teaching is mainly a matter of the training of perception.

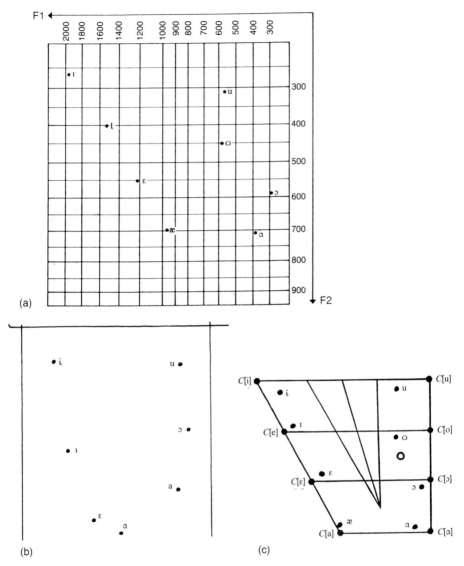

Figure 9. Vowel Space and the Significance of Formants: (a) Acoustic – The representation of the English steady vowels plotted according to the two lowest resonant frequencies of the vocal tract, F1 and F2; (b) Perceptual – The result of judgements of perceptual distances between vowels; (c) Phonetic – The vowel quadrilateral used in descriptive phonetics.

Figures taken from:

(a) Ladefoged (1982), Fig. 8.7; The vowels are for American English.

(b) Klein, Plomp and Pols (1970), Fig. 1.5.1; from a study of Dutch vowels. Their figure has been rotated and reflected about the central axis.

(c) Gimson (1980), Fig. 6; data on American vowels from Ladefoged (1982, Fig. 4.2) have been added.

Both F1 and F2 can range over about two octaves (adult male F1: 200–800 Hz; F2: 700 Hz–2.8 kHz). Formants can be about 40% higher for adult females, and still higher for children. Unfortunately, each formant does not scale uniformly with vocal tract length, so a child's formants will not be a fixed percentage increase on the adult male values quoted. But one would not expect a child's formants to be more than double those given above.

The basic decisions about vowels are:

1. F1 and F2 far apart vs close together ('front' vs 'back' vowels).
2. F1 high vs F1 low ('open' vs 'close' vowels).

Many of the world's languages can use the above decisions to produce a system using from three to five vowels. In English the perception can be modelled as based on five vowels: a 3-way decision on F1 and a 2-way decision on F2-F1, which yields six categories. This collapses to five because F2 is constrained when F1 is high.

But English has many more than five vowels! A second decision is added, based upon length, yielding 5 more vowels (there may well also be quality differences between the 'long' and 'short' members of a pair). Finally, if the formants move slowly diphthongs are produced, of which Southern British English has a particularly large number. Interested readers are referred to Gimson (1980) and Ladefoged (1982) for further details.

In Southern British English, perception is aided by constraints imposed upon vowels. Syllables can be divided into open (no syllable-final consonants) vs closed (ending in a consonant or cluster of consonants). ONLY long vowels can occur in open stressed syllables. In unstressed open syllables the reduced forms /ə/ and /I/ also occur. Thus whether a vowel is heard as long is governed partly by the syllable structure. If it is an open syllable it will be a long vowel, regardless of the actual acoustic properties of the vowel itself. This is one example of the many ways in which the sounds of speech are really a question of larger units (the syllable) and the whole system of contrasts.

Consonantal Contrasts

Consonants are by definition those sounds occurring in the syllable margins. It is conventional to divide consonants according to place and manner (of articulation) and voicing. This section will extend this description to the acoustic consequences of the place, manner and voicing taxonomy.

Voicing principally refers in articulatory terms to laryngeal activity, the presence or absence of vibration of the vocal folds. The acoustic consequence is ideally a periodic or aperiodic waveform. The actual acoustic cues to voicing depend upon the consonants involved (stops or fricatives or affricates), syllable stress, syllable position, and whether or not the consonant is part of a cluster. Manner categories are shown in Table III.

Manner	Speech Sounds
Stop	p t k b d g
Fricative	f θ s ʃ v ð z ʒ h
Affricate	tʃ dʒ
Nasal	m n ŋ
Approximant	w j r l

Table III: Manner categories

Place refers to the main place of constriction within the vocal tract, as shown in Table IV. These categories are the main positions for English, working from the front of the mouth to the back. For detailed phonetics more places and multiple articulatory gestures may actually be involved, but those given will suffice for a discussion of the system of contrasts.

Place	Speech Sounds	Examples
Bilabial	p b m	pie, buy, my
Labiodental	f v	face, vase
Dental	θ ð	thin, then
Alveolar	t d n s z	to, do, new, Sue, zoo
Palato-alveolar	ʃ ʒ tʃ dʒ	shy, measure, church, judge
Velar	k g ŋ	back, bag, bang
Laryngeal	h	hooray, Henry

Table IV: Place categories

Syllable Initial Consonant Contrasts

Decoding of consonants within the syllable-initial margin is considerably simplified by a very strong constraint: only ONE yes/no decision is required for each manner possibility for the whole cluster, and ONE voicing decision for the whole cluster. For instance, a cluster AS A WHOLE is either nasal or non-nasal. There is no possibility of combining nasals into clusters to require two or more decisions about nasality. The same simplification applies to all the manner contrasts, and to voicing.

Thus a syllable initial consonant cluster (as a whole) is either:

1 — nasal or not
2 — fricative or not
3 — stop or not
4 — approximant or not
5 — voiced or voiceless

Further there are usually only one or two and at most three initial consonants, and their sequence is subject to further strict constraints. The result is that, although there are about 24 consonants, there are nowhere near $24 \times 24 \times 24 = 13,824$ possible clusters involving three consonants. In fact there are less than ten (some variation according to dialect); they all begin with /s/, the second consonant is a voiceless stop, the third is an approximant, and nearly half of the stop+approximant pairs are not allowed (/tl/, /kl/, /pw/ and /tw/). Now these five manner and voice decisions can be discussed in turn.

NASAL. The main acoustic cue to nasality is presence of a relatively strong nasal formant at about 300 Hz. The F1 for the related non-nasal articulatory configuration is eliminated, and F2 and higher resonances decay more quickly because of the extra loss through the nasal tract. This extra loss can also be described as a widening of formant bandwidths and a reduction of formant amplitude. (See Ladefoged, 1962 for a discussion of loss and bandwidth.)

FRICATIVE. Acoustic cues to frication, on the other hand, lie in the frequencies above 1 kHz, and spreading as high as 8 to 10 kHz for /s/. Frication is the audible consequence of air turbulence at a constriction. This signal is aperiodic, though it may be added to a periodic signal from the larynx in the case of voiced fricatives. In either case, the presence of random noise above 1 kHz will be the cue to frication.

STOP. A stop has a temporal cue, an abrupt interruption or gap in the signal. This definition is sensible for words within an utterance, but not for the beginning of an utterance. Although no gap as such occurs in this position, the release from vocal tract closure is still cued by the abrupt onset (half a gap!), the rapid energy rise as the syllable begins. Also associated with stops is rapid formant motion as the vocal tract moves from an obstructed to a non-obstructed shape. In particular, F1 will rise. The change in F2, though ultimately of great significance, is related to place, and so can be ignored for the purposes of manner decisions.

An affricate is acoustically a stop with a slow release, so the gap is followed by frication produced at the same 'place' as the closure (homorganic fricative).

APPROXIMANT. An approximant is vowel-like but with slowly varying formants (but not so slow and not with the same pattern of motion as for diphthongs).

VOICING. Voicing in syllable initial position is complicated. There is no voicing contrast for nasals and approximants. Similarly many clusters have no voicing contrast. Fricative + stop is always 'voiceless', regardless of the actual articulation or acoustic manifestation. Similarly fricative + nasal has a 'voiceless' fricative. All that really remains are single stops, and stop + approximant clusters; even here a voicing contrast may not be required except on stressed syllables.

For unconjoined stops and stop + approximant clusters, on stressed syllables, in syllable-initial position, one must consider acoustic cues to voicing. The cue is generally characterized by *Voice Onset Time (VOT)*, which is the asynchrony between release of the closure and initiation of larynx vibration. In English the sounds /b,d,g/ begin to have laryngeal vibration at about the time the constriction opens (is released), or shortly (less than 25 msec) thereafter. If larynx vibration does not begin until well after release (well over 25 msec) the sound is categorised as a /p,t,k/.

The same holds for stop + approximant, except the VOT may become very long indeed and an entire /r/ or /l/ (for instance) may be produced without laryngeal vibration (as a voiceless fricative). The perception of this difficult contrast (a few milliseconds either way from 25 msec) is aided by concomitant effects: larynx activity produces low frequency (below 1 kHz) spectral content, so the tilt of the spectrum is a cue. Lack of low frequency energy means there is little excitation for F1, so absence (cutback) of F1 is a related cue.

Syllable Final Consonant Contrasts

Syllable final contrasts start off by following the same simplification as for syllable initial: only one manner and voicing decision for the whole cluster. Unfortunately this is then complicated by the affix system in English which can add markers for plural or possessive (/s/, /z/, /ə/) and for past tense and past participle (/t/, /d/, /əd/). Only one voicing decision still must be made, because these affixes 'agree' for voicing; but multiple fricative and stop combinations are introduced. Also longer sequences are possible (up to four), and fewer constraints upon combinations.

One simplification, however, is that the approximant possibilities are reduced to just /r/ or /l/ in English, and reduced even more (though with a compensatory increase in diphthong possibilities) to just /l/ in some dialects (non-rhotic; no /r/ sound).

The basis for fricative and stop decisions is essentially as for syllable initial position. For nasality (in clusters) and voicing, however, the decision has much to do with the preceeding vowel.

NASALITY. A vowel preceding a cluster involving nasality will itself be nasalized, and this will acoustically be cued by the 'nasal' formant at about 300 Hz and a general widening of the other formants. Whether an actual nasal consonant is produced is less important. 'Granted' will be heard the same whether pronounced /grãntId/ or /grãtId/. Of course if the pronunciation changes to /grãnId/ then the nasal consonant must occur; but then it is no longer a consonant cluster. One might even say that the vowel *always* carries the nasality information, and the /n/ is only required to mark the syllable as closed.

VOICING. The syllable final voicing contrast is almost a misnomer, because the periodicity of the signal during the final portion of the syllable is somewhat irrelevant. The strong cue is the length of the preceeding vowel: long for voiced, short for voiceless. The syllable initial VOT and the syllable final vowel length decisions are both temporal; thus decisions about the time domain must be made correctly in order to properly decode the 'periodicity' distinction voiced vs voiceless.

Differentiation Within a Manner Group: Place Contrasts

Speech perception is now almost complete. Given all the decisions about prosodic shape and stress pattern and syllables and syllable structure and the decisions about which manner categories are involved in consonant clusters, only differentiation within a manner group remains. This difference consists of place distinctions. It deserves note that there are strong visual place cues. In fact, the visual cue can be stronger than the acoustic cues for bilabial stops (McGurk and Macdonald, 1976).

At this lowest level the decisions are made which finally unambiguously decode the 'sounds' of English. These decisions do not 'recognize' sounds; they decide amongst a few alternatives. Once all the decisions about the structure of a syllable margin have been made (manner and voicing contrasts) only decisions within a manner group (roughly, decisions as to place) remain.

stop:	/ptk/ or /bdg/
nasal:	/mnŋ/ (just /mn/ syllable initially)
approximant:	/wjrl/ (just /rl/ or just /l/ syllable finally)
fricative:	/fəsʃ/ /vðzʒ/ (/h/)
(affricate:	/tʃ/ /dʒ/)

Affricate manner could be treated as detecting stop followed by fricative.

The status of /h/ requires discussion. It is only possible syllable initially, has no voicing contrast, and is acoustically similar to a fricative but produced by 'aspirant' turbulence at the larynx rather that fricative turbulence at another constriction. In articulatory and phonological terms it might be considered a separate manner, but for perception it is close to the other sounds produced by turbulence, the fricatives. So decoding /h/ can be considered part of the determination of place, along with /fəsʃ/ (presenting an asymmetry in that it has no voiced counterpart, owing to laryngeal 'place).

The differentiation within these groups will now be discussed in detail.

STOP. The F2 transition must now be used. Bilabial /pb/ lower F2, alveolar /td/ raise it. Because actual place of articulation varies according to the neighbouring vowel for /kg/ (closure may occur along the hard palate rather than at the velum), the acoustic cue for /kg/ is modified by vowel context.

These transitions are among the most difficult cues in speech. The durations can be less than 50 msec, and the amplitude is low, 30 dB or more below the level of an adjacent vowel.

NASAL. The same F2 transition cue as used for stops will separate /m/ from /n/. Syllable final /ŋ/ has the same variation according to neighbouring vowel as has /kg/. There is no syllable initial /ŋ/.

FRICATIVE. The sibilants /sʃ/ /zʒ/ and non-sibilants /fθ/ /vð/ have a sizeable amplitude difference. The voiceless non-sibilant fricatives are the weakest of the sounds of English, roughly 30 dB below the loudest vowel sounds. Separation by amplitude and voicing leaves the four pairs listed above.

All that remains is the decision within these pairs, which is mainly cued by the frequency at which the noise energy is concentrated. For the sibilants, /s/ and /z/ will have appreciable energy between 4 to 8 kHz, while /ʃ/ and /ʒ/ will have a lower frequency concentration. This distinction is very much a matter of a contrast between relatively higher and relatively lower; absolute values vary greatly across speakers.

Similarly, the dental fricatives /θ/ and /ð/ will have a higher frequency concentration of energy than for /f/ and /v/.

Finally, the aspirant /h/ does not have a characteristic energy concentration, and this fact becomes its distinctive cue. The energy will be determined by vocal tract shape, thus making the spectrum for /h/ very much conditioned by any associated vowel. Indeed in whispered (all aspirant) speech, the /h/ isn't really distinguishable from a neighbouring vowel in purely acoustic terms.

In all cases fricative energy is mainly above 1 kHz, and in many cases, as mentioned, the sound is quite weak. Thus problems with fricatives provide an early warning system for hearing impairment.

As with stops and nasals, visual cues are useful for partly differentiating fricatives: /θ/ and /ð/ are clearly different from /f/ and /v/; and liprounding is a cue to /ʃ/ and /ʒ/ vs /s/ and /z/.

APPROXIMANT. In general, the approximants have an amplitude somewhat below that for vowels. This is especially true for /r/ and /l/. A strong cue for /r/ is provided by F3. In a spectrogram a very clear dip in F3 is observed for an intervocalic /r/. Another clear cue to /r/ is liprounding. Both /r/ and /l/ produce a lowering of F2, though the significance of this effect varies according to the vowel involved (vowels with a high F2 are affected more than those with a low F2).

The 'semivowels' /w/ and /j/ are similar to diphthongs, with two differences:

1. formant motion is faster (though still slower than for stop and nasal transitions) and
2. formant motion is greatest at the beginning of the sequence (a /w/ or

/j/ followed by a vowel), whereas for diphthongs the motion is faster toward the end.

Note that cue (2) can only be used (in English) because /w/ and /j/ are restricted to syllable initial position.

With completion of the place decisions the decoding of the speech signal is complete.

Speech Perception

Auditory Space

The implications for speech perception are a main concern in hearing loss. It is common in audiology texts to summarise certain acoustic properties of the speech signal on a sort of audiogram (level vs frequency), with areas marked out for the various categories of speech sound. A typical diagram is Figure 10.

Such a chart is informative but incomplete. It is a map only of the short-term spectral content of speech superimposed on the auditory dimensions of response to the level and frequency of pure tones. It provides mainly a summary of the parts of 'auditory space' involved in vowel contrasts and place/manner decisions.

Pitch detection is usually neglected, or consigned misleadingly to the part in auditory space occupied by the 'laryngeal tone'. As has been discussed, strength of the fundamental is not the determiner of pitch, and a more informative diagram would show pitch related information as dependent upon the entire spectral content of the signal, although a voiced sound would ordinarily have most of its energy below 1 kHz.

The real problem with conventional auditory space, for pitch perception and generally for all of speech processing, is that the time dimension is neglected. Speech perception depends upon a three dimensional auditory space (amplitude vs frequency vs time), and the conventional diagram is just a slice through this space. The time we selected for Figure 10 is at the short-time end of the complete picture. Consideration of a time dimension is particularly relevant to pitch perception and sensory-neural hearing loss, because of the existence of a temporal mechanism for frequency discrimination.

Audiologists are familiar with the frequency selectivity along the basilar membrane within the cochlea. Hair cell loss or other damage impairs the capabilities of this frequency analyser. Stronger signals must be used to get a response. Minimum detectable frequency change is increased. The rate at which frequency changes can be followed is reduced. Finally, frequency selectivity is reduced (Moore, 1982).

But pitch judgements for speech do not have to depend upon this 'place mechanism' of frequency analysis, as a temporal mechanism is available for

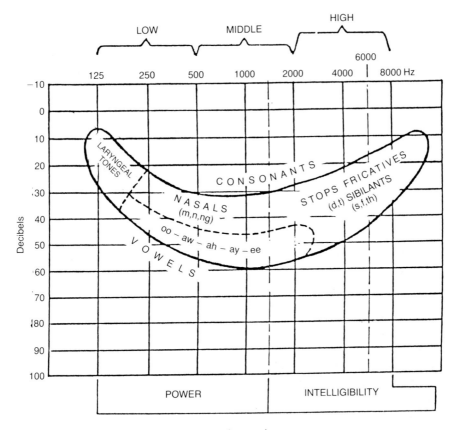

The frequency components of English speech sounds.

Figure 10.   Auditory Space. From Ballantyne, J. (1970) *Hearing*, 2nd Ed.

signals up to at least 1 kHz. Similarly, the various durational aspects of speech contrasts can also be handled by temporal processing. These temporal capabilities are not essentially properties of the cochlea, as is the place (on the basilar membrane) mechanism of frequency discrimination.

Figure 11 shows normal frequency discrimination. It is a plot of the minimum detectable change in the frequency of a pure tone as a function of frequency. Such a minimum change is referred to as the Just Noticeable Difference (JND). For auditory frequency discrimination, there are essentially two quite different areas on the graph.

1. Discrimination for frequencies below 2 kHz is nearly constant at about 2–3 Hz.
2. Discrimination above 2 kHz follows a ratio scale. The JND is a fixed ratio of about 0.2% of the frequency.

25

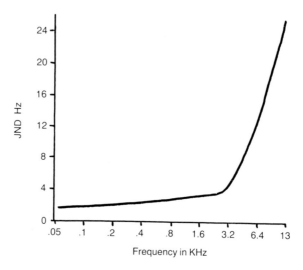

Figure 11.   Frequency Discrimination

The difference in slope for the two regions reflects the difference in mechanism. The implication for hearing impairment is that low frequency temporal processing, including the entire range for human voice pitch, may continue when place processing is lost.

Temporal Processing

The only decisions that have no temporal aspect are those relating to vowel quality. Even for vowels we can only establish (in English) five categories before we must consider the time dimension for 'short' vs 'long' and for diphthongs. Everything else directly involves time.

PROSODIC SHAPE. The first decisions require pitch and pitch motion to determine the major parts of the utterance, called tone groups. The pitch itself depends upon the temporal mechanism (periodicity) of pitch detection. The periods involved for the human voice range from 20 msec down to 2 msec. The minimum detectable change in period can be deduced from Figure 11, but is presented directly in Figure 12. It can be seen that the changes in period required to detect a frequency shift are relatively large at low frequencies (and large periods), whereas they are small at high frequencies (small periods). At 2 kHz a JND of 4 Hz represents a change in period of one microsecond. Obviously a temporal mechanism needs to be extremely accurate to work at 2 kHz, and would have to be impossibly refined for higher frequencies. Thus it is very reasonable for the place mechanism to take over for the higher frequencies.

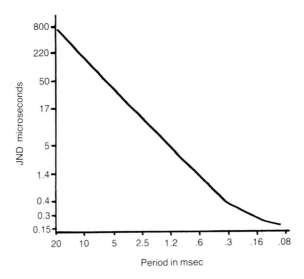

Figure 12. Period Discrimination

The size of a tone group can vary from a single syllable ("No!") to very many words ('I THOUGHT it was Miss Scarlet in the library with a piece of pipe').

INTONATION. The patterns of pitch change (and related loudness and duration changes) operate at the phrase or tone group level. Divisions may be made within a tone group, though this becomes very much a matter of the 'school' of intonation theory to which one adheres. The important fact is that intonation patterns never operate below the unit of the syllable. Thus the fastest motion we should expect (in terms of frequency change per unit of time) is about an octave over the duration of a single syllable (probably several hundred msec for so large an intonation marker). Ordinarily pitch motion will be rather less emphatic, and have lower rates of change.

STRESSED SYLLABLES. Stressed syllables have been defined in terms of their length and ability to carry an intonation marker. A syllable is roughly 100 to 500 msec. Durational differences between stressed and unstressed syllables are usually quite clear; a two-to-one ratio is typical.

SYLLABLES. Defining the syllable is fraught with difficulties. The easy case is a vowel surrounded by stops. The utterance /bebebeb/ is clearly three syllables, and each syllable division is marked by a 30 dB amplitude change over as little as 30 msec. At the difficult end are words like "power", and words where only the approximants /wrlj/ divide the vowels. For such words there may be no amplitude changes, but there will still be a change of spectrum vs time, occupying something like 50 to 100 msec in the ordinary

27

case. The hearing impaired person can be expected to have most difficulty with these spectral cues to syllable division.

VOICING. Voicing is the name for the contrast in English between two groups of stops and fricatives which otherwise have identical place and manner. The actual acoustic cues involve periodicity, spectral balance, and vowel length. These decisions are made only once per syllable margin (consonant cluster). Allowing for the open syllables and for those syllables not involving stops and fricatives, there is as a rough average one voicing decision per syllable. The duration of the cues themselves, however, can be very brief: 30 msec VOT difference between a definite /p/ and /b/. Vowel length differences for syllable-final voicing will be roughly twice this long, or more.

MANNER CONTRASTS. As with voicing, there is only one decision per syllable margin for each of the possible manners. So again the decisions are progressing at something like the syllabic rate, though there can be two stops or fricatives in a syllable final cluster (because of suffixes). The manner cues thus can be thought of as occupying the roughly 50 to 100 msec slot that we have allowed for syllable margins, and in worst case will be half that length. Manner cues tend to depend mainly upon lower frequencies, below 1 kHz. The exception is frication, which is characterized by random noise above 1 kHz.

PLACE CONTRASTS. Place contrasts operate at the segmental level, and thus have multiple decisions per syllable margin. The decision making is simplified by various phonological processes. Elision (deleting segments) and assimilation (making adjoining segments agree for place) reduce the number of place decisions. Thus though one might expect at worst to make five or six (or possibly seven) place decisions for a single syllable, the average is probably again something like one per syllable margin.

Place cues are the shortest speech cues, principally involving 20–50 msec transitions in the second formant. These cues will be in the 1 kHz to 3 kHz region, and will be transitions from or to low amplitudes for stops and nasals. Cues to fricative place will be more spread out, from 1 kHz up to 8 kHz or so, but will also be of low amplitude, as much as 30 dB less than the center of a stressed vowel. These temporal considerations are summarised in the three-dimensional auditory space diagram, Figure 13.

How To Use Speech in Speech Audiometry

Two important questions about various approaches to speech audiometry are: (1) the kind of speech to be used, and (2) the kind of results to be collected. The various answers produce a range of possibilities,which will be considered in turn.

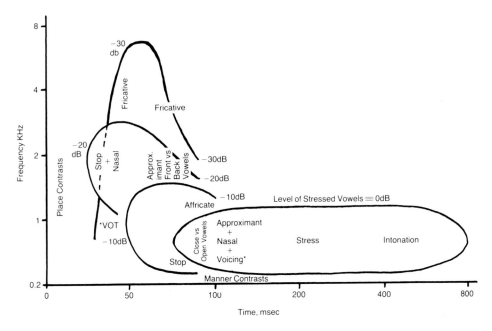

Figure 13. Auditory Space-Time

Speech Detection and Reception Threshold

The simplest possible approach is to:

(a) Dispense with all the linguistic levels except the very lowest and simply use isolated monosyllables.

(b) Ignore all questions of structure. Do not score anything about phonetic type or context. Just score items as right vs wrong.

(c) Ignore confusions between perception and production: the person taking the test 'simply' says what he or she hears. These are called open response tests, because the set of allowed responses is open rather than closed.

(d) Ignore all problems of constraints upon perception and production. Ignore differences in probability of various sounds and sequences; ignore the general tendency to 'grasp after meaning', to prefer a known word to a nonsense word. Ignore the difficulty of producing non-English sequences, even if they were perceived.

(e) Do not enquire into what the person hears. Simply concentrate on the acoustic level at which the sounds begin to be heard (speech detection threshold, SDT), or the level at which sounds are heard with a specified accuracy (such as 50% correct; speech reception threshold, SRT). This approach concentrates on questions of level

29

rather than questions of speech, which is convenient for reducing speech audiometry to something like pure tone audiometry.

Speech Audiogram

The next simplest form of speech audiometry is to make all the simplifications just mentioned, with the exception of testing at various discrimination levels. A graph can then be made of percent correct vs presentation level, Figure 14. In psychophysics such a graph is called a discrimination function, but audiology uses the term speech audiogram.

A speech audiogram improves upon a simple SDT or SRT measurement in that it recognizes that speech is more complicated than pure tones, and hence there are more questions to ask than simple detection threshold. But all the speech audiogram actually tests is multiple thresholds rather than single thresholds. The whole approach still reflects a preoccupation with levels.

Closed Response Tests

The problems of interaction of production with perception and the constraints of the language involved are largely overcome through 'multiple-choice' tests (see Stevenson and Martin, 1977 for a review). The subject selects from a small set of allowed responses. The selection is usually made by marking a response sheet. A written response simplifies the test, eliminating problems of speech production on the part of the person taking the test (and of perception of that production). Special 'pointing to picture' responses have been used with children.

Closed response tests were originally developed to assess the intelligibility of speech transmission systems (the Rhyme Test and its descendents; Hawley, 1977).

A very important benefit of closed response tests is control over 'errors'. The key to behavioural tests is to restrict the subject just to those decisions being investigated. With only a few error possibilities it becomes possible to analyse errors rather than simply to accumulate them. Such diagnostic tests (DRT, Voiers, 1977; FAAF, Foster and Haggard, 1984) can then be used to add a qualitative aspect to the audiometry. Such tests not only quantify the impairment, but point to specific problem areas.

Continuous Speech Tests

The concept of linguistic levels and their associated constraints can be introduced through the use of continuous speech, sentences and paragraphs. Unfortunately, continuous speech adds a whole new set of problems: responses can now be even more variable than for single words, scoring

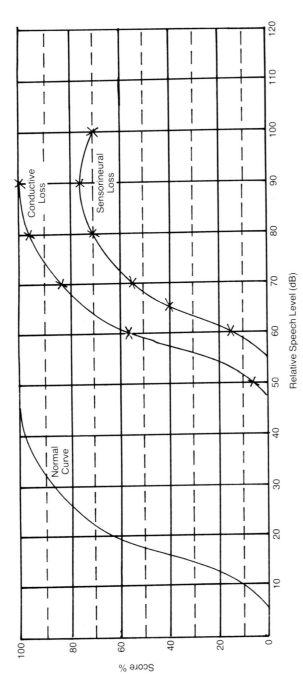

Figure 14. Speech Audiogram with the format recommended by the British Society of Audiology published in the British Journal of Audiology Vol. 9, 1975. A 20% change in score is equal to a 10dB change in level. The shape of the normal curve will depend upon the speech material used. The other two curves illustrate the results from two people one with a conductive hearing loss and the other with a sensorineural loss.

becomes almost impossible, and it is hard to control the difficulty level of materials.

Again, it improves matters greatly to use closed response tests. One particular development (the SPIN test; Kalikow *et al.*, 1977) really only extracts one bit of information out of the whole linguistic structure: how the same acoustic item is perceived in a highly constrained sentence (high predictability) vs a marginally constrained sentence (low predictability). Much research involves linguistic constraints, but very few clinically appropriate tests exist.

Synthetic Speech Tests

Systematic and detailed investigation of auditory time–space requires the use of synthetic stimuli. Much basic research has been performed, but little of direct clinical application. However the advent of the microcomputer and the proliferation of speech synthesis devices at much lower cost than was the case ten years ago eliminate the main technical difficulties with the use of synthesis.

Synthetic speech adds the missing dimensions to a speech audiogram. With synthesis an experimental continuum can be explored step-by-step. The result is a comparison with normal performance on a single acoustic cue to a single speech contrast. Thus in a methodical way the whole pattern of contrasts can begin to be tested. Further, the fact that synthetic speech requires a control computer can be turned to advantage and the stimuli can be computer generated according to the subject's response pattern. These adaptive tests can be made comparatively efficient.

Further, synthetic speech allows a form of speech audiometry which can be made suitable for use with the profoundly deaf, with persons who score at chance level on conventional speech tests. Such testing is very relevant to the screening of candidates for tactile and electrical prostheses, such as cochlear implants and wearable vibrotactile stimulators. (King, this volume; Fisher *et al.* (1983); Pickett *et al.* (1983); Hazan and Fourcin (1985).)

There are many difficulties with speech audiometry. Several have just been mentioned, and other chapters of this book will raise further problems. But we point to these problems in order to find solutions. It should be of great interest for the reader to see how the remaining chapters in this book attempt not just to find problems, but to solve them.

Chapter 2

Towards a Theory of Speech Audiometry Tests

P. Lyregaard

By and large speech audiometry is empirically based, which is not surprising given that our knowledge of the factors mediating speech intelligibility is rudimentary, particularly when a hearing impairment is involved. The present chapter outlines the framework of a theoretical approach to speech audiometry which, although incomplete in detail, nevertheless may be helpful, particularly for the development of new tests. The theory was developed in the wider context of speech intelligibility tests, for the purposes of handling the difficult problem of the international standardization of such tests. It largely draws on work performed at The National Physical Laboratory in Teddington (Lyregaard, Robinson, and Hinchcliffe, 1976).

Even if our knowledge of the detailed mechanisms of speech perception were profound, this would not imply that a theory of speech audiometry were readily available; this is partly due to the fact that a large number of practical factors also affect speech audiometry (e.g., manner of presentation, response technique, scoring method and interpretation of results), but even more important, the purpose for which speech audiometry is used in the audiological clinic is unclear. It would appear that speech audiometry is mostly being used as a general-purpose test, for such purposes as differential diagnoses, assessment of social handicap, monitoring rehabilitation progress, and hearing aid fitting. Needless to say it is highly inconceivable that one single test can be optimum for such diverse uses.

Inevitably, therefore, it is necessary to discuss some of the factors involved and how they affect the outcome of speech audiometry tests. Following this discussion the framework of a theory will be introduced, and its consequences discussed. The presentation will by and large be limited to monosyllabic words, since this is the most common type of material in use.

The Rationale For Speech Audiometry

Carhart (1951) has defined speech audiometry as follows:

> The technique wherein standardized samples of a language are presented through a calibrated system to measure some aspect of hearing ability.

Lyregaard *et al.* (1976) offer the following definition:

> Speech audiometry means any method for assessing the state or ability of the auditory system of an individual, using speech sounds as the response evoking stimuli.

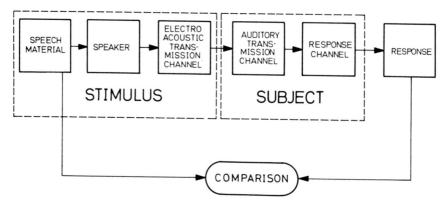

Figure 1.   Block diagram of the major components/variables in speech audiometry.

These definitions are broadly similar, and they both emphasize that the purpose of speech audiometry is to assess the auditory system. Speech audiometry forms a sub-group within the more general domain of speech tests, and the basic principle involved is illustrated in Figure 1: selected speech items, e.g. words, are presented through an electroacoustic system to the listener, who in turn indicates what he heard; these responses are compared to the original material, and percent correct responses is taken as the test result. In speech audiometry this test result would then typically be compared to results obtained in similar test conditions for a group of normal hearing individuals. Test validity hence requires that all factors other than the test subject be held constant. The auditory system of the individual test subject is therefore, as mentioned previously, the object under scrutiny. As illustrated in the table Figure 2 other uses of speech tests appear when the focus of attention is shifted to the other system components shown on Figure 1.

Speech audiometry tests are notoriously difficult to specify and standard-ize. What, then, is the rationale for using them in the first place? In other

Independent variable	Typical areas of utilization
Speech material	Linguistic research (grammar, semantics) Phonological research
Speaker	Phonetic research (articulation) Diagnosis of articulatory disorders Speaker identification research Speech synthesiser assessment
Electroacoustic transmission channel	Speech transmission systems Speech distortion and noise interference Acoustic environment in halls, offices, etc. Hearing aid design
Auditory transmission channel	Assessment of auditory handicap Monitoring audiometry Test of occupational fitness Monitoring improvements in the auditory training of hearing handicapped Diagnosis of auditory dysfunction Research in hearing and neurophysiology
Response channel	Psychological research (motivation, association, memory, etc.)

Figure 2.   Examples of areas where speech tests are used.

words, what are the advantages likely to accrue in speech audiometry, as compared to simpler audiometric tests? The answer is by no means clear-cut, given that speech audiometry is used for a variety of purposes. Partly it boils down to the fact that speech signals, being highly complex, are representative for sounds in daily life, that speech comprehension is an important human faculty in society, that the speech test situation is readily understood by test

35

subjects, and finally that the human auditory system is believed to be peculiarly geared to perception of speech. Speech audiometry has, in other words, a very high degree of face validity.

General Factors in Speech Audiometry

Speech intelligibility scores are affected by a large number of factors, and it is inconceivable that one would ever be able to establish a model dealing with all these. If feasible, such a model could, in an analytic formulation, be stated as:

$$R = f(a,b,c \ldots)$$

where R is the intelligibility score, and a,b,c . . . represent the different factors. Factors in this context are all parameters that, in one way or other, affect the result, such as the number of test items (e.g. words) in a list, the number of phonemes per item, the linguistic competence of the listener, and the level and spectrum of background noise. Some factors may be virtually unquantifiable, e.g. the degree of mismatch between the speaker's and the listener's dialect.

Consider the following reformulation:

$$R = f(a) \cdot g(b) \cdot h(c) \ldots$$

where one assumes that factors do not interact, and their effects, therefore, are independent of each other. While this simplification is probably not accurate in detail, the information available at present does not include interactions.

In considering the generation of a new speech test one is, implicitly or explicitly, forced to take decisions on all the relevant factors, and this is of even greater importance when comparing the merits of different tests.

A few preliminary comments on speech perception in general may be useful. Speech perception is here regarded as a pattern recognition process where the listener hears (perceives) certain acoustic cues and selects an 'appropriate' category in which the item 'fits'. Here the operative word is 'appropriate'. Thus this selection is based not only on acoustic/phonetic factors, but also on syntax, semantics and overall context. The choice, in other words, is governed by expectations, and the less cues the acoustical image provides, the more do expectations determine the response. It is this effect which can induce one to believe his name has been called out in what turns out to be only ambient noise, one's own name being a stimulus with high expectation. But note that even this strong 'halo' effect may be overridden; in speech audiometry the listener's name is virtually never among the responses given, because he 'knows' that in a formal testing procedure this particular stimulus is very unlikely. What constitutes an 'appropriate' response must therefore be seen in the light of all information, explicit and implicit, available to the listener.

Note also that recognition is regarded as a categorization process, thereby implying some underlying continuum, namely the multidimensional set of acoustic parameters. Consider, for instance, the listener engaged in a phoneme recognition task. Within limits, a speaker can vary the articulation of a phoneme but still elicit the correct response. In acoustical terms, one can appreciably vary the parameters (duration, formant frequencies, formant transitions), whilst maintaining the correct response, whereas a larger variation will cause the sound to resemble some other phoneme, and the response to change accordingly. A phoneme therefore corresponds to a subspace of the phono-acoustic space which is needed to describe the stimulus. This is illustrated in Figure 3, where, for simplicity, only two phono-acoustic parameters are included. Whereas each point in the plane in principle corresponds to a particular phone, the listener would, on hearing a phone, categorize it into one of a small set of phonemes (possibly with some ambiguity near the boundaries). In phonetic terms variations within such a subspace are known as allophonic variations, and it points towards the important distinction between a phonetic and phonemic description of utterances; the phoneme is an abstract concept, related to semantics, whereas its many possible realizations (phones) are the physical manifestations.

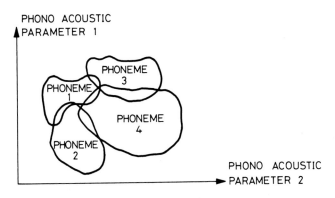

Figure 3.   Illustration of the phonemic categorization process in speech perception.

Factors Related to the Test Material

The test material consists of speech stimuli (items). Whether these items should be described in phonetic or phonemic terms is uncertain. Initially we will therefore consider the phonemic aspects, and subsequently the ramifications of the acoustic realization of the material.

37

But first a few remarks on the nature of items and lists, and their characteristics. An item is a response-evoking stimulus, typically a syllable, word or sentence. Quite apart from whether we consider the item to be a linguistic element or one of its many acoustic images, the term 'item' is used in a somewhat ambiguous way in the literature of speech tests. In fact it may refer to at least four different concepts, as suggested below:

ELEMENT OF INTEREST (or independent variable). For instance we might be interested in the effect of varying a phoneme, but nevertheless present words (containing the phoneme) to the listener.

STIMULUS ELEMENT. If, for instance, the elements of interest are words, they will occasionally be inserted in sentences (called carrier sentences), whereby the physical stimulus becomes a sentence rather than a word.

RESPONSE ELEMENT. Although frequently the listener is asked to repeat or identify the stimulus as heard, certain experiments will call for other types of response. The example mentioned above might for instance require the listener to respond only with the inserted word, not the whole sentence.

SCORING ELEMENT. Even when the response is in the form of a sentence one may opt to score certain key words only, rather than the whole sentence.

Where these distinctions are of minor importance we shall simply use the word 'item'.

Items may be construed as the fundamental unit of speech tests, just as an isolated tone burst is the fundamental unit in pure-tone audiometry. But just as presenting a pure tone once will not yield a statistically satisfactory result, one is forced to present a speech test item again and again until the statistical variation on the compounded score is reasonably low. Unfortunately, repeated presentation of a speech item is not a viable method, because memory effects will render the result meaningless. The alternative commonly employed is to select a number of *different* items, all within the speech material to be considered, and present each item of this subset once. If all items are equal with respect to the relevant properties, this subset (list) will yield a compound result (score) equivalent to that which would have been obtained if a single item could have been used again and again (Lyregaard, 1973).

A list is thus the set of items necessary to obtain a stable score for the conditions imposed (e.g. speech level, masking noise). In this respect it is akin to the set of pure-tone stimuli necessary to obtain an estimate of threshold at a given frequency. Because we may want to compare scores for different imposed conditions, several lists may be needed, all with exactly the same properties. Thus, irrespective of the particular set of conditions, scores obtained from any of the lists should be equal, save for random fluctuations.

In summary, the list concept is based on:

1. Statistical stability of scores (implying that items must be repeated, or a set of items presented)
2. Human memory (implying that items in the list must be different)
3. Interchangeability of lists (implying that lists must have equal relevant properties in all test conditions).

For some purposes these fundamental requirements are supplemented by others, for example, that the speech material should be representative of 'everyday' speech.

Given a frame of items and lists as described above, a strategy for filling in the frame (i.e. selecting the items) is needed. This problem divides into two:

From which population should the items be sampled?

Which method of sampling should be employed?

Selection of Speech Material

The type of material to be used would be one of the following, or a combination thereof:

Phonemes
Syllables
Words (mono-, bi-, or polysyllabic)
Sentences

These categories are not mutually exclusive, and there may be difficulties in defining their boundaries. It is of importance to bear in mind that the material to be selected is spoken rather than written. The differences between written and spoken English can be rather large, particularly in its more colloquial forms, and the syntactic structures proper to written English are often distorted in the spoken language, where prosodic features in part perform the role of syntax.

Selection of speech test material entails consideration of the following factors:

REDUNDANCIES. Phonemes are the least, sentences the most redundant type of item; and the less choice among alternatives, the more redundant are the items. This is reflected in the shape of the intelligibility curves for different types of items (Lehmann, 1962), suggesting that the higher the redundancy, the fewer the acoustic cues needed to recognise the stimulus. A test using sentences will therefore partly measure a hearing deficiency at the

39

peripheral level, and partly a combination of linguistic competence and general cerebral function.

SCORING OF RESPONSES. Responses to phonemes, and to some extent syllables, are difficult to score, in the absence of a phonemic transcription system familiar to the average patient. At the other end of the scale, sentences are equally difficult to score because a correct response would be one showing that the sentence was understood even though not repeated verbatim, minor errors in adverbs, prepositions, etc. being irrelevant. Attempts have been made to do this in Immediate Appreciation tests (Richards, 1973) and more oblique scoring methods have been devised in telephonometry, based on the time required for a complete information transfer to be accomplished, e.g. the reproduction, by the listener, of geometrical designs (Richards, 1973).

RELATION TO 'EVERYDAY' SPEECH. There is little doubt that, in terms of 'face validity', sentences (and possibly words) would rank high as prospective speech test material, and that results so obtained would be more easily related to speech hearing performance than would be the case with syllables or phonemes.

TEST DURATION. This plays an important role in clinical audiometry, and in this respect long items such as sentences are inefficient compared with other types of item, for a given target variance (reliability) of the compound test score. In other words, a given number of sentences will require much longer measurement time than would the same number of words, but the information yielded by the test does not increase in the same proportion.

Arguably the most important factor is that of redundancy. As stated by Fry (1961), the more specific the items, the more the test results will be predictable from the pure-tone audiograms, and thus reflect a measure of peripheral hearing. Conversely, linguistic competence and intelligence will substantially affect results of tests using more complicated items such as sentences, and the test will become a measure of both peripheral and central hearing processes. Various attempts have been made to control this redundancy in speech test materials. Telephone engineers, for example, have for a long time used logatoms to test electroacoustic systems. Logatoms are artificial words which, on the basis of their phonemic composition, could well have been meaningful words, but in fact are not, at least in the language in question. Examples of the CVC-type are 'GAV' and 'NED'. Quite a different approach has been used for the assessment of room acoustics, using artificial sentences consisting of real words linked together in syntactically satisfactory but meaningless sentences.

In the face of such conflicting requirements most designers of speech audiometry tests have opted for a compromise, in the form of monosyllabic meaningful words (CVC).

Selection of Tests Items

Having selected the type of material, it is then necessary to sample the items actually to be used in the test. Sampling is the principle utilized when one needs to measure a property of a large number of objects (the population), but can only manage to measure a few of them; the technique is to select a few hopefully representative objects such that, if the whole population had in fact been measured, the results would be rather similar to those obtained from the sample. Obviously the larger the sample, the better the fidelity. If one has no prior knowledge of the properties of items in the population, the selection (sampling) should be random, implying that all items have the same probability of being selected. Under these circumstances probable deviations on measures, as compared to the 'true' measures, can be estimated by standard statistical methods. On the other hand, if one already possesses some prior knowledge of the parameters to be measured, a more economical stratified sampling scheme may be adopted, generally leading to the sampling of a subgroup within the population rather than the whole population, but the statistical methods needed to estimate the results and their relation to population values may then not be as simple as before.

In what way does the choice of a particular sampling scheme affect the speech test?

Provided the population to be sampled is reasonably wide, the choice will make little difference to the test results *per se*; but results will, at least on the face of it, only be valid for the subgroup from which the sampling has been done. (In a series of tests using medical students as listeners and medical phraseology as items, a drastic change of scores occurred once the listeners realised the subgroup from which samples had been drawn [Quist-Hanssen, personal communication]. Thus too narrow a sampling can lead to entirely false results.) Thus any imposed phonemic balance scheme will not necessarily affect the scores, but only the validity of these as measures of some general speech-hearing ability.

The purpose for which the test is intended therefore becomes important, and the relevant distinction is primarily between assessment of communication ability, and diagnosis. Clearly the sampling aspects as stated above are crucial for speech tests for communication, results from such tests being ultimately used to assess a person's ability to hear and understand a spoken language. By contrast, such considerations are irrelevant for diagnostic speech tests because the merits of tests for diagnostic purposes must be evaluated in terms of ability to differentiate between different disorders. In this case items are to be selected so as to optimize a diagnostic distinction, irrespective of whether they correctly reflect the linguistic/phonetic properties of the parent population from which they are sampled. By way of example, assume that a particular disorder results in poor discrimination of the fricatives /s/ and /ʃ/ (as in SEE and SHE). In this case a sensitive test would consist of items containing a large proportion of fricatives, whereas if items had been selected on a basis of phonemic balance, the fairly small proportion of fricatives would diminish the diagnostic sensitivity for the disorder in question. Thus a good diagnostic test may prove unsuitable for assessing the ability to perceive speech in general, and vice-versa.

Although hypothetical, this example illustrates that item selection is linked to the purpose of the test, and that the current practice of demanding phonemic balance in diagnostic speech test materials may well result in a test of poor diagnostic sensitivity. In the following we examine in detail two frequently used selection criteria, namely phonemic balance and familiarity.

Phonemic Balance

This is normally, but erroneously, termed phonetic balance (or PB for short). It is realised by a test material having a phonemic composition equivalent to that of everyday speech, that is, the different phonemes should appear in the test material with the same relative frequencies as in everyday speech. The rationale is as follows: if the listener were totally unable to perceive a particular phoneme which occurs infrequently in normal everyday speech, the handicap he/she experiences is not as severe as it would have been had the phoneme been a more common one. In effect one may consider phonemic balance as a weighting:

$$S = W_1S_1 + W_2S_2 + \ldots + W_iS_i + \ldots + W_NS_N$$

where S is the total score, W_i the weighting factor for the i-th phoneme, S_i the score obtained for the phoneme i, and N the total number of phonemes. A score obtained in such a test would be analogous to a cost-of-living index, in that a loss (or price increase) is weighted according to how often it occurs (or how many pence the average family spends on the item in question). A number of points regarding PB should be mentioned:

Although phonemes in context differ markedly in respect of their sequential affinities, PB is normally based on a simple count, as if the phonemes occurred in isolation.

The very strong sequential and semantic constraints in normal words or sentences diminish the relevance of PB. In a way this is fortunate, because PB is not easy to achieve except in submorphemic material.

Phonemic (or phonetic) balance may be thought of as a relation between parent population and test material. In fact the same concept is relevant at the next stage, namely between test material and list. For speech audiometry test lists are regarded as interchangeable if each has the same phonemic balance. We should term this *phonemic equalization* as opposed to *phonemic balance*.

Assuming that the principle of phonemic balance is accepted, there remain two questions to resolve, namely:

Selecting a suitable phonemic alphabet.

Determining the relative occurrences of the phonemes in the parent population.

It may be useful at this point to reiterate the essential difference between phonemic and phonetic elements. Roughly speaking phonemes are abstract concepts related to semantics; phonetic elements (phones), on the other hand, are articulatory/acoustic manifestations of phonemes. Thus, a particular phoneme can manifest itself as a number of different phones, all of which would be interpreted as the same phoneme. To test whether two phonetically different elements relate to different phonemes one must insert the two alternatively in all possible words of a language. If, in any word, the alteration between the two phonetic elements results in a change of the semantic content of the word, they must belong to two different phonemes. Otherwise they would be regarded as allophonic variants of the same phoneme.

A common *phonemic* inventory is thus a prerequisite for communication, whereas differences in the *phonetic* inventory, such as found between different dialects of a language, will not necessarily impede communication. According to our fundamental view of speech perception it is phonemic rather than phonetic balance which is relevant.

Fortunately this makes for simplification, in that there are far fewer phonemic than phonetic elements to take into account, and a given phonemic balance is likely to yield an effect independent of the listener's dialect. In a given language phonemic elements are common, whereas phonetic elements may vary, for instance on a geographical, demographical or even idiosyncratic basis. If two different languages are compared, both phonemic and phonetic inventories may differ, thus inhibiting international work in this field. In fact the situation can be even more perplexing, as when two phones are phonemically distinct in one language, but not the other. By way of example the words MAN and MEN are readily distinguished by persons whose native language is English but not, for example, if it is Dutch.

The question of a suitable phonemic inventory is not as simple as it may seem. Whereas the consonants are fairly well defined, vowels give rise to considerable disagreement, to some extent related to dialectal differences. Likewise phoneme clusters are subject to arguments, centred on such questions as whether the consonant clusters /tʃ/ and /dʒ/ should be regarded as a single phoneme or not; whether diphthongs are to be regarded as single phonemes, and if so, how many diphthongs should be included in the phonemic alphabet; and whether more complex clusters like /ndl/ as in 'HANDLE' and /str/ as in 'STRUGGLE' should be admitted.

There is no simple answer to these questions, because phonemes (or rather phones) do not occur as individual units, but in an articulatory or acoustic stream, linked together in such a way that they interact, mainly due to the limitations of the articulatory musculature. This interaction is called coarticulation, and its effect is to smoothe out the distinctiveness of phones, thus making the distinction between single phones and clusters a matter of arbitrary decision. Figures 4 and 5 show a phonemic alphabet found suitable for standard British English (often termed RP, or Received Pronunciation). American English deviates from this in respect of the vowels.

CONSONANT	FRY (%)	DENES (%)
n	12·47	11·67
t	10·56	13·84
d	8·46	6·88
s	7·91	8·38
l	6·02	6·08
ð	5·86	4·93
r	5·77	4.56
m	5·30	5·42
k	5.08	4·77
w	4·62	4·23
z	4·05	4·10
v	3·29	3·05
b	3·24	3.43
f	2·95	2·85
p	2·93	2·91
h	2·40	2·75
ŋ	1·89	2·05
g	1·73	1·91
ʃ	1·58	1·16
j	1·45	2·52
dʒ	0·99	0·85
tʃ	0·67	0·61
θ	0·61	0·98
ʒ	0·16	0·08
TOTAL	**60·78**	**60·73**

Figure 4. Frequency-of-occurrence of consonants in British English (From Fry (1947) and Denes (1963)).

As regards the frequency of occurrence of phonemes there are at least a dozen different counts to choose from, mostly based on American English. A comparison of these counts has indicated that consonant frequencies are fairly stable (Wang and Crawford, 1960), and that vowel/consonant ratios are typically 2/3. Differences in the counts are mainly due to the following:

Different material (conversations, texts, plays, dictionaries)
Exclusion of certain parts of the material e.g. exclamations, articles)
Dialect in which the material is recorded
Differences in phonemic inventories
Random sampling error

VOWEL	FRY (%)	DENES (%)
ɔ	27·39	23·03
i	21·24	21·02
e	7·57	7·16
ai	4·67	7·25
ʌ	4·46	4·25
ei	4·36	3·81
i:	4·21	4·55
ou	3·85	4·45
a	3·70	3·89
o	3·49	3·90
o:	3·16	3·06
u:	2·88	3·62
u	2·19	1·95
a:	2·01	1·97
au	1·56	1·97
ɔ:	1·33	1·70
eə	0·87	1·10
iə	0·54	0·73
oi	0·36	0·22
uə	0·15	0·36
TOTAL	**39·22**	**39·27**

Figure 5. Frequency-of-occurrence of vowels in British English (From Fry (1947) and Denes (1963)).

Figures 4 and 5 include two counts of particular relevance to British conditions. Both are based on 'phonetic readers' and Southern British English, and they both make use of the same phonemic inventory. One set is based on some 17 000 phonemes (Fry, 1947), the other on 72 210 phonemes (Denes, 1963).

Even accepting that such counts are in fact representative of the parent population, practical implementation can lead to difficulties. Consider, for illustration, the construction of CVC monosyllables:

1. The most frequently occurring vowel is the unstressed e (/ə/, as in CON-SERVATION), however this vowel is virtually never found in monosyllabic words.
2. The phoneme counts are averages over all words and also over all positions in a word. But in fact the distributions of initial and final consonants are unequal (French *et al.*, 1930), e.g. no English word ends on /h/, or begins with /ŋ/.
3. Given that phonemic equalization of lists is needed, and only a rather limited number of words per list is contemplated (say 10–50), the very infrequent phonemes will not be represented at all. This, however, is

45

probably not a serious problem, because PB word scores could be obtained by weighting the responses on individual phonemes in lists with equal distribution of phonemes (Isophonemic lists), rather than use PB lists. Using this method each phoneme need in principle only occur once in a list, and all of them could be included.

In conclusion it appears that there is sufficient information available to ensure an approximate phonemic balance of English speech material. However, it is suggested that phonemic balancing is irrelevant for diagnostic purposes, and that its precise fulfilment for communication purposes is questionable, except perhaps for 'nonsense' material.

Familiarity of Material

Whereas the question of phonemic balance has little bearing on the actual test, but is possibly important for the interpretation of results, the familiarity of speech material is important for both test and interpretation. The notion of familiarity is rather vague, and implies that the more one is acquainted with a stimulus, the more readily will one recognize it. In order to quantify the familiarity of a word the assumption is often made that it is equivalent to the frequency with which a person has been exposed to the word, and that this in turn is approximated by the frequency of occurrence of words as found in a corpus of word material, sampled so as to ensure a good coverage of written or spoken material (e.g., Figure 6).

The work of Black (1952), Howes (1957), Pollack *et al.* (1959), Owens (1961), and Savin (1963) indicates that uncommon words have a lower intelligibility than common words, everything else being equal. The size of the effect, in terms of shift of SRT from common (2000 ppm) to uncommon words (1 ppm), is estimated at 15 dB (Howes, 1957). If, however, subjects are acquainted with the words before or during the experiments, no word-frequency effect is found (Pollack *et al.*, 1959). In the studies cited the

REFERENCE	SOURCE	LANGUAGE	TOTAL SAMPLE
Thorndike and Lorge (1944)	Literature, magazines, etc.	American	4 500 000
Carrol *et at.* (1971)	School texts	American	5 000 000
French *et al.* (1930)	Telephone conversations	American	80 000
Howes (1966)	Interviews	American	250 000

Figure 6. Selected word counts in English.

measured word-frequency effect has been somewhat confounded by intervening factors. Thus, there is a correlation between word-length and word-frequency effect, likewise phonetic similarities between correct and alternative response are of importance.

In practice most speech tests have, to a greater or lesser extent, allowed for the word-frequency effect. Normally very uncommon words are excluded from the test material, and sometimes the very common words are also omitted. In the testing of communication equipment it is common practice to familiarize the listeners with the test material prior to the start of the experiment. Tests based on a forced-choice methodology are insensitive to the word-frequency effect. Although familiarity (or, at least, frequency-of-occurrence) of the test words clearly has an effect on intelligibility, that in itself is no impediment to diagnostic speech audiometry, provided the effect is equal for all patients. Certain groups of patients (persons with minimum scholastic aptitude, children, and persons for whom English is a second language) will, however, tend to exhibit deviant frequency-of-occurrence effects, leading to depressed intelligibility scores that have no relation to their auditory capacity, and therefore confounding the diagnostic test. The difficulty is largely remedied if lists are composed of fairly common words only.

Selection of Speaker

The final factor to be considered in relation to speech material is the speaker. In many ways this is the most difficult to deal with, as it is all but unquantifiable. It is a serious impediment to standardization in that a listener may obtain different scores if the same list is read by two different speakers (Asher, 1958). Probably the best known example of this is the two different recordings of the PB-50 lists, by Rush-Hughes and Hirsh respectively. Not only do these two recordings give significantly different scores for normal listeners (difference 10–20%), but this difference is increased for listeners with sensorineural hearing loss (Carhart, 1965).

Male and female voices are sufficiently different to cause differences in intelligibility scores for the same material and listener, and, as one might expect, such differences are aggravated if the speech signal is low-pass filtered before presentation (Hirsch *et al.*, 1954).

It has been suggested that there is an element of familiarisation on score differences due to different speakers; in other words there is a 'tuning-in' period during which one may get accustomed to the peculiarities of a particular voice. A difference has been found where scores obtained with lists read by the same person throughout are compared with scores from lists where each word was read by a different speaker (Creelman, 1957). However, the effect is rather small, consistent with a phonemic rather than a phonetic mode of perception. The problem might be more serious if the speaker and listener have vastly different dialects, although there are ways of overcoming such difficulties. This is achieved merely by recording the material in a 'dialect' typical of broadcasting speakers, and subsequently pruning the material of any items that are sensitive to dialectal differences, either on phonetic, grammatical or semantic grounds. No doubt proliferation of radio and television will gradually erode dialectal barriers, at least for the listener, even though dialects persist in direct communication regionally. Nevertheless full generality is probably not achievable, and speech audiometry scores should therefore always be interpreted with caution if the listeners are of foreign origin.

Even a single speaker will not articulate words in precisely the same way on different occasions. Scores obtained by the same listeners, lists and speaker, but recorded on different occasions, yield differences of up to 10% (Brandy, 1966).

Statistics of Speech Audiometry Scores

The purpose of a list in speech audiometry is to provide convenient subsets of the total test material, each allowing the estimation of a score under the specified test conditions. By transmitting different lists at different speech levels one can determine sufficient points to estimate the intelligibility curve, provided the lists are interchangeable.

There remains the problem of deciding how many items, N, each list should contain. Essentially this is trade-off between precision and test duration. Test duration is linearly related to the number of items per list, and the relation between precision and N is found as follows (Lyregaard, 1973):

Assuming, for simplicity, that every word in the list has the *same* probability (p) of being perceived correctly by a listener, then the intelligibility score (i.e. the number of words perceived correctly) is a stochastic variable (I), the distribution of which is binomial. This distribution is discrete, and, as illustrated in Figure 7, the dispersion depends on the value of p. The probability of obtaining a score of S words is:

$$\Pr \{I = S\} = \binom{N}{S} p^{S} (1 - p)^{N - S}$$

Figure 8 gives the equivalent cumulative distribution for 50-word lists. Although the exact distributions could similarly be derived for lists containing other than 50 words, the method is clearly cumbersome. A closer inspection of Figure 8 reveals that, if extreme values of S and p are avoided, the distribution is approximately gaussian (corresponding to straight lines on the plot), with a mean value of $n \cdot p$, and a standard deviation of $(N \cdot p \cdot (1 - p))^{1/2}$. This

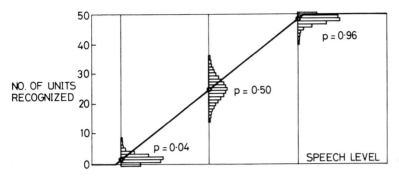

Figure 7.   Illustration of the binomial distribution of list scores (N = 50).

standard deviation is plotted on Figure 9, as a function of p. Using the gaussian approximation it is possible to estimate the number of words required to achieve a given precision (Figure 10). It is apparent that the statistical fluctuation is quite substantial in speech audiometry, and moreover that fairly long lists are required to bring it down to an acceptable level.

In practice every word in a list does not have the same probability of being recognized, and the simple binomial distribution must therefore be substituted by the more general *subnormal binomial distribution*. In this case a simple analytical expression is not feasible, but it appears (Lyregaard, 1973) that, if the distribution of *probabilities* is not too wide, the dispersion will only be slightly less than the one pertaining to the simple binomial.

There are ways of approaching the statistics of speech test data other than that given above. One such method effectively abolishes the list concept (Barfod, 1973). If test words are selected at random from a large dictionary of words, then the resultant distribution will be strictly binomial, even if the items have different recognition probabilities (Barfod, 1973; Lyregaard, 1973). At present the technical means of presenting words in a random order are, however, not available in routine clinical testing.

A good approximation to the variance of the subnormal binomial distribution is given as:

$$V(I) = N[E(p) (1 - E(p)) - V(p)]$$

where E(p) and V(p) are the mean and variance respectively of the probability distribution (Kendall and Stuart, 1958). Clearly a large dispersion of probabilities will tend to narrow the confidence limits; however, this is inevitably accompanied by a loss of information obtained (Lyregaard, 1973). Therefore this method of increasing reliability of scores is not attractive.

However, two other methods are in current use to achieve increased reliability: if the list items consist of monosyllabic CVC-words one might choose to score responses in terms of phonemes rather than words. On the

49

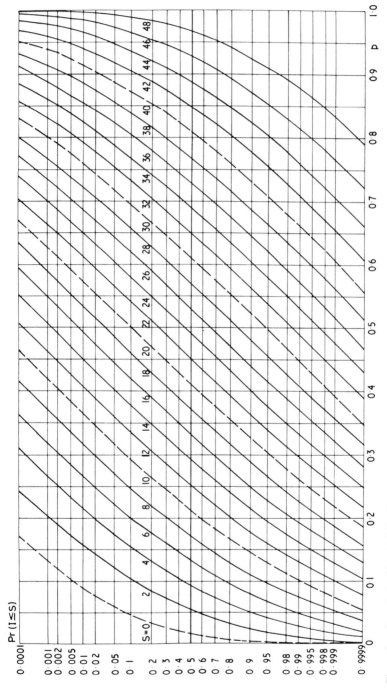

Figure 8. Cumulative binomial distribution from N = 50. Note that the ordinate is gaussian. There is for example a probability of 0.1 (10%) for obtaining a score of 20 or less correct words when p = 0.5.

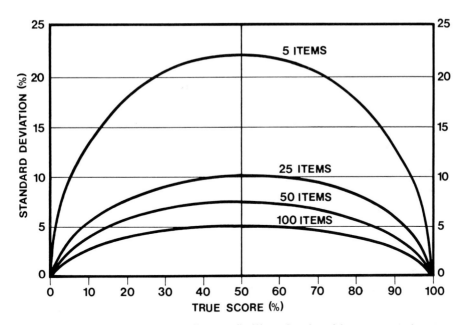

Figure 9. The standard deviation of a list score (in %) as a function of the mean score, for various number of items per list. A binomial distribution is assumed.

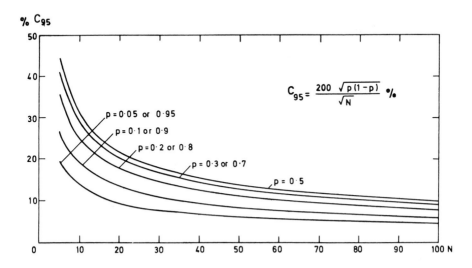

Figure 10. The 95% confidence interval (in %) for the binomial distribution, as a function of number of items per list.

face of it the number of scoring items would be multiplied by 3 and thus, for the same time and effort, yield a 3 times smaller variance of the intelligibility score. This interpretation would be correct provided the number of degrees of freedom were in fact multiplied by 3, but in general the advantage will be less than 3-fold due to sequential constraints between phonemes. As an example, take the word MOUTH/mauð/. If the final consonant and one of two remaining phonemes have been determined, only one English monosyllable will fit, and therefore the third phoneme conveys no new information. In this case the number of degrees of freedom is 2 rather than 3. Thus the effective number of degrees of freedom for phoneme scoring is higher than for word scoring, but not as high as the number of phonemes.

Word and phoneme scores will in practice differ, the latter typically being 20% higher, as shown in Figure 11.

The primary objective of speech audiometry is usually considered to be the determination of the *intelligibility curve*. This is conveniently done by determining list scores corresponding to different speech levels, and estimating the curve from these points, as illustrated in Figure 12. If the form of the curve were known beforehand, and therefore only a single point were needed to fix its position in the I-L diagram, the list scores could be compounded to yield an uncertainty estimate substantially better than each list score would yield on its own. If, on the other hand, absolutely nothing were known about the curve, no such improvement would occur. In practice the situation is somewhere between these two extremes, although there is no general agreement on how well the form of the curve is known. American practice tends towards considering the curve determined except for two parameters,so that two measurements are sufficient. These measures are the SRT and the maximum intelligibility attainable, the latter conventionally considered to occur at a speech level 30–40 dB higher than the threshold. European practice favours a determination of the whole curve, thus making fewer assumptions about its form. These assumptions are unfortunately difficult to quantify even for normal hearing. Consider, for example, the most elementary assumptions:

a) $I(L) \rightarrow 0\%$ $L \rightarrow -\infty$

b) $I(L) \rightarrow 100\%$ for $L \rightarrow \infty$

c) $\dfrac{dI}{dL} \geq 0$

d) absence of 'fine structure', i.e. the curve is 'smooth'.

Here, b) and c) are of doubtful validity and certainly violated in sensorineural cases.

This analysis presupposes that the intelligibility curve is indeed the result we seek to determine. Clearly any decision on the length of a list depends on what one sets out to determine, but having made such a decision, an estimate of reliability, and hence length of test, may be made.

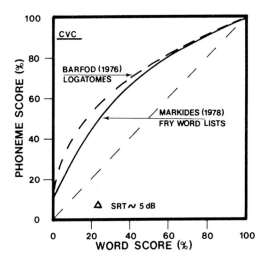

Figure 11.   Average relation between word and phoneme scores for CVC monosyllables.

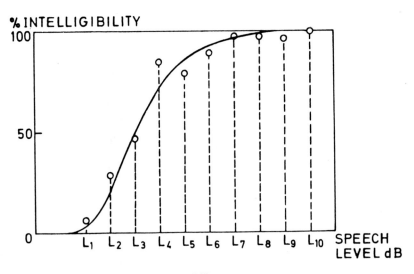

Figure 12.   Illustration of the speech intelligibility curve.

Theory of Speech Audiometry

Consider the following question: What responses are to be expected in speech audiometry, when words are used as stimuli, and the listeners are instructed to repeat what they believed they heard? Is it perhaps possible to predict the actual responses recorded in speech audiometry, rather than solely how many correct and how many incorrect? If so it might be hoped that deviations from expectation would be of clinical interest, indeed useful in assessing rehabilitational progress, and therefore worth clarifying; furthemore such knowledge would allow one to assemble new word lists according to a clear rationale rather than on the more or less random basis normally adopted. The latter would in turn enable speech materials more sensitive than at present to be assembled, because each single word would be 'pulling its weight' rather than perhaps being redundant.

Figure 13 tabulates the responses obtained for the stimulus word NUN /nʌn/, in a typical speech audiometry situation involving listeners with normal hearing. All the different responses obtained are listed in the first column, with the responses most similar to the stimulus word at the top, and the most dissimilar ones at the bottom. The five different data columns (A,B,C,D and E) refer to different level and masking conditions; for present purposes they may be considered simply as defining a generalized speech level axis, the level ascending from A to E. At first glance there is not much of a pattern to be seen, but closer examination reveals that, whereas the vastly dissimilar responses occur only at low speech levels, the more similar responses are found at low as well as at high speech levels. This trend is generally seen in all speech audiometry data, and the pattern of probabilities of words being responded, versus speech level, is as shown in Figure 14. At high speech levels, 100% correct responses are obtained (disregarding distortion effects at excessively high levels, or a sensorineural hearing impairment), and as the level is decreased a few error words start intruding, these tending to sound fairly similar to the stimulus word. As the speech level is decreased further, more and more different words occur, and these tend to have less phonetic similarity to the stimulus word. At very low levels one approaches a condition of random choice amongst a very large number of alternatives, most of them without much resemblance to the stimulus word. The latter does, however, assume that listeners are forced to respond; failing that the probability of not getting a response at all will quickly dominate.

A few other observations concerning word response patterns are worth noting. Whether or not the listeners are instructed in what type of material to expect, their responses will nearly always be of the type used. In other words, if the words presented are monosyllabic, the responses will be predominantly monosyllabic words, even if listeners are asked to respond to just that part of the word they actually heard. Furthermore responses will seldom if ever include uncommon words. Finally, in using monosyllabic words, it is observed that errors in one of the consonants are much more frequent than errors in the vowel.

To generalize these observations based on experiments conducted with monosyllables, errors in speech audiometry seem to have the following properties:

They nearly always have the same number of syllables as the stimuli.
They tend to be phonetically similar to the stimuli, particularly at high

RESPONSE	TYPE	A	B	GROUP C	D	E
NUN	111	2	11	5	3	5
NUMB	110	1	1	2	3	—
RUN	011	2	4	3	—	—
HUN	011	—	1	—	—	—
ONE	011	—	1	—	—	—
NINE	101	—	1	—	—	—
NOW	100	—	1	—	—	—
AGAIN	001	1	—	—	—	—
BONE	001	—	1	—	—	—
LINE	001	—	1	—	—	—
MUM	010	—	1	2	—	—
COME	010	—	2	—	—	—
YOUNG	010	—	—	1	—	—
LUNG	010	—	—	1	—	—
LOVE	010	1	—	—	—	—
ENOUGH	010	1	—	—	—	—
RUNG	010	1	—	—	—	—
THUMB	010	1	1	—	—	—
DRUG	010	1	—	—	—	—
UP	010	1	—	—	—	—
DANCE	000	—	1	—	—	—
LONG	000	—	2	—	—	—
ROW	000	1	—	—	—	—
FILL	000	1	—	—	—	—
WRONG	000	2	1	—	—	—
LAMP	000	1	—	—	—	—
MORE	000	—	2	1	—	—
—	—	5	2	1	—	—
		22	34	16	6	5

Figure 13. Responses to the word "NUN", classified according to the type of phoneme error (column 2). The bottom two rows indicate no-response and total number of responses respectively.

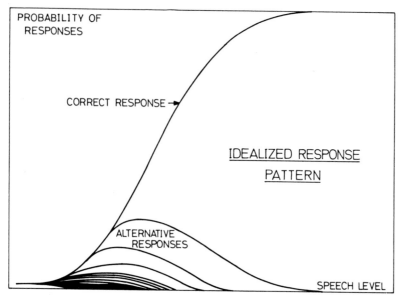

Figure 14.   Illustration of the pattern of correct/incorrect responses, as a function of speech level.

speech levels/favourable listening conditions.

They are meaningful words, and predominantly common ones.

Consonants are more easily missed than vowels.

It therefore seems that the probability of word B being mistaken for word A depends on (a) how common word B is, (b) how similar words A and B are phonetically, and (c) whether word B is a viable response word, given the knowledge the listener has regarding the test.

All these effects are well-established in the literature, but, with a few exceptions, they have been investigated separately, although they will always coexist. A suitable model must take them all into account.

The Model

For a given listener and a given recorded word material, presented in fixed acoustical conditions, the probabilities of different responses are conveniently described by a word confusion matrix (WCM) as shown in Figure 15.

This matrix gives the probability of obtaining a response W_j for the simulus W_i. As we shall mainly consider the free-response situation (which is the most normal in speech audiometry, but unfortunately also the most difficult to deal with theoretically), W_j may be any conceivable word, whereas

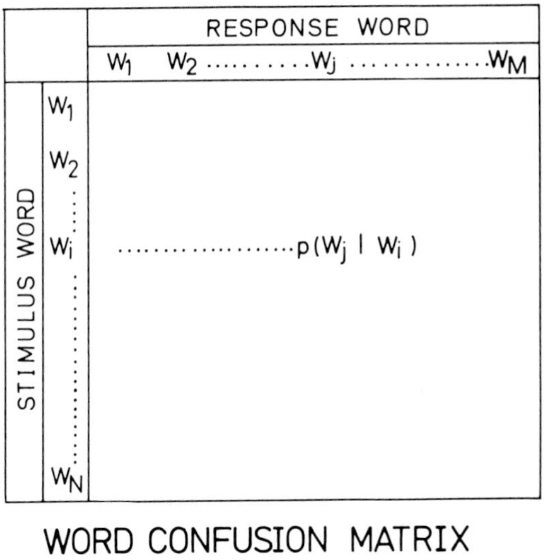

WORD CONFUSION MATRIX

Figure 15. Word confusion matrix (WCM), indicating the probability of word W_j being responded when the stimulus is W_i. The WCM depends on the test conditions, particularly the speech level.

W_i is restricted to the words contained in the word material. If we can assume that the probabilities are time-invariant and statistically independent, the WCM furnishes a complete description of the speech audiometry test (Lyregaard, 1973). Obviously the probabilities are normalized, hence:

$$\sum_{j=1}^{M} p(W_j|W_i) = 1$$

and the expected (i.e. mean) test score is:

$$E\{I\} = \sum_{i=1}^{N} p(W_i|W_i)$$

However, bearing in mind that the number of response alternatives is in principle equal to the number of words in the English language, this probability matrix is too large to be of any use, let alone determined experimentally. Therefore simplifications are called for, and it is proposed to consider only monosyllabic words, both as stimuli and responses. To simplify the problem further we consider each probability as a product of three independent probabilities:

$$p(W_j \mid W_i) = \alpha(W_j \mid W_i) \cdot \beta(W_j \mid W_i) \cdot \gamma(W_j \mid W_i)$$

57

where α reflects the influence of acoustic factors, β the linguistic factors, and γ the phonetic factors. Briefly they may be described as follows:

α is the probability of obtaining a response at all, and depends therefore on such acoustic factors as speech level and/or signal-to-noise ratio, but also on the methodology. Thus in a forced-response situation α will always be unity. In the free-response situation it will depend on the speech level and thus the stimulus word in question, but not on the response word. In fact we hypothesize that it will be equal to the psychometric function of the word, regarding the word as a physical stimulus (i.e. the probability that the listener will *hear* the word). The α-curve therefore depends on the definition of speech level. Indeed, one might argue that an optimum method of measuring speech level in speech audiometry is one that ensures that α is similar for all words.

Just as α takes account of the response probabilities in respect of the acoustic characteristics of the stimuli, β deals with the linguistic properties. Words (at least in one's native tongue) are perceived as entities rather than on a phoneme-by-phoneme basis. Therefore recognition may be regarded as a matching of the incoming acoustic/phonetic pattern with stored word images, and the question of which images are available, and even how available they are, becomes important. The availability or expectation is accounted for by β, and it may be thought of as the probability that a given word appears as response in the limit where no input stimulus at all is presented. Clearly the expectation is affected by any explicit or implicit limitation of choice, and in this sense β depends on the method used. Even if two words were both allowed as responses, and they were exactly alike in terms of acoustic/ phonetic features (as could be achieved with homophones such as BEAR and BARE), we would not expect their probabilities to be equal. This has been described as the frequency-of-occurrence effect, which asserts that, on average, uncommon words have a lower probability of recognition than common words. Evidently β will depend on the response word and the listener, but not on the stimulus word or speech level. Experiments with the frequency-of-occurrence effect seem to suggest that listener-to-listener differences are not large and we shall therefore, as an approximation, disregard listener variations. The estimation of β can then be based on frequency-of-occurrence data (Lyregaard, 1976), as shown in Figure 16.

The γ factor describes the phonetic similarity (and thus the confusibility) of the stimulus and response word. As it depends on both stimulus and response it forms a matrix of the same dimensions as the WCM. However, by introducing the following simplifications: (1) that phonetic similarity is the same as phonemic similarity, meaning that the abstraction of a word can be considered rather than its physical manifestation, and consequently that speaker-to-speaker variations may be disregarded, and (2) that consideration can be limited to monosyllabic stimuli and responses of the CVC-type, one can write:

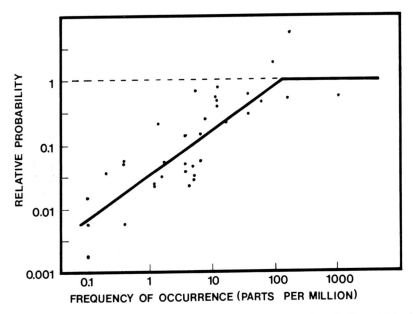

Figure 16. Estimate of β, based on the frequency of occurrence of words. Data obtained in an open-choice speech audiometry test using homophones (Lyregaard, 1976).

$$\gamma = p(W' \mid W) = p(C'_1 V' C'_2 \mid C_1 V C_2) = p(C'_1 \mid C_1) \cdot p(V' \mid V) \cdot p(C'_2 \mid C_2)$$

on the assumption that the latter probabilities are uncorrelated. Due to well-known sequential constraints (Shannon, 1948) this assumption may not appear warranted; however, since a large proportion of phoneme combinations do not form meaningful words in English, their contribution to the overall phoneme correlations may be disregarded if only meaningful responses are considered.

The simplification achieved by the delineation above is substantial, as the phoneme confusion matrices are of a manageable dimension (typically 20×20). But some difficulties remain, for instance the extent to which consonant clusters should be regarded as single phonemes; also vowel probabilities are intrinsically higher than consonant probabilities, due to the higher speech level of vowels relative to consonants. These problems are tractable, but further experimental evidence is necessary in order to resolve them.

Interpretation of Model

Although some of the factors still remain to be quantified, it is possible to consider implications of the model qualitatively.

Free Response

If the stimulus is a common word (high β), and there are no other common words nearly similar to it, then the intelligibility curve of this word will approximate the psychometric function (α). In fact the psychometric function is the limiting curve for any intelligibility curve, and if all words in a list approximate it we should expect a good agreement between average pure-tone thresholds and SRT.

If, on the other hand, there are many alternatives with a high degree of similarity to the stimulus, and especially if the stimulus is an uncommon word, pure-tone audiometry and speech audiometry results will not agree. In other words the α-curve describes the intelligibility when the only possible response is the stimulus word, and the extent to which this curve deviates from the actual intelligibility curve is an indication of the number and degree of 'intrusion' of erroneous responses. It is precisely this deviation which the β- and γ-factors describe, and which accounts for the difference between pure-tone and speech audiometry. The excess loss of intelligibility is not due to the listener not hearing the word, but due to his confusing them with likely alternatives.

Forced Choice

Here the model is simplified because both α and β are constant (the listener is forced to respond, and the alternatives are known). Therefore a forced-choice technique will essentially limit speech audiometry to depend on the phonetic factor. Here the form of the intelligibility curve for each item, and thus for the whole list, can be dramatically modified simply by manipulation of the alternatives/foils allowed.

Limited Free Response

An explicit or implicit limitation of acceptable responses will change the listener's expectations, thus β for response words outside the limits will be zero. The net effect is a shift of the intelligibility curve towards lower speech levels (nearer to the α-curve), a shift that is observed when for instance digits are used as words.

Discussion

Pending experimental evidence the ramifications of the model presented here can be summarized as follows, bearing in mind that only CVC-monosyllables have been implicated:

> It provides a framework for a rational interpretation and comparison of different methodologies, and an understanding of the results obtained.

Because responses are, in a statistical sense, predictable, there is a vast fund of information available in speech audiometry, namely the deviations from predicted errors in response. This information is even available in currently used tests without extending the test duration, but it is at present discarded.

In assembling new speech audiometry materials, or modifying already existing ones, the model allows one to select words such that error intrusion is controlled, thereby ensuring that the words have a prescribed distribution of correct-response probabilities. In particular it is possible, without resorting to extensive experimental work, to ensure approximately equal probabilities throughout the list, thereby avoiding words that do not contribute any information to the list scores. The model is particularly useful in selecting foils in the forced-choice method; without having to resort to experimental work one can predict the most probable alternatives, and thus ensure a maximally sensitive test.

It seems plausible that auditory disorders may be interpreted in terms of the factors of the model. Thus a conductive hearing loss will only affect α. A sensorineural loss may be interpreted as consisting of a conductive loss component and a 'distortion'; whereas the former only affects α, the latter will only implicate γ. Whether or not specific types of 'distortion' lead to specific confusion patterns remains to be investigated; if it were so more discriminating speech tests would clearly be feasible. The β factor is implicated in cortical disorders such as aphasia and to some extent in presbyacusis.

The model also has good prospects for the difficult question of international standardization of speech tests. The main problem here is to ensure that materials prepared in different languages are in fact equivalent, and this could be managed by specifying the probability factors discussed here. Such specifications could then be translated into words and word lists in each language. Such an approach is still some way off, but certainly appears to be feasible.

Chapter 3

Speech Tests in Quiet and Noise as a Measure of Auditory Processing

M. E. Lutman

Understanding of speech is fundamental to verbal communication and depends on many characteristics of the auditory system. This chapter aims to describe the more important aspects of auditory performance which are necessary for satisfactory speech processing and how these are affected by hearing impairment. The chapter also outlines methods which are commonly used to assess speech intelligibility in the individual and how the measures thus obtained may be used to estimate the disability or handicap experienced.

A Model of Speech Processing

The ability of the ear to unravel the complexities of speech depends on many aspects of hearing, including sensitivity as measured by the pure-tone audiogram. Over the past decade, much interest has been focused on the role played by frequency resolution (the ability of the ear to detect a target signal at one frequency in the presence of a competing sound at a different frequency). Some of this research is reviewed briefly in a later section in this chapter. Information has also become available to implicate temporal resolution (the ability to resolve detail in the waveform envelope of a signal), suppression (the increase in threshold at one frequency due to presentation of a sound at an adjacent frequency) and intensity discrimination (the ability to distinguish between two similar sounds at different intensities). It is known that all of these properties of audition are influenced adversely by hearing impairment, particularly of the sensorineural type.

In order to develop a tractable model of speech processing, Plomp and Duquesnoy (1982) have simplified the above by lumping all of the above characteristics, other than sensitivity, under a category termed 'distortion'. Their model expresses speech performance in terms of different levels of sensitivity and distortion. A series of experiments were undertaken to validate the model in which speech intelligibility was measured at various intensity levels. The measure of speech intelligibility they used was the speech intensity required for 50% correct score on sentences when presented together with a competing noise. Measurements were made at various noise levels in order to plot the speech level as a function of the noise level. Using decibel scales, if the speech were to be correctly identified at a constant signal-to-noise ratio, the plotted function would be a straight line with a slope of 45 degrees. Figure 1 illustrates the form of the relationship that was found in four groups of subjects categorised respectively as (i) normal sensitivity, normal distortion, (ii) normal sensitivity, increased distortion, (iii) reduced sensitivity, normal distortion and (iv) reduced sensitivity, increased distortion.

All of the curves are flat at the left-hand side. This is due to the effect of absolute threshold. Obviously, the speech must be above absolute threshold to be heard, independent of noise level, and the speech levels at which the flat portions of the curves occur are strongly influenced by threshold sensitivity.

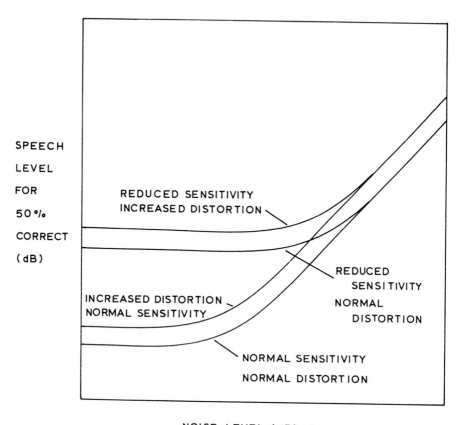

Figure 1. The form of relationship found in four groups of subjects when categorised by sensitivity and distortion.

Once the noise level exceeds a certain point, the curves increase in slope to the predicted 45 degrees. The effect of distortion in both sensitivity groups is to uniformly shift the curves upwards by a few decibels. Expressed in another way, increased distortion results in an increase in the signal-to-noise ratio required for correct identification, regardless of intensity level. Notice also that the curves of groups (i) and (iii) and of groups (ii) and (iv) converge at the higher intensities. Thus, at high intensities the only determinant of speech intelligibility is distortion; sensitivity is not a factor as long as the speech is audible.

Relationship Between Speech Intelligibility and Pure-Tone Sensitivity

The model described above was obtained under experimental conditions using subjects who had been selected to form discrete groups for the purpose of the study. Such neat groupings seldom occur in practice and there is a wealth of data on speech intelligibility in which the effects of sensitivity and distortion were hopelessly confounded. In the vast majority of studies, no measures of distortion had been made, but it is well established that most aspects of distortion are correlated with sensitivity. Typically such studies have measured speech reception threshold (SRT) and/or discrimination score (DS) for speech in quiet, although a smaller number have used speech in noise. Noble (1978) has extensively reviewed this literature. As a very general rule fairly high correlations have been found (circa 0.8) between SRT and auditory sensitivity and slightly lower correlations (circa 0.7) between DS and sensitivity. Best correlations with SRT are generally obtained when sensitivity is averaged over frequencies in the 0.5–4 kHz range.

When speech is presented with noise, the correlations tend to be some-what lower (e.g. Festen and Plomp, 1983; $r = 0.38$) but not in all studies (e.g. Tyler and Smith, 1983; $r = 0.84$). Presumably the direct effect of sensitivity is removed for speech-in-noise and the correlation reflects an indirect relationship mediated through distortion.

The relationship between speech intelligibility and sensitivity has been used as the basis of formulae for predicting speech performance from the pure-tone audiogram. Much attention has been focussed on the relative weights that should be attached to each audiometric frequency in the formula, although such an exercise can be misleading. The frequencies which correlate best with the speech identification scores are highly dependent on the test materials used (frequency spectra of speech and noise) and may not be the same for different materials, as pointed out by Haggard *et al.* (1987). For example, if all subjects had noise-induced hearing losses, there would be little variance in sensitivity at 500 Hz amongst the subject group, leading to a low correlation between speech performance and sensitivity at 500 Hz.

65

Studies of self-reported speech disability in the general population are not prone to the same biases and Lutman *et al.* (1987) suggest that the actual choice of frequencies in the range 500 Hz to 4 kHz in a prediction formula does not influence its accuracy very much. Averages including sensitivity at 500 Hz, however, were very slightly better correlated with self-reported disability than those composed only of the higher frequencies.

Relationships Between Speech Intelligibility and Measures of Distortion

Several studies have shown that frequency resolution is related to speech test performance (e.g., Leshowitz, 1977; Bonding, 1979; Dreschler and Plomp, 1980). With respect to temporal resolution, Tyler *et al.* (1982) have shown an effect, whereas Festen and Plomp (1983) did not. In all studies of this type, subjects tend to vary in auditory sensitivity, frequency resolution and temporal resolution, as well as age, and all of these factors tend to covary. Therefore, it is extremely difficult to identify whether one parameter is fundamentally related to speech performance, or simply varies with another parameter which is fundamentally related (so-called collinearity). Lutman and Clark (1986) have attempted to account for such collinearity and have shown that in hearing-aid users with sensorineural hearing impairment, age and sensitivity at 2 kHz are sufficient to account for the variation in performance in a speech-in-noise task, without the necessity to include frequency and temporal resolution measures. This does not mean that the distortion parameters are unimportant; rather they can be predicted by the measurement of sensitivity.

A factor that has not been investigated adequately is the dependence of the form of any relationship between distortion measures and speech performance on the severity of the hearing loss. It might be expected that different factors would be important in normal and mildly-impaired subjects than in moderately or severely impaired subjects. In fact, recent data (Lutman, 1987) suggest that frequency resolution is the major factor for mild impairments; and sensitivity at 2 and 4 kHz and temporal resolution are most important for moderate impairments.

Effects of Type of Hearing Loss on Speech Discrimination

The dependence of speech-in-quiet and speech-in-noise scores on pure-tone sensitivity and measures of distortion has already been described. A further factor is whether the hearing loss is primarily conductive or sensorineural. From a database of conventional speech-in-quiet test results, Gatehouse and Haggard (1987) obtained word identification scores for a heterogeneous clinical population with sensorineural, conductive and mixed hearing losses. They derived iso-performance contours plotted against axes of mean air-conduction threshold and mean air-bone gap. For a given air-conduction threshold, increasing air-bone gap was associated with poorer performance at all but the highest intensities used for speech (i.e. peak SPLs of 95, 100 and 105 dB). Thus, the presence of a conductive impairment led to worse discrimination for a given air-conduction hearing loss when the speech was at low and moderate speech intensities. It was only at speech intensities at and above 95 dB that sensorineural losses exhibited worse discrimination. These authors argue that their findings result from recruitment in the sensorineural cases which has the beneficial effect of conferring greater loudness on supra-threshold signals, compared with non-recruiting ears having equal loss of sensitivity at threshold. At the very high intensities (and as a consequence of the speech audiometry procedure, predominantly in the more impaired ears), the greater distortion accompanying a sensorineural impairment becomes the over-riding factor. A similar disadvantage for conductive cases seems to be evident in the everyday experience of hearing impaired subjects in that self-reported disability is greater in people with conductive or mixed losses greater than about 35 dB than those with comparable sensorineural losses (Lutman *et al.*, 1987).

Effects of Age and Socio-Economic Group

It is normally extremely difficult to separate the effects of age and socio-economic group on speech test performance from the effects of hearing loss since they tend to be heavily confounded. However, there are indications that age and manual versus non-manual occupation *per se* have effects in the expected direction (greater age and manual occupation associated with poorer performance), as described by Davis (1983).

Summarizing the information presented so far, it can be stated that sensitivity and distortion factors interact in a complex fashion to determine speech intelligibility. Sensitivity measures alone can predict speech intelligibility nearly as well as a combination of sensitivity and distortion measures, although the predictive accuracy is not high, particularly for speech in noise. Other parameters not included under the umbrella of sensitivity and distortion also affect intelligibility, such as type of hearing loss, cognitive factors and aspects of central processing including those reflected by age. Thus, there is a need to measure speech performance directly which cannot be met by other tests of auditory dysfunction.

Objectives of Speech Testing

Theoretically, it is possible to design speech tests to measure any specific aspect of auditory processing. However, other than those used for diagnostic purposes, speech tests are generally intended primarily to be representative of everyday speech used for communication and the tests aim to give an indication of disability. Studies of the relationship between self-reported disability and speech tests have often found a poor correspondence, even when using speech-in-noise tests which would suggest themselves as preferable to speech-in-quiet for this purpose. None the less, speech testing gives the most practicable performance measure of disability and avoids the difficulties, inherent in self-report methods, of personal opinion and bias.

The use of speech-in-noise tests has an additional advantage over speech-in-quiet when testing a heterogeneous population of subjects. The signal-to-noise ratio of the test can be set to achieve a suitable range of scores in advance. This means that the absolute level of the materials can be set at a moderately high intensity which is easily audible to all subjects (within reason). In this way, it is possible to reduce or avoid the problems of 'ceiling' and 'floor' effects where the score obtained by a subject is curtailed by the 100% or 0% absolute limits available.

Choice of Materials for Assessing Speech Processing Ability

Some experimental studies of communication systems or speech processing have used isolated phonemes or nonsense syllables. These items have the advantage of minimal semantic content, thus effectively eliminating differences between subjects in education and vocabulary. However, it requires considerable training to achieve stable performance on the tests and they are not really suitable in a clinical context. At the other extreme, running speech contains all the semantic, contextual and prosodic features of everyday speech and therefore has great face validity as a material for disability measurement. None the less, it also requires some training for the subject to repeat running speech and it is difficult for the tester to score responses accurately.

The most common compromises which are used for practical clinical tests are lists of either single words or sentences. The latter have greater external validity for representing everyday situations, but they are more difficult to incorporate into tests because of the limitations imposed by grammar and syntax. Also, sentence materials tend to have a steep psychometric function (i.e. the curve relating score to intensity or signal-to-noise ratio). This latter characteristic makes sentences more suitable for a speech-in-noise task where the signal-to-noise ratio can be pre-set to a level which achieves the desired level of performance and avoids 'ceiling' and 'floor' effects.

Word lists are not subject to the influence of cognitive factors in the subject's use of context and syntax to determine the correct response, as are sentences. This may be an advantage or disadvantage, depending on the purposes of the test.

For all types of materials, the efficiency of the test depends on the relative difficulty of items within the test. Ideally, all items should be equally difficult and therefore none will be redundant. Clearly, if an item is significantly easier than others, it will nearly always be identified correctly by all subjects and thus not contribute any information. A corresponding effect occurs if an item is relatively more difficult than the remainder. A great deal of pilot work is necessary to obtain an efficient set of materials which is appropriate to the subjects with whom it is intended to use the test.

Speech-in-noise tests require the selection of a suitable noise. In general, this should have significant energy at all frequencies present in the speech signal. Typically, a noise may be generated to have a frequency spectrum which approximates the long-term spectrum of the speech. Alternatively, the voice of another speaker or several speakers may be used. When speech from several speakers is amalgamated to form the noise it is referred to as 'speech babble' or 'cafeteria noise'. When the speech signal and noise have different frequency spectra it is difficult to define the signal-to-noise ratio in any meaningful way. For example, if the difference in dB between the overall level of the signal to the overall level of the noise is taken, this may differ quite markedly from the signal-to-noise ratio in any specific frequency band. It is usually the most advantageous band signal-to-noise ratio which determines intelligibility and thus the overall signal-to-noise ratio may not relate at all well to intelligibility.

Because speech is a spectro-temporal code, containing information in both the frequency and the time domain, the temporal structure of the noise is also a factor. Steady noise is less likely to mask the amplitude modulations of speech than a noise with similar amplitude modulations to those in speech. Therefore either 'babble' or amplitude modulated noise tends to have a greater masking effect than steady noise. Furthermore, modulated noise has a relatively more deleterious effect on intelligibility than steady noise in subjects with a sensorineural hearing loss (Tyler and Smith, 1983). These authors also showed that a sentence-in-noise test using modulated noise was more highly correlated with self-reported disability than the same sentence lists, against a background of steady noise with the same frequency spectrum as the modulated noise.

Whatever speech or noise materials are used, calibration and setting of levels is extremely important. For speech-in-noise tests, variations in signal-to-noise ratio of as little as 1 dB can have marked effects. Therefore, accurate documentation of the levels used for each subject is essential. It is most important that descriptions of signal-to-noise ratio define exactly what has been measured as there are no accepted standard methods available. More specific details of equipment and calibration are covered in Chapter 4.

Method of Subject Response and Scoring

For identification tests, the subject may simply repeat or write down what he has heard. In clinical practice it is common for the subject to repeat what he has heard and for the tester to score the response. This means that the tester must be able to hear the subject clearly, either directly or using a microphone/amplifier system. Scoring (and instructions to the subject) must take account of the possibility that subjects may be lax in their use of plurals or tenses in their reply, even though they may have correctly understood the item.

When the speech test offers a limited set of alternative responses (e.g., four-alternatives in FAAF test) scoring may be by pencil and paper using a pro-forma worksheet completed either by the subject or the tester. In the latter case, given that the alternatives in such closed-set tests usually sound very similar, there is a possibility of the tester mis-hearing the response. Alternatively, electronic or computer-recorded scoring using push-buttons may be used. Clearly, closed-set tests in this general format require that the subject can read, although an equivalent two-alternative picture-pointing version has been used for children.

Adaptive Speech-In-Noise Tests

It is virtually impossible to design a fixed signal-to-noise ratio test that will cater for a wide range of patients without ceiling or floor effects. For example, using the SIiN test which involves sentences against a background of noise, a signal-to-noise ratio which gives scores in the region of 80% in normal ears is unusable in patients with hearing impairments greater than about an average of 45 dB because they score less than 20%. Increasing the signal-to-noise ratio would cause some of the normal subjects to reach the ceiling of 100%.

One method to overcome this problem is to adjust the signal-to-noise ratio adaptively during the test to achieve a predetermined level of performance (e.g. 50% correct or 71% correct). This approach has been used conventionally for speech-in-quiet tests to measure the SRT. For speech-in-noise, Plomp and Mimpen (1979) have developed a test which uses a fixed level of noise. The signal is composed of Dutch sentences which are presented initially at a relatively high-intensity. If the subject repeats the sentence correctly, the speech intensity is reduced. When he makes a mistake, the speech level is increased. This procedure continues and it is possible ultimately to estimate the intensity at which he scores 50% correct for the given noise level. Thus, the outcome measure is the signal-to-noise ratio for 50% correct.

A similar principle is used in the adaptive version of the FAAF test which involves a closed set of single-syllable words, each trial having four alternatives. The adaptive test has been described by Lutman and Clark (1986) and involves a fixed level of speech and a variable level of noise, both speech and noise having the same long-term frequency spectrum. The criterion level of performance can be pre-set, levels of 50 and 71% being used in practice.

In general, adaptive speech-in-noise tests have the advantage of widespread applicability in a clinical context and some control of error patterns and would seem to be a favourable choice for assessment of speech processing ability.

Error Patterns

For most speech tests, it is possible to score the type of error as well as simply whether the item was identified correctly. For example, the error might be plosive instead of fricative, as in 'pan' instead of 'fan'. Tests such as the FAAF have been designed to contain specific contrasts between alternatives within a single trial and therefore give the opportunity for specific error types. Thus, scoring of the test can be focussed on analysis of the error patterns as well as the overall performance. These data can be used to infer how information from different regions of the frequency spectrum is being used.

In general, errors of place of articulation (e.g., the contrast between 'gay', 'day' and 'bay') are sensitive to even mild hearing impairment or noise masking. Place of articulation information is carried predominantly in the higher frequencies. Manner of articulation (e.g., the contrast between 'tick', 'lick' and 'pick') and voicing (e.g., 'bay' versus 'pay') are relatively robust. As a consequence, in speech-in-noise tests, subjects scoring highly will probably be making only place of articulation errors, whereas those scoring poorly will be making all types of error. An advantage of adaptive testing when comparing individuals is that subjects will all tend to be making similar error types. The disadvantage is that this limits further analysis of error type.

Lip Reading

Hearing and lip reading are elegantly complementary (Summerfield, 1983). The place of articulation information in speech (e.g. 'gay', 'day', 'pay') which is so easily removed by hearing loss or background noise is most easily inferred from lip reading. Additionally, the timing information obtained from a combination of lip reading and hearing provides extremely useful (audio-visual) cues, as exemplified by the relative onsets of lip opening and voicing in 'mole', 'bole', 'pole'.

Audio-visual tests involving lip reading are difficult to devise for a heterogeneous population because they are extremely prone to floor and ceiling effects. Research into a method of modulating lip reading information for possible use in an adaptive test is in its early stages of development at the Institute of Hearing Research in Nottingham.

Despite these difficulties, audio-visual tests of speech identification have seemingly a high face validity for disability assessment, but require further research to support this contention.

Practical Speech Tests

The following are some of the speech test materials used in the UK which are potentially available for measurement of speech processing using English (not American) speakers. Availability is by arrangement with the organization named for each test.

Speech-In-Quiet

Arthur Boothroyd word lists (Boothroyd, 1968). Fifteen lists of 10 consonant-vowel-consonant words isophonemically constructed. Normally scored as phonemes correct out of 30. AB(s) recordings have 'Standard British Southern' pronunciation using a male speaker. Tapes containing the 12 most equally difficult AB(s) lists may be purchased from the Institute of Sound and Vibration Research, University of Southampton.

BKB Sentence Lists for children. Twenty one lists of 16 sentences, each list containing a total of 50 key words to be scored. Restricted to vocabulary of partially-hearing children (Bench and Bamford, 1979). Recorded by female speaker with southern English accent. Tapes available from Audiology Unit, Royal Berkshire Hospital, Reading, Berks.

Speech-In-Noise

Sentence-Identification-in-Noise (SIiN) based on BKB recordings against modulated noise. Noise has same long-term spectrum as speech and is modulated with the same amplitude envelope. Tapes available through Institute of Hearing Research, University of Nottingham.

Two example sentences from the Sentence-Identification-in-Noise Test (SIiN) follow. Scoring is based on key words which are in capitals. Based on BKB word lists.

The BATH TOWEL was WET
The MATCHES LIE on the SHELF

Four-Alternative-Auditory-Feature (FAAF) test. Four-alternative forced choice test based on a vocabulary of 80 consonant-vowel-consonant words in 20 sets of four, composed like rhyme tests on the binary feature principle. Items presented in the carrier phrase 'Can you hear . . . clearly' and against a steady noise background with the same long-term frequency spectrum as the speech. Male speaker with resonant voice and 'Standard British Southern' accent. Scoring may be total correct or by error types. Computer program assists in analysis of error types.

Two example trials from the Four-Alternative-Auditory-Feature Test (FAAF) follow.

BAD BAG BAT BACK
GAB DAB TAB CAB

Two-Alternative Picture Pointing. Tests described by Haggard, Wood and Carroll (1984). Recording of 48 consonant-vowel-consonant words, against a background of steady speech-spectrum-shaped noise, by a female speaker with a North Midlands regional accent using vocabulary of 24 minimal pairs, each pair differing only in the initial phoneme. Illustrates corresponding to the 48 words allows forced-choice picture-pointing response suitable for use with 5-year-old children. Scored as percent words correct. Materials available by arrangement with Institute of Hearing Research, University of Nottingham.

Audio-Visual Tests

Four-Alternative-Disability-And-Speechreading-Test (FADAST). Similar in principle to the FAAF test, but recorded on Sony U-matic video cassette and displaying head and shoulders of speaker. No carrier phrase is incorporated, but visible cues warn of onsets of words. Four alternative responses also displayed as caption and differ in vowel as well as either initial or final consonant.

Two examples from the Four-Alternative-Disability-And-Speechreading-Test (FADAST) follow.

HEEL SEAL HAIL SAIL
SUCK SUNG SACK SANG

Chapter 4

Equipment for Speech Audiometry and its Calibration

H. Fuller

The basic requirements for speech testing are a source of speech, a means to control the level of the speech received by the patient and a record of the patient's response. At its very simplest level, a test may be performed by asking questions in a quiet, a normal or a loud voice, to which the patient will provide an appropriate answer if enough is heard for the question to be understood. Such a speech test has many uses, but it does not warrant the name 'speech-audiometry' since there is too little control over both the level of the speech reaching the patient and the amount of the stimulus which has to be understood for a response to be made.

The term 'speech audiometry' is reserved for a test in which a representative sample of speech is presented to the patient under measurable conditions and the response is given in a form which indicates how much of the stimulus has been understood. In speech audiometry, it is necessary to be able to measure the stimulus, to measure the response and to relate the two to those of normal hearers and to groups with known pathologies. At all stages the emphasis is on control, measurability and reproducibility.

It is because of the need to measure and control the stimulus that, whether for live-voice testing or for tests using pre-recorded material, speech audiometry usually makes use of an audiometer or an independent amplifier to feed the stimulus signal to the patient via earphones or a loudspeaker.

Figure 1, derived from Lyregaard *et al.* (1976), shows the information flow in a speech audiometry test in which the result is a discrimination curve constructed by comparing the stimuli and responses at different measured levels of presentation. The choice of equipment to perform such a test is wide and its selection will often be determined by what is already available. Some of the considerations which might play a part in equipping a speech audiometry test facility are outlined here together with the measurements and calibrations which are needed to ensure that the test results have meaning and can be compared with those made at other centres.

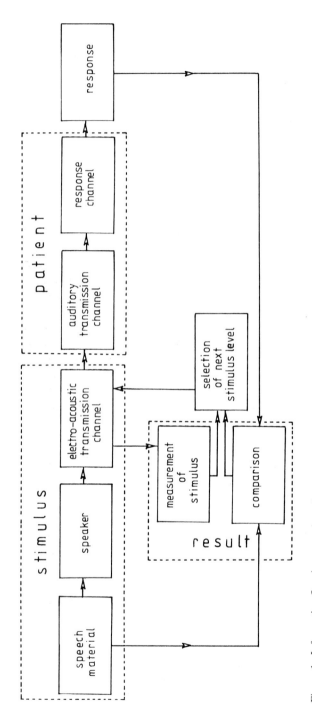

Figure 1: Information flow in a speech audiometry test

Audiometers

Many audiometers are designed so that they can be used for speech tests as well as for pure-tone audiometry. If this is the case, the audiometer will be equipped with a speech or audio channel, which will take the signal from a tape recorder or microphone, and with a wide-band masking facility.

The masking is used to ensure that when one ear is tested, there is no significant contribution caused by a more sensitive non-test ear picking up the test signal by bone conduction or by cross hearing. The noise provided will either be white noise or speech spectrum noise. White noise has equal amounts of energy at each frequency and speech spectrum noise is white noise which has been shaped so as to approximate to that of an idealized average speaker, falling by 12 dB per octave between 1 and 6 kHz (IEC 645). Masking by either kind of noise is equally effective, but the speech spectrum noise has the advantage of cutting out the unnecessary energy at the higher frequencies. For research purposes, a masking noise is sometimes used which conforms exactly to the spectrum of the voice speaking the test words, but the use of such a masker requires non-standard equipment and for most applications the broad band masking noise facility built into the audiometer is quite adequate.

The calibration of audiometers should form an important part of the routine of any test centre. Although a full workshop test, adjustment and re-calibration of the equipment will be necessary if the audiometer develops a major fault, routine checks and calibrations should be made in the clinics at regular intervals. If the audiometer has to be sent out of the clinic to the manufacturer or to a specialized laboratory for a routine calibration, the inconvenience is likely to prove a substantial barrier to this important activity. It would be a great advantage, therefore, if each clinic had either the equipment necessary to carry out its own audiometer calibrations or had access to a mobile calibration service visiting at regular intervals.

Since speech audiometry is usually carried out using a facility on a pure-tone audiometer, all of the checks recommended to ensure that the audiometer is working correctly are applicable to the speech audiometer. Some of these checks and procedures should be carried out at weekly intervals (or more frequently) and do not require any specialized equipment. For example, the audiometer and its ancillary equipment can be checked for any signs of wear, ensuring that the correct earphones are used with the audiometer and that they and their headbands are in good condition. Making use of the fact that one of the best means of checking the audiometer is the audiologist's own ears (if they are near normal), the output of the audiometer can be checked approximately by listening to all frequencies at a hearing level of 10 or 15 dB. Listening at a high level, all the functions of the audiometer, including the speech circuits, can be checked to ensure that there are no distortions, clicks etc., whilst listening at low levels the equipment can be checked for hum and for breakthrough between channels. It is also possible to check the quality of the tones and speech signal, which should not change when masking is introduced, and the attenuators, which should attenuate over their whole range without introducing mechanical or electrical noise.

Objective calibration of the audiometer, which does require special equipment, should ideally be carried out every 3 months and should comply with IEC publication 645. The minimum equipment which would be needed is given below:

> precision sound level meter with 1 inch condenser microphone
> octave or 1/3 octave filter set
> artificial ear or acoustic coupler
> mechanical coupler (artificial mastoid) only required for bone conduction measurements
> digital frequency meter (audio frequencies)
> oscilloscope

The aspects of the audiometer performance which should be measured include the frequencies of the pure tone signals, the output of the earphones and bone vibrators, the levels of the masking noise, the attenuator steps and the harmonic distortion of the whole system. For speech audiometry, the accuracy of the level indicator should also be checked, together with the performance of any ancillary equipment such as a tape recorder. Table I shows the British Standards and their IEC and ISO equivalents which are relevant for the calibration of audiometers.

British Standard	IEC Publication	ISO Standard	Topic covered
5966	645		Audiometer equipment specification
2497		389,7566	Reference zero for the calibration of pure tone audiometers
4009	373		Mechanical coupler for the calibration of bone vibrators
4668	303		Acoustic coupler for the calibration of audiometric earphones
4669	318		Artificial ear for the calibration of audiometric earphones

Table I Standards relevant to the calibration of audiometers

Tape Recorders

There are considerable advantages in using recorded speech rather than the live-voice for audiometric purposes. The use of a recorded stimulus ensures that the test material is always the same and allows the editing of the master recording, so as to approach the ideal of a set of test materials of equal difficulty which give reproducible discrimination curves. The original speech audiometry test lists were recorded on 78 rpm records, but these have long ago been discarded in favour of tape recordings.

The advent of the domestic hi-fi market means that the electronic specifications for suitable tape recorders will easily be met by any good domestic equipment. The tape recorder should be capable of handling the dynamic range of speech (about 30 dB), it should have a harmonic distortion of less than 1% and the flattest possible frequency response over the major speech frequencies (250 Hz to about 4 kHz) and it should have an output impedance which is matched to the input impedance of the audiometer. In practice none of these requirements is very severe. The impedances will cause no problems as the audiometer speech channel will have been built to accept a signal from a tape recorder and many recorders have a good dynamic range with very flat frequency responses and low distortion well beyond the range needed for speech reproduction.

Cassette recorders, when they were first introduced, gave relatively poor performance compared with reel-to-reel recorders, but with the introduction of noise reduction systems and better quality tape, they are now capable of excellent performance. Many of the recorded lists which were originally available only on 6.3 mm tape have now been transcribed onto cassettes, with the result that the audiologist is free to choose equipment from the very wide range which is available. Robustness, convenience, ease of use and cost all play an important part in the selection of the right recorder, and a recent survey of National Health Service audiology clinics in the UK showed that approximately half of the clinics now use cassette recorders for speech audiometry (Fuller and Moss, 1985).

The performance of the tape recorder should be measured when the audiometer is calibrated, but as with other audiometric equipment, listening to the quality of its output provides a useful day-to-day check that nothing is seriously wrong. The frequency response, harmonic distortion and tape speed should all be checked during routine calibrations or after a major repair (IEC publication 94). In addition, the tape heads should be cleaned regularly by gently wiping them with a cotton bud impregnated with alcohol or a proprietary head-cleaning fluid. The frequency with which this will be necessary will depend on the extent to which the recorder is used and on the quality of the tape, as some tapes shed more of the oxide coating than others, but it should become part of the regular routine of equipment care in the clinic.

Measurement of Word Level

For the audiologist using pre-recorded material, the level for the presentation of a word list to the patient can easily be set using the calibration tone recorded at the beginning of each list or at the beginning of the whole tape. Once the level of the tone is set, adjustments to the level of the whole list are made with the audiometer attenuators which are, in turn, checked as part of the audiometer calibration procedure.

For those who are practicing live-voice testing or are recording new test material, however, the measurement of the levels of the individual words is important and is by no means a simple matter because of the nature of the speech signal. A plot of amplitude against time for a single word shows the difficulty.

It can clearly be seen that most of the acoustic energy in the word is in the vowel, yet much of the information is in the consonants and, in addition, the vowel has a very short rise time which might affect the measurement made. The problem is not quite as great as might at first appear because there is a natural pattern to the relationship between the different phonemes of a word and this will not be broken as long as the speaker does not deliberately try to distort the word by, for example, speaking more 'clearly' than usual.

Fuller and Whittle (1982) made a study of the measurement of word levels for audiometric purposes. They took as their criterion the Speech

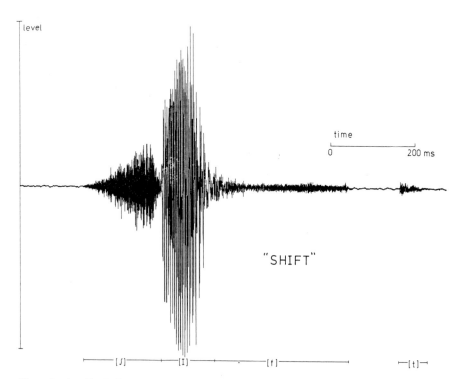

Figure 2: Amplitude (instantaneous voltage) plotted against time for the word 'SHIFT'

Detection Threshold (SDT) that is, the level at which the listener can just detect that a stimulus is present but cannot recognize the word, and investigated which of a number of different physical measures gave the best prediction of the subjectively determined SDT for normal hearing subjects. They included a wide range of instruments and measures in their study, including the VU meter, Peak Programme Meter (PPM), measures of the total energy, the peak level, the RMS level measured with fast and slow meter characteristics and the maximum impulse level. The differences between the predictive ability of the different measures was comparatively small, but the correlations jumped from 0·7 to 0·9 when the A-weighting network was added to each of the measures. Brady (1971) also made a study of the measurement of word level and showed that there was considerable variability in measurements made with a VU meter by non-expert observers.

This works suggests that whilst the VU meter, which is the indicator usually fitted to an audiometer, gives an adequate objective measure of the subjective level of a word, it would be better to use a meter which is more easily read. A meter giving an RMS (fast) reading and with the ability to switch in A-weighting would be a better choice for this purpose.

When recorded lists are being prepared, it is possible to avoid total reliance on measurements of the levels of the words and to produce lists which have been subjectively equalized. The technique is to make a first recording with an experienced speaker using equal vocal effort or feedback from a monitoring meter to get the levels approximately equal. An iterative process is then begun, testing normal hearing subjects close to threshold, to determine which items of the list are particularly easy or difficult to perceive. The levels of these words are then adjusted by lowering those of the easy items and raising the difficult ones until the words are all of approximately the same difficulty. In a similar manner the different word lists of a set can be examined to ensure that the whole corpus of recorded material is homogeneous.

The process of selecting material and setting the recorded levels of individual words by subjective testing is tedious and demands considerable investment of time, but if the resultant material is to have widespread use, the effort is well worthwhile. Hood and Poole (1977) spent considerable time studying one set of British recordings (MRC, 1947) and found that they were able to improve them markedly by adjusting the levels of the words. In the USA, Hirsh *et al.* (1952) made a classic study using subjective measurements during the development of the CID lists and this led to reduction in the total number of test items from 84 to 36. Similarly Markides (1978) performed a normative study on a set on recordings of the British Boothroyd lists (Boothroyd, 1968) recorded at Southampton University. This led to 3 of the 15 lists being omitted from the final tapes because they gave results which were significantly different from the other members of the set, but it meant that the rest of the recordings could be confidently used as a coherent set.

The final step in the preparation of recordings for use in speech audio-metry is to preface each tape with a calibration tone which can be used to set up the audiometer and to check the level of reproduction of the word lists. The duration of this tone should be sufficient to allow ample time for the adjustment of the audiometer, which means that it should be at least 60 s long. In practice, if the recordings have been edited so that the lists on a particular tape have been equalized, it is unlikely that there would be any advantage in recording a separate calibration tone before each list. The stability of the equipment should be more than adequate to allow for a complete test of both ears to be made, and a tone before each list would only be an encumbrance to the audiologist.

For the purposes of setting up the audiometer, a single pure tone at a frequency of 1 kHz should suffice. If a check is to be made of the response of the whole system, however, then a separately prepared tape containing a series of carefully recorded pure tones should be used. For speech audi-ometry, the range up to 8 kHz should be covered and tones at frequencies of 125, 250, 500, 1 k, 2 k, 4 k and 8 kHz are recommended.

It is important that care should be given to the choice of the level of the calibration tone recorded on a speech audiometry tape and to its relationship to the recording levels of the word lists. Ideally, the calibration tone should either be recorded at the mean level of the words or should bear a fixed relationship to it. The definition of the mean level will be dependent upon the method which has been used to equalize the constituent parts of the word lists, but as an example, if it is the peak levels of the words which have been equalized, it would be advisable to record the calibration tone at a level of 3 dB below the peaks.

Two factors need to be balanced in choosing the recording level used; the need to avoid the possibility of overloading the amplifier by having too high a level and the danger that if too low a level is used, problems may arise through the introduction of excessive background noise. The available dyna-mic range will vary with the equipment which is being used, but a good compromise would seem to be to record the calibration tone at such a level that, when the hearing level control on the audiometer is set to zero, the level produced by the calibration signal is 20 dB SPL.

Earphones

In contrast to the choice of a tape recorder, where the hi-fi market provides highly suitable equipment, the choice of earphones for speech audiometry should properly be confined to those designed specifically for audiometric applications. The performance figures quoted by the manufacturers for domestic circum-aural earphones are often excellent, but they suffer from two major drawbacks. It is very difficult to measure the sound pressure levels developed at the ear drum, which will be affected by the use of the circum-aural cushions (Tillman and Gish, 1964 and Stein and Zerlin, 1963) and no audiometric standards relate to the use of domestic earphones. There is no guarantee of constancy between different types of earphones which might be used in different clinics and since the comparability of results is one important aim of all audiometry, the argument must be to use audiometric earphones set in supra-aural cushions, choosing those models which have the flattest frequency response over the speech frequencies.

The standard types of audiometric earphones have all been studied extensively and they have the advantage that their performance can be measured on an artificial ear or reference coupler. An artificial ear consists of a condenser microphone set inside an enclosure whose impedance character-istics approximate to those of the human ear. The frequency response of the earphones should be measured as part of the routine audiometric calibration procedure. For pure-tone audiometry, frequencies between 125 Hz and 8 kHz are measured and, because the frequencies are tested singly, it is a relatively simple matter to make allowances for any small deviations of the earphone frequency response from the ideal. In speech audiometry the frequencies lying between 200 Hz and 4 kHz are particularly important and as all frequencies are present in the speech stimulus, it is very much more difficult to compensate for earphone frequency response. The audiologist has to rely, therefore, on the earphone response being as flat as possible over the important frequencies and should also select a pair of earphones which are as closely matched as possible from those available for use.

Two earphones in particular, the Telephonics TDH-39 and TDH-49 are both widely used and are suitable for pure-tone audiometry. The TDH-39 however, shows a marked resonance at 6 kHz (Rudmose, 1964). This frequency is just above the main speech frequencies, but the TDH-49, which was designed to have more built-in damping and a flatter frequency response to higher frequencies, would probably be the preferable earphone of these two for speech audiometry work.

Loudspeakers

There is sometimes occasion to conduct speech audiometry as a free-field test, though speech material is more frequently used in this way in order to test patients using hearing aids. This latter form of testing is not strictly audio-metry, but the tests form a useful part of the audiologist's repertoire and the considerations applying to the choice of equipment are the same in both cases.

In free-field testing where the stimulus is presented to the patient via a loudspeaker, it is desirable that this should show low distortion and as flat a frequency response as possible over the speech frequencies. In addition it is necessary to ensure that the loudspeaker will generate sufficient levels for the loudest presentations which will be used. As with tape recorders, good domestic equipment will be perfectly adequate for speech testing. Many loudspeakers have excellent frequency responses up to and well beyond 6 kHz and a good power handling capacity, but the placing of the loudspeaker in the test room and the position occupied by the patient will interact to affect the received signal (Stream and Dirks, 1974). The measurement of the sound field generated at the position of the patient's head needs some care.

The majority of audiometric test rooms, although acoustically treated, are not anechoic and for this reason problems arising from standing waves will occur if measurements of the loudspeaker output are made using pure tones. To avoid such difficulties, it is necessary to create a more uniform distribution of the sound in the room and this can be achieved with either bands of noise or warble tones — pure tones which are frequency modulated about a centre frequency. Using a condenser microphone placed at the position which will be occupied by the patient's head, the output of the speaker can be measured using speech spectrum noise or white noise, whilst the relative frequency response of the loudspeaker in the room is measured with either warble tones or narrow bands of noise centred at $\frac{1}{3}$ octave intervals over the frequencies of interest. It should be remembered, however, that the presence of the patient in the room will affect the sound field slightly and that free-field testing is not, generally, as well controlled and monitored as testing using earphones.

A number of studies have been carried out to compare thresholds of hearing obtained under earphones and free-field conditions. These have shown that the unaided free-field thresholds are about 6 dB better than those measured using earphones, a difference which is probably accounted for by physiological noise (Anderson and Whittle, 1971). This difference in threshold should be remembered when interpreting the results of any free-field measurements (Tillman *et al.*, 1966).

Test Rooms

All audiometry must be carried out in quiet conditions because of the masking effects of extraneous noise. The perception of the test signal is affected by noise which is within the same critical band as the stimulus and it is thus not sufficient to measure only the overall noise level. The background noise in the test room must be measured in $\frac{1}{2}$-octave bands in order to ensure that it is not excessive at any frequency. The maximum permissible ambient noise levels for audiometry are given in ISO 6189 and are reproduced in Table II. These levels are for audiometric tests of 250 Hz and upwards, where the least hearing level to be measured is 0 dB (re ISO 389).

The background noise in the test room should be measured under normal working conditions, that is with test doors closed and with normal ventilation

$\frac{1}{3}$-octave band centre frequency (Hz)	Maximum SPL (dB re 20μPa)	$\frac{1}{3}$-octave band centre frequency (Hz)	Maximum SPL (dB re 20μPa)
31.5	78	630	18
40	73	800	20
50	68	1000	23
63	64	1250	25
80	59	1600	27
100	55	2000	32
125	51	2500	35
160	47	3150	38
200	42	4000	40
250	37	5000	38
315	33	6300	36
400	24	8000	39
500	18		

Table II Maximum background sound pressure levels for audiometric tests of 250 Hz and upwards (ISO 6189).

systems functioning. Intermittent sources of noise which might affect the test room, such as structure-borne noise from other parts of the hospital, should also be taken into account as the figures in the table represent the maximum desirable levels when testing is taking place.

Effective Masking Level

When all the equipment used for speech audiometry has been adjusted and objectively calibrated, two further subjective measurements are necessary — the determination of the effective masking level of the audiometer's broad band noise and the establishment of a normal response curve.

In speech audiometry, as in pure tone audiometry, it is necessary to ensure that the non-test ear does not contribute significantly to the results. A signal applied to one ear will be transmitted to the other by bone conduction through the head with a loss of about 40 dB in level. If the pure tone audiogram suggests that this bone-conducted signal will be heard, a masking noise must be applied to the non-test ear, using the wide-band noise facility of the audiometer (Liden, 1971). Because of the existence of critical bands, the masking noise is most efficient when its energy is in frequencies which are close to those being masked. The audiometer will probably provide either white or speech spectrum noise, neither of which is exactly matched to the spectrum of the particular voice used for the tests. It is therefore necessary to determine the effectiveness of the audiometer's masking noise for the test-voice used (Coles and Priede, 1974).

85

Using a group of about 20 normal-hearing adults, the audiometer is set at a level where at least 95% of the test lists are correctly heard. The masking noise is then added to the SAME ear as the speech and, using a different word list each time, the masking level is increased by 5 dB steps until the discrimination score just drops below 10%. The difference between the settings for the masking noise and for the speech is then equal to the effective masking level of the audiometer. If the effective masking level is +10 dB, this means that a masking noise set at 10 dB above the speech signal will just mask out the speech. It is good practice to balance the design of these measurements, using the lists in different orders and at different levels to eliminate any systematic effects. It is also important that the chosen subjects should have no familiarity with the test materials.

Normal Response Curve

Differences in the test lists used, in the acoustic conditions of testing, in the accent of the local population and in the instructions given to the patients, may all affect the results of speech tests. For this reason it is necessary to establish a normal response curve with which the patients' results may be compared.

In order to do this, a group of normal-hearing adults, who are representative of the population from which the patients will be drawn, are tested using the equipment, test lists, pattern of presentation levels and instructions which will be used with patients. Following the presentation of a number of word lists at different levels, the results are scored in the same way as they would be for the tests and the results are pooled to give an average response curve for normal-hearing subjects.

Ideally the response curve should be established using a minimum of 20 people, but certainly no less than 10. In practice the normal listeners are often drawn from members of staff of the hospital concerned, but if this is the case, it is important that they are native to the local area and are not already familiar with any of the test material. As when measuring the effective masking level, it is important to balance the order of presentation of the lists when establishing the normal response curve so that any slight differences do not distort the shape of the curve obtained. Fuller and Moss (1985) noted that audiologists differ in the extent to which they elicit responses from patients when the stimulus is difficult to hear and the score is low. If different audiologists within the same clinic use markedly different instructions for speech audiometry, it would be advisable to establish a separate normal response curve for each audiologist, but if the instructions are fairly uniform this extra step is unlikely to be necessary.

Computer-Controlled Audiometry

With the rapid development of small and relatively cheap computers, interest is growing in their possible applications in the field of audiometry. Campbell (1974) and Berry *et al.* (1979) are amongst those who have explored the possibilities for computerized pure-tone audiometry, but in speech audiometry the prospects are particularly interesting.

Computerized applications of speech audiometry give the opportunity to examine other aspects of the patients' responses in addition to the rather crude right/wrong markings applied in the conventional test. In an early piece of research, Stevenson (1973) demonstrated some of the advantages of the sophisticated control and marking aspects of a computerized system. Using a tape recorder and a computer together as a hybrid system, he was able to examine the use of additional measures such as the recognition times and the particular confusions made at different levels of presentation.

Developments since Stevenson's work was carried out mean that it is now feasible to dispense with the tape recorder, storing the test words in digital form and using the computer to replay the stimuli, record the patients' responses and mark the test. Many of the improvements offered by such a system can readily be seen, although the possibilities need to be explored and evaluated carefully before they can be introduced into clinics for regular use — important preparatory work which is only just beginning.

The great advantage of a computer over a tape recorder-based system is flexibility. The speed at which a conventional test is performed is very largely determined by the timing of the words as they are recorded on the tape. This has to be chosen to be suitable for average patients and may be too fast for those who find the test difficult, or frustratingly slow for those who could cope with a faster pace. It is very simple to arrange for a computer to repeat words on demand, to present a test word only when a response has been made to the previous item and to adapt to the preferred pace of the patient.

Multiple choice tests, giving the alternatives either in written form or as pictures, offer automatic marking of the tests and open up the further possibility of adaptive testing. In computer-controlled adaptive tests, the level of each stimulus or group of stimuli is determined by the patient's responses to the previous items — increasing the level if the previous items have been mis-heard and decreasing it if they have been correctly perceived. Items can also be selected to test more closely any particular discriminations which the patient finds difficult. In this way the speech reception threshold, optimum discrimination score and the presence of roll-over effects at high levels can all be explored without necessarily needing to use a whole word list at each level or to plot the whole of the discrimination curve. A shorter test conducted in this way would, of course, differ significantly from the current tests and the effects of both the multiple-choice items and the adaptive paradigms would have to be carefully studied and the results normalized before such testing could be introduced.

At the moment, the main disadvantage in using computer-controlled testing is that the storage necessary to hold a sufficient number of words in digital form is considerable and is expensive. A cheaper alternative would be to use computer-synthesized speech, that is speech which is generated according to a series of rules. In that case only the rules and not the full digital representation of the speech are stored by the computer, but at the time of writing the quality of the speech produced is not sufficient to replace the digital storage of material generated from spoken words. The technology is improving so quickly, however, that computerized audiometry will be an economically viable alternative to the current equipment in the near future and it is important that the normalizing studies are undertaken so that the full potential of computerized testing can be exploited as soon as the technology becomes available.

See Appendix to this Chapter, pp. 287, for Equipment for Speech Audiometry: A Draft Standard.

Chapter 5

The German Path to Standardization in Speech Audiometry

K. Brinkmann

Speech audiometry is widely used in the Federal Republic of Germany as a basis for the assessment of auditory handicaps and the selection of suitable hearing aids. It was recognized early on, however, that the results of speech audiometric tests carried out at different times, at different places and with different equipment were comparable to each other only if

— equivalent word lists,
— equivalent copies of the same recording of these word lists, and
— speech audiometers with equivalent characteristics for the reproduction of the recorded speech

were used. A comprehensive concept of standardization in the field of speech audiometry has, therefore, been elaborated in Germany mainly in the decade from 1968 to 1977. Its principles are summarized below.

Standardization of Speech Material for Intelligibility Testing

Lists of Numerals and Monosyllabic Nouns

As early as 1961, as a first step, word lists for hearing tests using speech were laid down, in the German Standard DIN 45621 based on previous basic research work of Hahlbrock (1957). These lists comprise ten groups, each containing ten polysyllabic numerals, and twenty phonetically balanced groups, each containing twenty monosyllabic nouns. Examples of both tests are:

Numerals
Group 1: 98[1], 22, 54, 19, 86, 71, 35, 47, 80, 63

Monosyllabic nouns
Group 1: Ring Spalt Farm Hang Geist Zahl Hund Bach Floh Lärm Durst
Teig Prinz Aas Schreck Nuß Wolf Braut Kern Stich

[1] pronounced 'acht — und — neun —zig' with uniform pitch

89

The numerals are easy to understand if their level is high enough to detect at least the vowels contained in them. The sound pressure level corresponding to a 50% intelligibility of numerals for otologically normal subjects under monaural listening conditions is intended to form the reference level for the hearing loss (hearing level) scale for speech in Germany.

The monosyllabic nouns usually require a level which is about 10 to 20 dB higher than that of numerals to achieve the same intelligibility among subjects of normal hearing. Very often, subjects with impaired hearing will not reach a 100% intelligibility even at very high sound pressure levels. In Germany, the minimum discrimination loss (or the maximum intelligibility) in % and the sound pressure level at which it occurs are considered the most important outcomes of hearing tests with monosyllables.

Lists of Sentences

Besides the single polysyllabic and monosyllabic test words mentioned before, a speech test consisting of short meaningful sentences developed by Niemeyer (1967) was standardized in Germany (DIN 45621-2). This test comprises 10 phonetically balanced groups, each containing ten sentences of four to six words. Each group thus consists of fifty words. An example is as follows:

Group 1:
1. Geld allein macht nicht glücklich.
2. Böse Menschen verdienen ihre Strafe.
3. Mittwoch kommt uns Besuch passend.
4. Ich bin nicht naß geworden.
5. Uns're Eltern tanzen Wiener Walzer.
6. Lärmt nicht, Jungs, Vater schreibt.
7. Wer weiß dort genau Bescheid?
8. Er geht links, sie rechts.
9. Leider ist dies Haus teuer.
10. Dienstag wieder frisch gebrannte Mandeln.

The intelligibility of these sentences is between that of numerals and that of monosyllabic nouns. The redundancy of information inherent in sentences can be used to compensate for a discrimination loss that may occur with monosyllables if subjects with impaired hearing are tested or if hearing tests are performed in noisy environments. Speech audiometry with sentences, therefore, provides additional information on the ability of subjects to understand speech in daily life and has proved to be a useful tool especially for the selection of a suitable hearing aid.

Word Lists for Intelligibility Testing in Paediatric Audiology

Special word lists, which are in use for testing the hearing of children, have recently been standardized in the German Standard DIN 45621-3. Two alternative tests are specified: Test A compiled by Biesalski *et al.* (1974) consists of three parts for, (1) the age group below 4 years (2) the group from 4 to 5 years and (3) the group from 6 to 8 years. Speech Test B developed by Chilla *et al.* (1976) is intended for use with 3 to 6-year-old children.

Tests With Different Speech Audiometers — Basic Ideas For Further Standardization

In spite of the early standardization of word lists, the technical level of speech audiometry was still unsatisfactory in the late sixties as far as the comparability of the equipment used and the methods applied for calibration were concerned. At that time, German audiologists asked the German national institute for metrology, the Physikalisch-Technische Bundesanstalt (PTB), to evaluate the technical level of speech audiometry and to make suggestions for a new recording of the word lists, for an objective calibration procedure and for future standardization.

A series of investigations with seven different models of commercial speech audiometers were therefore started at the PTB, the results of which led to following main conclusions.

Sound Pressure Level of Speech

Various recordings of word lists according to DIN 45621 were in use at the time of the investigations above. According to the judgements of otologically normal test subjects, all of them showed large fluctuations in the loudness of the recorded words. A correlation analysis was performed in which the subjectively perceived loudness level of individual monosyllabic test words and their sound pressure level measured objectively using different devices such as a peak level indicator, a volume unit meter, a sound level meter with time weighting 'fast', and an impulse sound level meter were compared (Brinkmann *et al.*, 1969a). The outcome of this investigation was that the indication of devices with a short integration time, such as the impulse sound level meter, correlated best with the results of subjective loudness estimates. It was therefore decided to define the level of an individual word to be the sound pressure level (re 20 μPa) in dB as indicated by an impulse sound level meter according to DIN 45633-2[1] without any frequency weighting[2] but with an additional 'hold' circuit, and to use this well-specified instrument for the purpose of equalizing word levels in the course of the planned new recording of word lists (see below). Consequently, for the purpose of standardization in speech audiometry, the term 'sound pressure level of speech' was defined to be the mean impulse sound pressure level of all individual words of a test word group according to DIN 45621 and/or DIN 45621-2.

The Concept of Free-Field Calibration of Earphones

Speech audiometry is equally performed in a sound field using loudspeakers as sound sources and by means of earphones (and sometimes bone vibrators). To make test results comparable, a common basis must be established both for the determination of the absolute sound pressure level of speech and for equivalent specifications of frequency responses of the transmission system.

Listening tests with loudspeakers are most frequently carried out under quasi free-field conditions with frontally incident sound waves. Reference to the sound pressure level in the undisturbed free sound field at a specified distance from the loudspeaker therefore seems quite logical. Sound pressure level measurements and frequency response specifications are then straightforward.

But how can earphone (or even bone vibrator) sensitivity be referred to free-field conditions? Acoustic or mechanical couplers, artificial ears or ear simulators usually applied in earphone and bone vibrator measurements are apparently unsuitable for this purpose. Acoustic couplers can only simulate the median acoustic impedance of the human ear (as do artificial ears for supra-aural earphones according to IEC 318 and occluded-ear simulators for insert earphones according to IEC 711) and can correctly measure the sound pressure level generated by the earphone at a well-defined point inside the human ear canal and under well-defined conditions (as an occluded-ear simulator does with respect to the ear drum under no-leakage conditions of the earphone). However, they neither take into account leakage effects (which occur especially with supra-aural earphones on human ears) nor are they basically designed to represent sound diffraction effects caused by the head of a test subject under free-field listening conditions in a sound field.

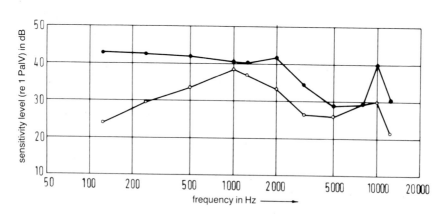

Figure 1.   Free-field sensitivity level (○——○) and coupler (IEC 303) sensitivity level (●——●) of a supra-aural Beyer DT 48 earphone

Mechanical couplers can only simulate the mechanical impedance of the human headbone and can correctly measure the force exerted by a bone vibrator. However, they are not designed to include sound diffraction effects at the human head and the transfer function of the external and middle ear (Richter and Brinkmann, 1976).

The frequency response of earphones (or bone vibrators) can, however, be referred to free-field conditions if instead of the coupler (or artificial ear or ear simulator) sensitivity level the so-called free-field sensitivity level is determined. The free-field sensitivity level is 20 times the logarithm to the base ten of the ratio of the free-field sensitivity factor to the reference factor 1 Pa/V. The free-field sensitivity factor at a given frequency and for a number of test subjects of normal hearing is defined as the quotient of the sound pressure of an undisturbed plane progressive sound wave impinging vertically from the front on the respective subject, and of that voltage of equal frequency which must be applied to the terminals of the earphone (or bone vibrator) in order that the test subjects appraise on the average the sound wave and the sound produced by the earphone (or bone vibrator) as being equally loud, both sounds being received in the same ear.

Test methods for the determination of the free-field sensitivity level are described in textbooks (e.g. Zwicker *et al.*, 1967) and specified in the German Standards DIN 45619-1 and DIN 45619-2 and, more recently, in the IEC Standard 268-7 (where the term is called a free-field comparison frequency response). The method can be applied to all kinds of earphones (whether they are of the supra-aural, circum-aural or insert type) and even to bone vibrators (Richter and Brinkmann, 1976). Similar methods were used long ago when reference equivalent threshold sound pressure levels had to be established for new types of earphones (see ISO 389).

Once the free-field sensitivity level has been ascertained for a specified type of earphone, it can be determined in a simple manner for all other earphones of the same type without the necessity to always repeat the extensive loudness comparison measurements. For this purpose, any suitable coupler or artificial ear or ear simulator may be used. The coupler sensitivity factor is defined as the quotient of the sound pressure generated by the earphone in the coupler and the voltage applied to the terminals of the headphone and can be determined without sophisticated measurement arrangements. For two earphones of identical design, the difference of their free-field sensitivity levels equals the difference of their coupler sensitivity levels. Consequently, if for a definite type of earphone and for each frequency, the difference between free-field sensitivity level and coupler sensitivity level is known, the free-field response can be determined for each earphone of this design by measuring the coupler response.

Free-field and coupler sensitivity levels were determined for various types of earphones (Brinkmann *et al.*, 1969b) and bone vibrators (Richter and Brinkmann, 1976). A typical example is shown in Figure 1, which contains both the free-field sensitivity level and the coupler sensitivity level (as measured with an acoustic coupler according to IEC 303) of a Beyer DT 48 earphone with flat cushion. Great differences between the two sensitivity levels can be seen both at low frequencies (mainly due to leakage effects at real ears) and at medium and high frequencies (due to insufficient acoustic impedance simulation and resonance effects in the coupler and due to sound diffraction effects inherent in free-field listening conditions).

The concept of free-field calibration of earphones described above has been accepted for the purpose of standardization in speech audiometry and has proved its utility in later investigations (see below).

A survey of frequency responses of speech audiometers available at the time of testing showed typical deviations in the free-field responses of loudspeaker and earphone branches (Brinkmann *et al.*, 1969b). Earphone free-field responses are typically less flat than loudspeaker responses, especially in the frequency range from 2–6 kHz which is important for the correct discrimination of consonants. It could be proved by the listening tests described in the following paragraph that this fact must be given special attention in the standardization of speech audiometric equipment. At least with present audiometric earphones, special equalizing networks will have to be introduced in speech audiometers in order to obtain comparable results when performing hearing tests with earphones.

Outcome of Listening Tests

Listening tests with a large group of otologically normal persons were carried out with five different types of speech audiometers both via loudspeakers in a free sound field (binaural listening) and via earphones (monaural and binaural listening). The sound pressure level of the recorded speech material was directly measured in the field at the listener's position or referred to free-field conditions following the principles described in the preceding section. The results of these tests can be summarized as follows (Brinkmann and Diestel, 1970):

On average, a 2.5 dB lower sound pressure level of speech was sufficient for binaural listening conditions to achieve the same intelligibility as for monaural hearing. The result was the same whether polysyllabic numerals or monosyllabic nouns were used as test material.

On average, identical free-field sound pressure levels were needed to achieve an intelligibility of 50% for numerals both in the case of binaural earphone and binaural loudspeaker listening conditions which shows that the concept of referring the sound pressure levels generated by earphones to the free sound field as described before yields reliable results.

However, on average, a 5 dB higher free-field sound pressure level of monosyllabic test words was necessary to achieve the same intelligibility under binaural listening conditions when the speech material was transmitted via earphones instead of loudspeakers. This result seems to be in contradiction with the findings with numerals; however, the reason for this discrepancy was easily found: the free-field frequency responses of the earphones used with the audiometers showed pronounced dips in the frequency range from 2–6 kHz. These dips cause effects in the case of monosyllabic words (which contain much information in consonants) while they do not influence the intelligibility of numerals (which contain most of their information in their vowels).

With a sound pressure level sufficiently high to achieve 100% intelligibility, the response of test subjects are quite rapid. If the sound pressure level is, however, reduced, the answers are given with noticeable hesitation. The testing time thus becomes longer the lower the intelligibility is. To obtain comparable results, the sequence of words on a sound carrier must therefore also be given attention and it must be standardized (Brinkmann *et al.*, 1969a).

New Recordings of Word Lists and Sentence Lists

Based upon the results of the investigations described above, the word lists according to DIN 45621 and the sentence lists according to DIN 45621-2 were newly recorded and further improved in 1969 and 1973. Both recordings were performed in a studio of the North German Broadcasting Corporation by the same professional speaker.

In the case of the word lists, the levels of all individual test words, i.e. 100 polysyllabic numerals and 400 monosyllabic nouns were adjusted to the same level by means of a sound level meter with time weighting I. The pauses between the test words were adjusted in such a way that in the final version, the test words follow each other at regular intervals of 5 s (numerals) or 4 s (monosyllables).

In addition, a technical part was added consisting of three check tones of frequencies 125 Hz, 1 kHz and 8 kHz and a speech-simulating noise as recommended in G 227 of the Comité Consultatif International Télégraphique et Téléphonique (CCITT). The spectrum level of this noise has its maximum at about 800 Hz and falls off at a rate of about 5 dB per octave at lower frequencies and of about 12 dB per octave at higher frequencies.

The tones may be used for a simple check of the frequency response of the speech audiometer in use. The 8 kHz tone may also serve to adjust the recording head alignment of a tape or cassette recorder. The noise signal is mainly intended for calibration purposes as will be dealt with later in more detail. It may, however, also be used as an easy means of checking a given sound carrier with regard to the frequency spectrum characteristics (see below).

The actual levels of test words and calibration signals were measured later on various commercial copies of the mother tape (Brinkmann, 1974a). A typical result is represented in Figure 2: the levels of all 500 test words are equal to within about ±1 dB. The average level of the speech-simulating noise deviates from the total mean level of the test words by not more than 0.1 dB. The noise level, however, shows fluctuations with time of about ±0.5 dB. The levels of the three check tones are (18.0 ± 0.5) dB below the level of the noise.

In the case of the sentence lists, during the recording the speaker's voice level was monitored by means of a peak level indicator to obtain an optimum with respect to both a constant speech level and a natural melody of speech. In the final version, the standard deviation of the impulse sound pressure levels of all 500 words was only 2 dB and the mean levels of the ten groups did not differ by more than 1 dB from each other (Brinkmann, 1974b). It was therefore decided not to perform any further level adjustments.

A speech simulating noise and three check tones were added to the recording which had identical level relations with regard to the sound pressure level of speech as in the case of the recording of the word lists. Copies of both test recordings can therefore be used alternatively on a speech audiometer without any recalibration.

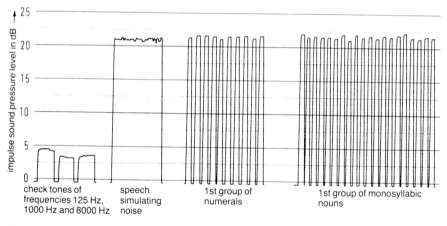

Figure 2.   Levels of calibration signals and test words of the new recording of word lists according to DIN 45621

Hearing Tests with the New Recordings

Extensive hearing tests were carried out with the two new recordings using large groups of otologically normal test subjects in order to determine the intelligibility reference curves and to evaluate the intelligibility of individual test words and groups of words and sentences (Brinkmann, 1974a and 1974b).

Equipment Used

In the case of word lists the tests were performed monaurally by means of laboratory speech audiometric equipment which included a high quality studio record player having a flat frequency response, a specially designed filter network with attenuation unit, a power amplifier and two supra-aural Beyer DT 48 earphones. The filter network was dimensioned so that the overall free-field sensitivity level of the earphones including the network had a value almost independent of frequency within the frequency range from 80 Hz to 12.5 kHz. This means that speech replayed via this equipment sounds as if it were replayed via a loudspeaker having a flat frequency response in an anechoic room.

The frequency response of the entire equipment referred to the free field was tested with a frequency measurement record. In the range between 100 Hz and 10 kHz it does not deviate by more than ±1.5 dB from the reference value at 1 kHz. Below 100 Hz and above 10 kHz, the sensitivity level decreases in a monotonous way, the −3 dB frequencies being 80 Hz and 12.5 kHz. Furthermore, the upper and lower frequency limit of the filter network could be altered in such a way that the sensitivity level of the equipment had already decreased by 3 dB at the frequencies 110 Hz and 7.5 kHz.

The individual frequency responses have been plotted in Figure 3: curve (a) represents the frequency response of the free-field sensitivity level of the earphone itself (the same as in Figure 1), curve (b) the free-field frequency response of the entire equipment without additional band limits and, finally, curve (c) shows the same with the band limits switched on.

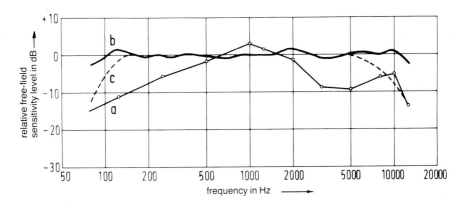

Figure 3. Frequency response (referred to the free sound field) of the equipment used for the determination of the speech intelligibility reference curves
a: relative free-field sensitivity level of the earphone used (from Fig. 1)
b: relative overall free-field sensitivity level of the speech audiometer (cut-off frequencies: 80 Hz and 12.5 kHz)
c: as b, but with additional bandwidth limitation (cut-off frequencies: 110 Hz and 7.5 kHz)

In the case of sentence lists monaural tests were carried out with similar equipment, but with a studio tape recorder instead of the studio record player. Additional hearing tests were performed binaurally using a high-quality electrostatic loudspeaker in an anechoic room. The overall frequency response of this equipment was frequency-independent within ±2 dB in the frequency range from about 80 Hz to about 15 kHz, except for two narrow dips near 120 Hz and 6 kHz.

Speech Intelligibility Reference Curves

A group of 97 test subjects (157 ears) took part in the basic intelligibility tests on numerals and monosyllabic words. They had fulfilled the criterion of having a hearing threshold level below 10 dB at each audiometric frequency up to 4 kHz; at either 6 kHz or 8 kHz a maximum hearing threshold level of 15 dB was allowed. The subjects were for the most part employees of the PTB (workshop and laboratory apprentices, as well as scientific, technical and administrative personnel). Apart from a few exceptions, the participants had no previous experience in the field of hearing tests.

All participants were tested at the same pre-set free-field sound pressure levels of speech using four out of 10 groups of numerals and four out of 20 groups of monosyllabic words chosen at random. In addition, a limited number of subjects (35 ears) were also tested in a corresponding manner with the audiometric equipment set at a limited bandwidth (curve (c) in Figure 3).

The arithmetic average values of intelligibility versus free-field sound pressure level of speech together with the corresponding standard deviations are plotted in Figure 4 for the case of the broader bandwidth of the equipment. The curves are extrapolated beyond the range of the sound pressure levels tested and have the typical S-form. The sound pressure levels of speech corresponding to a 50% intelligibility of numerals or monosyllabic nouns for monaural listening conditions are 18.4 dB and 29.3 dB, respectively. As could be expected, the slope of the curve for monosyllables is somewhat less steep than that for numerals.

The curves of the arithmetic average values in Figure 4 join almost asymptotically the 0% and 100% intelligibility lines. In general the curves of individual listeners continue somewhat more steeply than the average value curves, not only in the range of the lower sound pressure levels but also in the range of the higher ones. For practical speech audiometry the curve of an 'average normal listener' is therefore more relevant than the curve of the arithmetic average of a large group of listeners. For this reason, median instead of mean curves as shown in Figure 5 are proposed as speech intelligibility reference curves.

The range corresponding to approximately 68% of the individual intelligibility curves of otologically normal subjects has been indicated by shading.

98

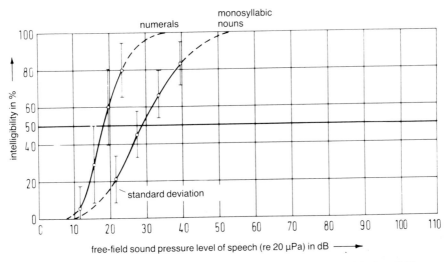

Figure 4.   Intelligibility of test words according to DIN 45621 as a function of the free-field sound pressure level of speech for monaural listening conditions (mean values and standard deviations of 157 otologically normal ears)

Parallel to the basic scale of 'Free-field sound pressure level of speech (re 20 µPa) in dB', a second scale has been entered at the level of the 50% intelligibility line referred to as 'Hearing level for numerals in dB', the origin of which is located at the sound pressure level of speech which otologically normal listeners need on an average to understand approximately 50% of the numerals, i.e. 18.4 dB.

Due to the concept of earphone calibration in terms of free-field sensitivity levels, the reference curves are valid for monaural test word presentation both via any type of earphone or via any type of loudspeaker in a free sound field, on the premise of sufficiently flat free-field frequency responses. Figure 6 shows that a slight limitation of the frequency range (lower cut-off frequency 110 Hz instead of 80 Hz, higher cut-off frequency 7.5 kHz instead of 12.5 kHz) has only a minor effect on the intelligibility curves. These results are based on tests with 35 ears. The curves valid for numerals are slightly shifted towards smaller sound pressure levels, presumably due to a reduction of the sound pressure levels of the test words at the same intelligibility level (influence of low-frequency cut-off). The shifting of the curve valid for monosyllables towards higher sound pressure levels is, on the other hand, probably a result of the high-frequency cut-off and the poorer discrimination accompanying it. Conclusions based on these results with respect to speech audiometer specification will be drawn later.

The results for the sentence lists were derived in a similar way to those for the word lists and are presented in Figures 7 and 8. Figure 7 contains two curves: the right-hand curve represents the arithmetic mean intelligibility

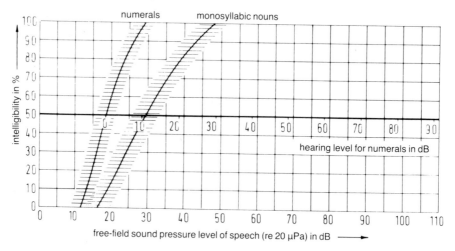

Figure 5. Speech intelligibility reference curves for monaural hearing
≡ spread on the basis of a 68% probability

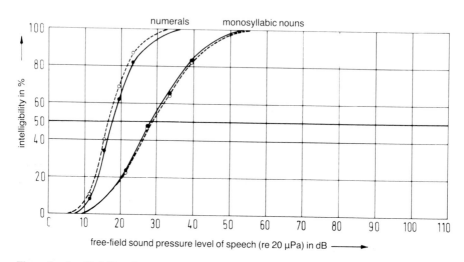

Figure 6. Intelligibility of test words according to DIN 45621 as a function of the free-field
sound pressure level of speech for different bandwidths of the speech audiometric equipment
used (mean values of 35 otologically normal ears)
audiometer cut-off frequencies: ●——● 80 Hz and 12.5 kHz
○——○ 110 Hz and 7.5 kHz

versus free-field sound pressure level based on tests with 59 subjects (91 ears)
with normal hearing under monaural earphone listening conditions, the left-
hand curve represents corresponding results based on tests with 15 subjects
with normal hearing under binaural loudspeaker listening conditions in a free
sound field. Both curves are almost parallel. The sound pressure levels of

speech corresponding to a 50% intelligibility are 21.0 dB (for monaural listening) and 18.6 dB (for binaural listening). This proves very clearly two facts: first, the speech volume increase with binaural hearing compared with monaural hearing is almost equal to 2.5 dB, a value formerly shown to be valid for speech with binaural earphone listening versus monaural earphone listening. Secondly, and more important, the calibration of speech audiometers based on free-field sound pressure level leads to correct and comparable results both for speech audiometry tests in a sound field and via earphones.[3]

The absolute response of the discrimination curves for sentences is also reliable. This can be seen by a comparison with the equivalent curves previously obtained for numerals and monosyllabic words. In Figure 8, instead of mean values, the median curves are plotted in each case for the reasons given above. As could be expected, the sentence curve runs well between the two other curves. All three discrimination curves have almost the same standard deviation with respect to the sound pressure level.

In principle, the free-field sensitivity level of bone vibrators can be determined in quite a similar way to that of earphones as was shown by Richter and Brinkmann (1976). Based on these measurements, speech audiometric equipment was set up using a Präcitronic KH-70 bone vibrator as a sound transducer. By means of an equalizing network, the frequency response of this equipment referred to the free sound field could be adjusted to be frequency-independent within ±3.5 dB in a range from 125 Hz to 8 kHz when the bone vibrator was applied to the test subjects' foreheads. Binaural intelligibility measurements by means of this equipment were initially carried out with a group of 12 otologically normal test subjects (Richter and Brinkmann, 1977) the number of which was later on increased to 20. The same group was also tested binaurally by means of earphone equipment almost identical to the one described above. In each case the same recording of monosyllabic words was used. The two resulting intelligibility curves are almost parallel and deviate by only 1.3 dB at a 50% intelligibility (Figure 9). This shows that the concept of free-field calibration of speech audiometers is even applicable to bone vibrators.

In a later, more extensive study concerned with the bone-conduction pure-tone threshold (Brinkmann and Richter, 1983) the remaining discrepancy between earphone and bone vibrator measurements could be explained to be most probably due to the influence of vibro-tactile sensation in the course of bone vibrator calibration.

Intelligibility of Individual Test Words and Groups of Test Words

The exact adjustment of the sound pressure level of individual test words to the same value does not necessarily result in all test words being equally understandable. On the contrary, considerable differences in intelligibility

101

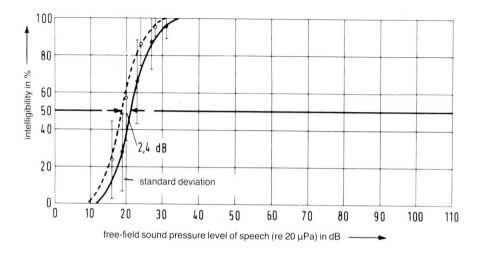

Figure 7.   Intelligibility of test sentences according to DIN 45621–2 as a function of the free-field sound pressure level of speech for different listening conditions

●——● monaural hearing via earphones (mean values of 91 otologically normal ears, 59 test subjects)

○– – –○ binaural hearing via loudspeaker in a free sound field (mean values of 15 otologically normal subjects)

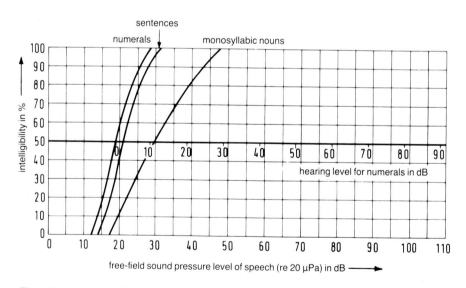

Figure 8.   Speech intelligibility reference curves for different test materials and monaural listening conditions

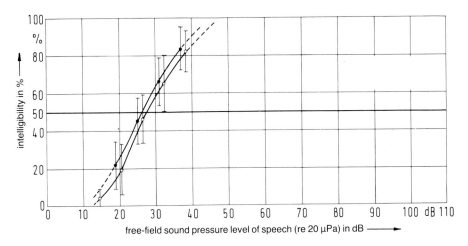

Figure 9. Intelligibility of monosyllabic nouns according to DIN 45621 as a function of the free-field sound pressure level of speech for different listening conditions (means and standard deviations of 20 otologically normal subjects)
●——● binaural hearing via loudspeaker in a free sound field
○– – –○ binaural hearing via a bone vibrator applied to the forehead

were found not only for monosyllabic words but also for the polysyllabic words when the results of the tests described previously in the chapter were evaluated. Some words were understood by almost all participants even at very low sound pressure levels while others were almost never repeated correctly even when presented at a level about 20 dB higher. This shows that not only the sound pressure level of a single word affects its intelligibility but also other factors, such as the articulation by the speaker, the specific extent to which a word is known in each group of subjects or the possibility of confusing it with similar words.

These large differences in intelligibility within the standardized word lists are the main reason why the words have been adjusted to equal sound pressure level instead of equal intelligibility. For equal intelligibility, the differences between the sound pressure levels would have been so great that the definition of an average speech level of the words in a group would have been very questionable.

For practical use of the recorded test words it is of particular importance to know whether the individual test word groups can be interchanged, i.e. whether they can be understood equally well when being played back at the same level. The results of the hearing tests were therefore also evaluated in this light. The greatest intelligibility difference between any two groups of numerals amounted to 10% (corresponding to one out of ten words), while between any two groups of monosyllables differences of up to 15% may occur (corresponding to three out of twenty words). It may be concluded that the existing differences are not very severe and that the interchangeability of the groups can be guaranteed for tests with the usual accuracy.

Similar evaluations were carried out regarding the sentence tests. Maximum deviations in intelligibility were found to be about 10% between any two of the ten sentence groups.

Standardization of the Recordings of Word Lists and Sentence Lists

In order that the new recordings described above are widely accepted and to provide suitable means for checking the electro-acoustical characteristics of a commercial copy, the technical specifications of sound carriers for hearing tests using these recordings have been laid down in the German Standards DIN 45626 (for the recording of word lists) and DIN 45626-2 (for the recording of sentence lists). Both standards contain the following basic information:

— the location of the mother tape of the recording,
— the frequencies and the levels of the check tones at the nominal frequencies 125 Hz, 1 kHz and 8 kHz with tolerances,
— the frequency spectrum and the level of the speech simulating noise with tolerances,
— the levels of the test words (or sentences) with tolerances,
— the minimum signal-to-noise and cross talk ratio,
— the reference intelligibility curves for the recordings as determined by the PTB (see Figure 8) for monaural hearing.

Together with the standards DIN 45621 and DIN 45621-2 containing the actual word and sentence lists, the two parts of DIN 45626 form the basis of a complete harmonization of speech audiometry in Germany.

Sound carriers according to these standards are commercially available in the form of records, tapes, tape cassettes and, quite recently, in the form of compact discs.

Recordings of the word lists for intelligibility testing in paediatric audiology according to DIN 45621-3 are also available on the market. However, their standardization is not yet being planned.

Standardization of Speech Audiometer Facilities

Parallel to the standardization of speech material recordings, specifications for speech audiometers have been evaluated and laid down in the German Standard DIN 45624. They are mainly based on the results of the investigations described in the preceding sections.

Basically, DIN 45624 deals only with instruments which use recordings of the test speech on a sound carrier for speech reproduction. Reproduction may be via earphones, loudspeakers or bone vibrators. Requirements for the transmission of live voice are not included since standardization of the equipment alone would not contribute very much to a reduction of the very large uncertainties inherent in live voice speech audiometry.

First, DIN 45624 defines two basic terms, i.e. the sound pressure level for speech and the hearing level for numerals in a way already presented above.

The specifications given are systematically referred to the free sound field, independent of whether they concern frequency response, sound pressure level accuracy or harmonic distortion. They are thus equally valid for both loudspeakers and earphones (bone vibrators are not yet considered).

The tolerances for the frequency response, for instance, are +2 dB and −5 dB in the range from 125 Hz to 4 kHz and +2 dB and −8 dB above 4 kHz and up to 8 kHz, both referred to the sensitivity level at 1 kHz. This must, of course, be considered a compromise between the physically desirable tolerances (based on the information given above) and those technically feasible. With regard to audiometric earphones at present available, these specifications require special equalization networks. However, no alternative can be seen if comparability of speech audiometric results with different sound transducers is aimed at.

Detailed information is given on how speech audiometers can be tested for compliance with these requirements. This information includes specifications of suitable reference tapes, reference tape cassettes and reference records, specifications of test signals and test methods for earphones using couplers (or artificial ears, or ear simulators) if the free-field minus coupler sensitivity level of the type of earphone is known from basic loudness comparison measurements.

The tolerance for absolute calibration in terms of the sound pressure level of speech is ±2 dB. The calibration must be carried out using a calibration signal which is recorded on the sound carrier used and whose level in relation to the level of the test words is known. The use of speech simulating noise with the same level as the test words is to be preferred for reasons which will be explained in more detail in the following section.

Finally, harmonic distortion figures are also specified in terms of free-field related values which again offers the possibility of comparing loudspeaker and earphone requirements (Richter 1976). Again, test methods are described in detail.

Testing and Calibration of Speech Audiometers

In the case of free-field speech audiometry via loudspeaker, testing and calibration are quite simple for the user: Testing mainly requires a sound level meter with known free-field sensitivity (together with some filter equipment if distortion measurements are to be included) and any suitable reference tape or record. The calibration in terms of the sound pressure level of speech is carried out in two steps: first, the amplification of the speech audiometer is adjusted to achieve a specified reference level indication of the calibration signal recorded on the sound carrier used on the monitoring instrument incorporated in the audiometer. If this is well done, the audiometer is expected to produce the sound pressure level of speech indicated at the level control setting at a specified distance from the loudspeaker.

This can be easily checked by means of a sound level meter using the recorded calibration signal. The use of the speech simulating noise is clearly preferable for this purpose, mainly because calibration errors can be widely avoided in non-ideally anechoic rooms and due to loudspeaker sensitivity irregularities at single pure tone frequencies. Moreover, because of its simple level relationship to speech (see above), the reading of the sound level meter equals — for exact calibration — the setting of the audiometer level control when speech simulating noise is used.

Testing and calibration of earphones of speech audiometers are as simple for the user as usual pure tone audiometer testing and calibration. If it is borne in mind that the frequency-dependent difference between the free-field and the coupler sensitivity level of an earphone only depends on the type of earphone but not on the specific unit (see above), all necessary measurements may be performed using a coupler (or artificial ear). The target values for coupler sound pressure levels both for testing the frequency response and for absolute calibration must be specified by the manufacturer of the audiometer: he (or the responsible national institute for metrology) must determine the free-field sensitivity level of the earphone in question, the user is only concerned with simple coupler measurements (as in the case of pure tone audiometers). Again, the use of a speech simulating noise instead of a pure tone as a calibration signal is to be preferred.

Final Remarks

The concept of standardization in speech audiometry described above and realized up to now in the Federal Republic of Germany guarantees comparable results if the various standards are really complied with by the equipment actually used and if test rooms fulfil certain minimum requirements with respect to sound field conditions and backgroud noise. Specifications of audiometric test rooms are at present being discussed by the responsible ISO working group and will certainly be included in German national standardization in an appropriate form. In Germany, regular testing and calibration of speech audiometers together with pure tone audiometers will, on the other hand, be covered by legal metrology in the very near future.

Notes

1. The requirements of the former German Standard DIN 45633-2 are almost identical to those of IEC Standard 651 for type 1 instruments providing time weighting I.
2. Recently, Fuller (1983) came to a similar conclusion regarding the suitable time weighting for measuring the level of single words. The apparent discrepancy between her results and those of the PTB with respect to frequency weighting (A versus linear) can easily be explained by the fact that she used earphones for the reproduction of the test words having a real ear response with high pass filter characteristics due to leakage effects (see Figure 1) while the tests at the PTB were carried out via loudspeakers with an almost flat frequency response down to low frequencies.
3. It is emphasized that this statement is valid for the case of frontally incident sound waves in free-field speech audiometry. Any other angle of sound incidence would require different frequency response specifications and a different calibration of the equipment due to the well-known sound diffraction effect of the human head as a function of the angle of sound incidence.

Chapter 6

Speech Audiometry for Differential Diagnosis

P. I. P. Evans

For over one hundred years (Wolf, 1874, cited in Lyregaard *et al.*, 1976) speech has been used in a systematic way to assess hearing ability. Undoubtedly for very much longer than that, and to the present day, it has been the basis of informal tests for hearing impairment by parents, general practitioners, teachers and others. Two factors predispose speech to this rôle. First is the common but arguable assumption that the primary function of human audition is that of communication with our fellows, that is the reception of speech. Thus, speech has face validity as a 'natural' and 'meaningful' stimulus for assessing auditory function. It is supposed that, if we can hear speech normally then our hearing is not significantly impaired. The second factor is the ready availability of speech as a stimulus, with no need for equipment to produce it. These two factors combine to perpetuate the use of a technique which is unscientific in principle and unreliable in practice as a test of auditory sensitivity. Speech is a stimulus of high redundancy because the information in it is conveyed in several ways simultaneously. The complexity of the human neural system enables it to make optimum use of the information arriving at any time. The listener extracts the message by analysis of both acoustic and linguistic features, application of learned phonological and syntactic rules, interpretation of contextual clues (including, where available, non-auditory information) and prediction and deduction on the basis of semantic probabilities. It is likely that these mechanisms operate in parallel (Cutting and Pisoni, 1978). This makes the recognition of speech a rapid information-processing procedure which is resistant to corrupting influences. Thus, the normal auditory system has little problem with moderately degraded speech material and an impaired system often copes well with good-quality speech in good listening conditions. A hearing loss involving only part of the auditory frequency range may go undetected in an informal speech test which is not carefully controlled. Even a mild or moderate hearing loss of end-organ origin, involving the majority of the auditory range, may not cause noticeable difficulty with speech identification if the test is carried out at normal

109

conversational levels in quiet, low-reverberent conditions (such as a doctor's surgery or a typical suburban living room).

Yet, speech audiometry, properly carried out with calibrated equipment and standardized recorded speech material can be a useful tool for audiological diagnostic testing. It can give a reasonably accurate prediction of the best hearing threshold levels in the mid-frequency region of the auditory range. It may also provide useful 'site-of-lesion' information about an auditory impairment, to aid diagnosis.

Acoustically, speech is a complex auditory stimulus, the correct identification of which depends fundamentally (but not only) on satisfactory frequency resolution, frequency discrimination, intensity discrimination and temporal resolution. Psychoacoustic tests of such auditory analytical functions exist but they are time-consuming, difficult and tedious for both subject and tester. Tests using speech material are generally regarded as clinically more acceptable for identifying patients with poor auditory analytical capability and they have been found to be powerful tools for distinguishing patients with various types of auditory disorders.

Terminology

The clinical use of speech materials to aid diagnosis involves the testing of the patient's ability to accurately identify samples of speech or speech-like stimuli. The frequently-used description 'speech discrimination testing' is usually not accurate as the patient is rarely asked to discriminate between two or more auditory stimuli or between a small number of possible responses. The term 'speech intelligibility', arising from communications research, is more accurate but, in the clinical context, it needs to be carefully distinguished from the intelligibility of the subject's own speech to others. The same confusion can arise with 'speech testing', the common use of which is to be deprecated. The term 'speech audiometry' is, itself, rather unsatisfactory as the procedure does not measure auditory sensitivity (or any other fundamental psychoacoustical function) alone. The test result depends not only upon the condition of the peripheral auditory system and its primary central neural projections, but also substantially upon the nature of the speech material, the availability of visual cues, the extent of contextual information and the size of the response set (which is partly determined by the linguistic competence of the patient). Nevertheless, as the term 'speech audiometry' is so deeply entrenched in audiological terminology, it will be used here also, but with the foregoing reservations in mind.

Objectives

In the clinic, speech audiometry is most often used diagnostically to place the patient into one or more of a number of 'auditory function' categories, namely:

Normal auditory function
Non-organic hearing loss
Conductive hearing loss
Sensory or end-organ disorder
Peripheral-neural (NVIII) disorder
Central auditory disorder

Although a characteristic pattern of response (or rather a characteristic deviation from a normal response) may be found in *conductive hearing loss* (Figure 1) speech audiometry is rarely of value in such cases. Carefully masked air-conduction and bone-conduction pure-tone audiometry, combined with acoustic immittance and stapedial reflex measurements, is a more appropriate way of identifying and investigating middle-ear disorders. Speech audiometry cannot be relied upon to give an accurate prediction of everyday hearing ability following middle-ear surgery. However, it may be useful for identifying unusually poor speech identification capability in a patient in whom the conductive component overlies a sensorineural hearing loss with considerable involvement of the acoustic nerve.

The identification and differentiation of *central neural disorders* cannot readily be achieved with the use of conventional speech materials. The effects of central neural disorder on speech recognition are usually subtle and frequently different in kind from those of peripheral disorders. Several

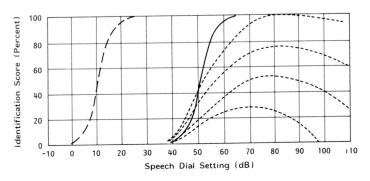

Figure 1.   Typical speech identification functions for monosyllabic words in subjects with normal hearing (— —), conductive hearing loss (——) and sensorineural hearing losses (----). In conductive hearing loss the effect is largely one of reduced sensitivity. In sensorineural disorders with similar pure-tone thresholds, the identification function tends to be flatter and the maximum score may be reduced, with greater reductions generally associated with NVIII lesions.

special techniques have been devised in an attempt to identify central auditory neural dysfunction and to distinguish cortical and brainstem disorders. They will be considered later in this chapter.

Materials and Parameters

There are usually two measures sought in the use of speech audiometry for diagnostic purposes in the clinic. The first is a 'threshold' for the identification of the speech material to provide an estimate of auditory sensitivity, as measured by pure-tone audiometry. The second is the maximum speech identification score achieved at supra-threshold intensities under optimum conditions.

In the United States, different speech materials are generally used to achieve each of these measurements with maximum accuracy. For measurements of maximum speech identification performance, lists of monosyllabic words are widely used. Initially 'phonetically-balanced' (PB) word lists were developed at the Harvard Psychoacoustic Laboratory (Egan, 1948) for the testing of communications systems. They became popular for clinical audiological use, as the W-22 word lists (Hirsh, 1952), after modification at the Central Institute for the Deaf to restrict the vocabulary to commonly-used words. In addition to meeting the criterion of word-familiarity, the lists were constructed to be of equal difficulty and equal phonetic (actually phonemic) composition, approximately corresponding to that found in everyday speech. More lists have subsequently been produced by other workers in the United States, but the W-22 lists have remained the most widely-used by clinical audiologists there. The maximum discrimination score achieved by a subject is generally referred to as 'PB$_{max}$' (Figure 2).

Spondee word lists were developed (Hudgins *et al.*, 1947; Hirsh *et al.*, 1952) for speech threshold determination, as the identification functions are steeper than for monosyllabic words (Figure 2) due to the higher linguistic redundancy or predictability of spondees. On average, normally-hearing listeners achieve 100% correct identification at an intensity 20–30 dB lower than for monosyllabic words (Rupp and Stockdell, 1980). The 'speech reception threshold' (SRT) is defined as the lowest intensity at which the listener correctly identifies 50% of spondee words. It is a reliable measure which correlates well with the pure-tone threshold average.

Jerger and Jerger (1976) pointed out several advantages of calculating a speech identification 'threshold' using monosyllabic word lists, though they found that the appropriate norm, with which to compare the patient's performance, depended upon the PB$_{max}$ achieved. Their results suggested that monosyllabic word lists are comparable with spondees in the accuracy with which they can be used to predict average pure-tone thresholds. Nevertheless, Rupp (1980) noted that the 'Guidelines for Determining the Threshold

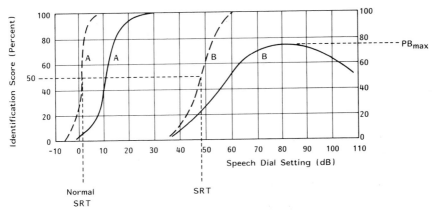

Figure 2. Typical speech identification functions for spondees (— —) and monosyllabic words
(——).
(A) Average functions for normal subjects; (B) Functions for a patient with a sensorineural
hearing loss.
SRT = speech reception threshold; PB_{max} = maximum identification score.

Level for Speech', published by the American Speech and Hearing Association in 1977, specify spondees as the standard test materials for speech
threshold measurements.

In the United Kingdom, considerations of time availability in the clinic
have led to monosyllabic word lists being used for both threshold estimation
and measurement of identification ability. Only a few word lists have been
published and used extensively in the UK. The MRC lists (1947), derived
from the Harvard lists for the determination of an 'optimum' hearing aid
frequency response, are generally thought to be too long and to contain too
many uncommon words to be suitable for clinical diagnostic use. The Fry lists
(Fry, 1961), with 35 words per list, are also often regarded as too time-
consuming. The isophonemic word lists of Arthur Boothroyd (Boothroyd,
1968) have achieved widespread clinical use in the UK. Boothroyd published
and recorded 15 lists, each comprised of ten consonant-vowel-consonant
(CVC) monosyllables, with the same 30 phonemes appearing in each list in
different combinations. Phonemic balance, consistent with that in everyday
spoken English, is precluded by the small number of phonemes in each list,
but is not of great importance for diagnostic application (Lyregaard *et al.*,
1976). The original recording by Boothroyd was felt by many to be unsuitable
for use across the whole of the UK, because of his strong northern English
accent. The lists were re-recorded in a 'standard' southern English accent on
at least two occasions, at the Institute of Sound and Vibration Research
(ISVR) in the University of Southampton and at the Royal National Institute
for the Deaf, who inserted two non-scoring practice words at the beginning of
each list. Original normative studies carried out at the ISVR, showed that the

113

intelligibility (and hence the degree of difficulty) of three of the original 15 lists (nos. 9, 10 and 15) in the Southampton recording differed significantly from the remainder and they were therefore discarded. Hood and Poole (1977) described a procedure for improving the reliability of the MRC word lists. A similar exercise was carried out at the ISVR on the re-recorded Boothroyd word lists. They have subsequently been used widely for clinical purposes in the UK and are generally referred to as the Arthur Boothroyd lists — Southampton recording: AB(S).

Markides (1978) showed that the test/retest reliability of the AB(S) word lists is reasonably high, with correlation coefficients for identification scores ranging from 0.34 at near threshold levels to 0.79 at supra-threshold intensities. He presented normative data for children aged 6–11 years and for adults. As the words are less familiar to children than to adults, the slope of the identification function becomes shallower and the intensity for 50%

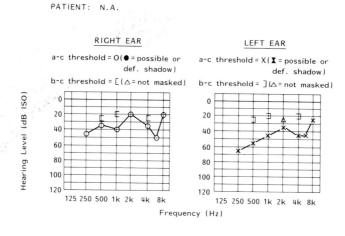

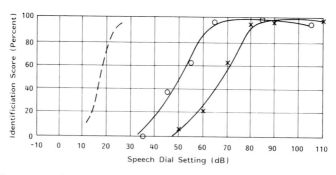

Figure 3.   Pure-tone audiograms and speech audiograms of a 30 year-old woman from Bangladesh with no knowledge of English. Speech audiometry was carried out with AB(S) word lists, phoneme scoring (— — average normal curve for equipment used).

recognition rises with decreasing age of the subject. However, the differences between adults and children are not great. Clinicians with extensive experience with the word lists know that they can be used even with subjects whose knowledge of English is minimal (Figure 3). In such cases the identification functions become still less steep, approximating those for nonsense words, where the linguistic redundancy of the material is minimal. The maximum identification score will, however, usually reach 100%.

Figure 4 shows the parameters of a speech identification function obtained with monosyllabic word lists. The term 'optimal discrimination score' (ODS), proposed by Coles *et al.* (1973), is synonymous with PB_{max} but acknowledges that the maximum score is obtained or estimated at the optimum speech presentation level indicated by the identification function. It is also more appropriate in cases where the identification function rises throughout the measured intensity range and appears likely to reach a maximum score at an intensity above the maximum output of the equipment.

As the identification function of monosyllables has a considerably lower slope than that for spondees, particularly for patients with sensorineural hearing loss, the SRT (the level at which 50% correct identification is achieved) does not always agree as well with the pure-tone threshold average. Coles *et al.* (1973) proposed the use of the 'half-peak level' (HPL), which is the intensity (in arbitrary dial-level units) at which the listener achieves 50% of his maximum score. The 'half-peak level elevation' (HPLE) is then the difference between the patient's HPL and the average normal HPL. The measure has the advantage that it can be applied to identification functions in which 50% correct identification is never achieved.

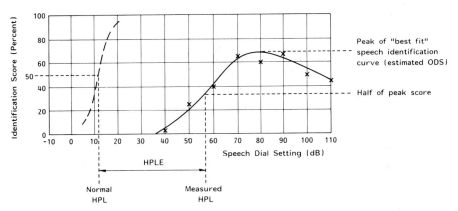

Figure 4. Speech identification functions and measurement parameters for monosyllabic word lists — — Average normal curve —— Pathological
HPL = half-peak level; HPLE = half-peak level elevation; ODS = optimal discrimination score (The ODS should be measured at the optimum speech dial setting indicated by the "best fit" identification curve).

In determining the presentation level at which the maximum identification score of the patient is likely to occur, it is important that a full identification function is obtained by presenting word lists at various supra-threshold levels. Several authors (e.g. Coles, 1972; Rupp and Stockdell, 1980; Hood, 1981) note the error of attempting to measure the maximum score with a single presentation level. Boothroyd (1968) estimated that, for his ten-word lists, a single-list phoneme identification score of about 50% would have associated confidence limits of ±20%. Therefore a 'best-fit' curve should be determined by eye, according to the theoretical expectation of a sigmoid psychometric function, rather than joining up individual list scores, each with its associated measurement error. When measuring the maximum discrimination score at the peak of the identification function, it is important to present sufficient items to ensure adequate reliability of the score. For the Boothroyd lists, three lists are recommended for ODS measurement (Priede and Coles, 1976), giving 90 test items (phonemes).

Method

A suggested systematic procedure for obtaining a speech identification function using monosyllabic word lists, is outlined in Appendix I. For accurate and reliable results the word lists should be recorded and played back to the subject through earphones driven by an audiometer or an amplifier with variable attenuation. Live-voice presentation, even when monitored with a sound level meter, gives rise to unacceptable variability of intensity both within and between lists and to variations in pronunciations between different presentations of the same list (Brandy, 1966). Wide-band masking should be applied as necessary to the contralateral ear (Coles *et al.*, 1973).

The requirements for calibration of recorded material will be found elsewhere in this book (Chapters 4 and 5) but it is important to realize that it is necessary for normal parameter values to be obtained or calculated for each set of play-back equipment used. Two items of calibration should be available for every combination of word-list recording and playback equipment:

   (i) The attenuator setting for the speech channel, which gives an average of 50% correct identification in a group of normally-hearing subjects (the normal half-peak level or SRT) and

   (ii) The effective masking level of the equipment (i.e. the relationship between the dial levels for wide-band noise masking and the speech material should be known, for a specified decrement in speech identification in normally-hearing subjects, when ipsilateral masking is introduced).

Each recording of the word lists will usually have a calibration tone at the beginning, allowing the input level of the audiometer to be adjusted to the same level on each occasion of use, thus ensuring that the dial settings are consistent and that the normal parameter values apply.

It is important that the patient understands the requirement of the test. The scoring of the word lists should be carried out on a *phoneme* basis (Figure 5) to improve the reliability of the test by increasing the number of test items (Lyregaard *et al.*, 1976). The patient should be instructed to respond to any parts of the word he or she hears. Suitable instructions are suggested in Appendix III. It is not important that the exact wording be adhered to, as long as the main points are covered.

STIMULUS WORD: "FISH"

Verbal response	Marking	Scoring
"FISH"	FISH ✓	3
"FIT"	FIS̶H̶	2
"WISH"	F̶ISH	2
"FOSH"	FI̶SH	2
"FLIT"	F̶I̶S̶H̶	1
"FAT"	FI̶S̶H̶	1
"DASH"	F̶I̶SH	1
"FISHED"	FIS̶H̶	2
"DEBT"	F̶I̶S̶H̶	0
(no response)	F̶I̶S̶H̶	0

Figure 5.   Examples of phoneme scoring.

Clinical Applications

Threshold Estimation

Coles *et al.* (1973) compared speech HPLE values (for Fry's word lists) with pure-tone thresholds in a large number of subjects with normal hearing or acquired sensory hearing loss. They found that, with a high degree of reliability, the HPLE lay within ±10 dB of the 'best-two-average' (BTA) of pure-tone thresholds for 500 Hz, 1 kHz and 2 kHz, with corrections for greater high-frequency and low-frequency threshold elevation as follows:

4 kHz threshold 11–20 dB poorer than BTA, add 1·0 dB to BTA.
4 kHz threshold 21–30 dB poorer than BTA, add 2·0 dB to BTA.
4 kHz threshold 31–40 dB poorer than BTA, add 3·0 dB to BTA.

4 kHz threshold over 40 dB poorer than BTA, add 4·0 dB to BTA.
500 Hz threshold 11–20 dB poorer than BTA, add 3·0 dB to BTA.
500 Hz threshold 21–30 dB poorer than BTA, add 10·0 dB to BTA.

The high correlation between HPLE and BTA (0.5–2 kHz), corrected for high-frequency losses, was similar to the relationship predicted by Fletcher (1950) for spondee SRT values. Priede and Coles (1976) showed that the relationship applied similarly to patients with hearing losses apparently of NVIII origin (Figure 6). Hood and Poole (1971) agreed with the general principle of a linear relationship between BTA and speech SRT for conductive hearing loss, but showed that it did not apply in patients diagnosed as having Meniere's disease. As Hood and Poole used monosyllabic word lists to test their subjects, their SRT measurements were not strictly comparable with

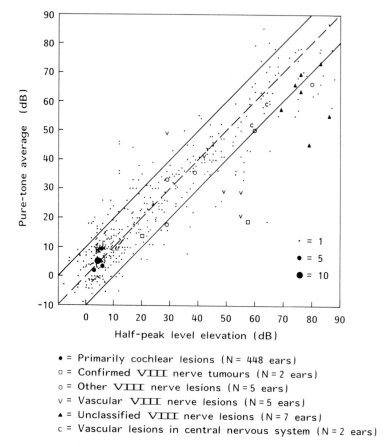

• = Primarily cochlear lesions (N = 448 ears)
□ = Confirmed VIII nerve tumours (N = 2 ears)
o = Other VIII nerve lesions (N = 5 ears)
v = Vascular VIII nerve lesions (N = 5 ears)
▲ = Unclassified VIII nerve lesions (N = 7 ears)
c = Vascular lesions in central nervous system (N = 2 ears)

Figure 6. Relationship between pure-tone average threshold (see text) and speech identification half-peak level elevation in patients with cochlear and eighth nerve lesions. (From Priede and Coles, 1976, by permission)

spondee SRT values measured by Fletcher. Nevertheless, in such a restricted group of patients, which is characterized by variable, but often poor speech perception, it is likely that Hood and Poole would have obtained similar results with spondee word lists. However, Hood (1981) rightly noted the limitation of the SRT parameter in patients whose maximum speech identification score is less than 50% and informal examination of Hood and Poole's (1971) group average data suggests that, if the HPLE value is taken as the speech identification 'threshold' (rather than the SRT), a reasonably good agreement with the BTA would be obtained, as Coles *et al.* (1973) predicted.

Markides (1980), using Boothroyd's isophonemic word lists with hearing-impaired children aged 9–14 years, calculated correlation coefficients between speech HPLE values and a variety of single-frequency and multi-frequency measures of pure-tone sensitivity. Of the two pure-tone threshold descriptors which gave the highest correlations with HPLE, the simplest formula was the best-two-average hearing level in the frequency range 250 Hz–4 kHz, which estimated the speech HPLE within ±10 dB in every case. Markides pointed out the importance of low-frequency hearing levels in predicting the speech identification threshold, but also warned that, for children with atypical audiometric configurations (e.g. predominantly low-frequency or U-shaped losses) the simple formula may not be reliable.

The speech HPLE for monosyllabic word lists is useful as a check on the reliability of pure-tone audiometric thresholds and has been shown to be a powerful measure for identifying non-organic hearing loss in clinical populations. Priede and Coles (1976) found that over 80% of patients with proven non-organic components in their hearing losses gave pure-tone average thresholds which were more than 10 dB greater than their speech half-peak level elevations (Figure 7). Aplin and Kane (1985) found similar discrepancies between pure-tone average thresholds and half-peak level elevations in experimental subjects who were asked to simulate hearing loss. Sophisticated subjects (staff or post-graduate students of a university audiology department) were no more successful in matching their HPLE values to their average simulated pure-tone thresholds than were unsophisticated subjects. Like Priede and Coles (1976), Aplin and Kane found that their subjects frequently, but not always, gave consistent speech half-peak level elevations which suggested some degree of hearing loss, albeit considerably less than indicated by the simulated pure-tone audiograms. This conflicts with the widely-held assumption that unsophisticated subjects (presumably including the majority of clinical non-organic cases) are unable to simulate a consistent hearing loss in speech audiometry, because the fluctuating nature of the speech signal makes it difficult for the listener to maintain a chosen performance level reliably. Indeed, both Coles (1982) and Aplin and Kane (1985) identified anomalous patterns of responding in speech audiometry by non-organic cases, which enabled them to maintain artificially elevated half-peak

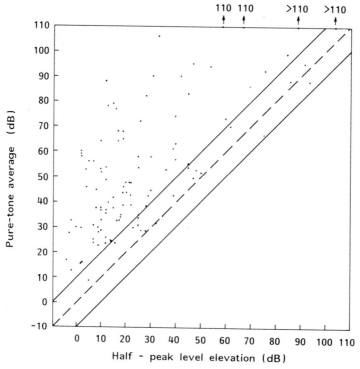

Figure 7. Relationship between pure-tone average threshold (see text) and speech identification half-peak level elevation in patients with non-organic hearing loss. (From Priede and Coles, 1976, by permission)

level elevations. These include giving few partly correct responses ('all-or-none' responding) or making systematic errors such as responding only to every second or third test word or omitting the third phoneme in all or most of the test words. Priede and Coles (1976) described a procedure for speech audiometry, based on the loudness alteration technique advocated by Fournier in 1956, in cases of suspected non-organic hearing loss. By alternately lowering the intensity of the speech by 20 dB and raising it by 15 dB on successive lists, it is possible to confuse the patient and cause him to respond at progressively lower intensities, often to a level within normal limits.

Differentiation of Sensory and Peripheral Neural Disorders

Lidén (1954) was one of the earliest authors to identify poor speech recognition as a characteristic of retrocochlear disorder. Prior to that time (e.g., Dix *et al.*, 1949) and for several years afterwards (e.g. Hood and Poole, 1971), poor speech recognition was held to be a consequence of loudness recruitment, which was indicative of end-organ pathology, in contrast to the good discrimination evident with high intensities in conductive lesions. Hood and Poole (1971) acknowledged that lesions of the acoustic nerve can cause discrimination losses well in excess of those typically found in cochlear lesions with similar pure-tone thresholds, but pointed out that '. . . the speech audiogram can have little practical diagnostic value unless it can be interpreted within the content [sic] of the predictability of speech curves encountered in cochlear hearing loss'. Priede and Coles (1976) took a similar view in plotting optimum speech discrimination scores against average pure-tone thresholds, corrected as recommended by Fletcher (1950), for cochlear and eighth nerve lesions. They found that the 90th percentile curve for cochlear ODS values approximated to the 10th percentile curve for neural cases. That is, the curve effectively separated 90% of the end-organ disorders from 90% of the eighth nerve lesions. The original data were obtained using Fry's word lists (Fry 1961) but a 90th percentile curve was later calculated for the Boothroyd lists (Boothroyd, 1968) and both curves are published in notes accompanying recordings of the AB(S) word lists available from the Institute of Sound and Vibration Research (Figure 8). Priede and Coles (1976) suggested that the disproportionately greater speech 'discrimination loss' of neural lesions might be a result of temporal distortion of the neural signal arising from variable conduction velocities of the nerve fibres. This notion was supported by Borg (1982) who showed that speech discrimination scores in patients with acoustic neuromata were well correlated with features of the

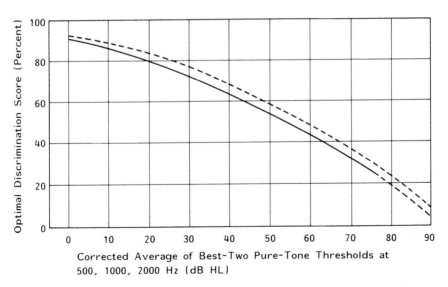

Figure 8. Criterion curves for distinguishing cochlear and eighth nerve lesions. When the non-test ear is properly masked, 90% of cochlear cases lie above the relevant criterion line and approximately 90% of neural cases fall below it. —— AB(S) word lists (three lists) ---- Fry's lists (one list)

auditory brainstem electric response which are dependent upon temporal coding within the nerve. No such correlation was found in cochlear hearing loss.

Hood (1981), while continuing to point to poor speech discrimination in patients with Meniere's disorder, stated that 'Speech audiometry, however, can be of particular value in the differential diagnosis of cochlear and nerve fibre lesions since the latter *invariably* [my emphasis] exhibit poorer speech discrimination than the former.' Such is clearly not the case, as the data of Priede and Coles (1976) demonstrated, with evidence of wide variations and some overlap of the ODS values for cochlear and eighth nerve lesions with similar pure-tone audiograms. White (1980) cited several studies which also showed variability of speech discrimination scores in retrocochlear disorder. Jerger and Jerger (1971) found similar variations in PB_{max} scores obtained with PB-50 word lists in cochlear and retrocochlear cases, but noted a tendency in retrocochlear disorders (particularly eighth nerve lesions) for speech discrimination to deteriorate markedly at high speech stimulus intensities. They termed this phonomenon 'roll-over' and recommended the use of a 'roll-over index' of:

$$\frac{PB_{max} - PB_{min}}{PB_{max}}$$

where PB_{min} is the lowest discrimination score recorded for stimulus intensities above that at which PB_{max} is obtained (up to a maximum of 110 dB SPL). Jerger and Jerger (1971) found that the roll-over index separated cochlear and eighth nerve cases without overlap. They acknowledged that many other investigators had not found the roll-over phenomenon to be diagnostically useful but noted the importance of recording a full speech identification function in order accurately to measure PB_{max} and PB_{min}. Dirks *et al.* (1977) supported the use of the roll-over index, but emphasized the necessity of deriving a new diagnostic criterion value if speech materials other than the PAL PB-50 words (Egan, 1948) are used. In the UK, the roll-over index is not widely used, probably due largely to the influence of British authors (e.g. Hood and Poole, 1971; Priede and Coles, 1976; Hood, 1984) who have reported the occurrence of roll-over in certain cases of cochlear disorder, as well as eighth nerve lesions. Nevertheless, in the United States, the roll-over index continues to be advocated (White, 1980) as a means of increasing the sensitivity of speech audiometry to retrocochlear disorders.

Evaluation of Central Auditory Nervous System Disorders

The reported effects of central auditory nervous system (CANS) lesions upon auditory perception are highly variable. With bilateral lesions of the auditory cortex (e.g. Jerger *et al.*, 1969) it is possible for the patient to experience severe auditory impairment, particularly with respect to the discrimination of speech. Such cases are rare, however, and most central neural lesions appear to give rise to varying but often relatively subtle perceptual disabilities (compared with lesions of the cochlea or acoustic nerve). Standard monosyllabic word recognition tests are generally insensitive to cortical disorders and Hurley (1980) summarized results from the literature showing that brainstem lesions give inconsistent results with such tests.

A large number of special test procedures have been suggested for the investigation of CANS disorders, using speech or non-speech stimuli. Although non-auditory variables, such as intelligence and linguistic competence of the subject can substantially affect the results of speech-based tests (Davis *et al.*, 1976) the familiarity of speech encourages patients into more consistent and reliable performance than is usually observed with non-speech stimuli.

Brainstem Lesions

Speech-based tests of brainstem function generally investigate aspects of binaural interaction which arise from the binaural representation of auditory information through crossing neural pathways at various levels. They include the binaural fusion of speech presented dichotically with the test material split either spectrally (e.g., Matzker, 1959), or temporally as in the RASP test (discussed by Lynn and Gilroy, 1977). In brainstem disorders, identification of the dichotic signal is often not significantly better than that achieved with monaural presentation of each part of the divided speech material.

The phenomenon of binaural release from masking, or masking level difference (MLD), giving improved signal detection and recognition when either the signal or the masking noise (but not both) is made anti-phasic between the two ears, has been widely used as a test of brainstem function. A similar improvement in recognition is observed with masked speech stimuli (Olsen *et al.*, 1976). The MLD effect is disrupted by brainstem disorder, but also unfortunately by cochlear or eighth nerve impairment, so that its reliable application may be limited to patients with normal auditory sensitivity.

Cortical Disorder

Owing to the complexity of the central auditory neural system, a limited impairment of cortical function may have little effect upon the perception of good quality speech, analysed by an intact peripheral auditory system. Most tests of cortical dysfunction therefore rely upon a reduction in the redundancy of the speech material to improve their sensitivity. This may be achieved by degrading the acoustic signal conveying the speech information, in terms of spectral content or temporal structure (see Hurley, 1980 for a review of these procedures). Speaks and Jerger (1965) aimed to reduce the redundancy of speech material linguistically as well as acoustically. They developed third-order synthetic sentences which give an advantage over monosyllabic words in having temporal variations in frequency and intensity that approximate 'real' sentences, while conveying minimal contextual and syntactic clues. For assessment of CANS dysfunction, competing running speech is presented simultaneously with the synthetic sentences, to either the ipsilateral or contra-lateral ear. Keith (1977) reviewed results showing the Synthetic Sentence Identification (SSI) test to be effective in differentiating acoustic nerve, brainstem and cortical disorders and in identifying the site of the lesion, though he emphasized the need to consider SSI results in conjunction with those of other auditory tests. Hurley (1980) however, reported that the test was not in wide use in the United States.

Probably the best standardized and most evaluated test of CANS function is the Staggered Spondaic Word (SSW) test (Katz, 1962). Katz (1977) and Brunt (1978) described the application of the test and reviewed a sizeable body of data available. Although the test uses dichotic binaural presentation of partially overlapping spondees, it appears to be most sensitive to cortical disorder.

Although tests of CANS dysfunction continue to be used and further developed in other countries, they have generally fallen out of favour in the UK over the last ten years. This is largely because of lack of confidence in the specificity and reliability of such tests, coupled with the rising popularity of auditory brainstem response measurements. Undoubtedly, much of the early published research data on CANS behavioural tests were of doubtful value because of the poor anatomical and patho-physiological specification of the central lesions being studied. Certainly, also, the tests are highly susceptible to the effects of concomitant peripheral auditory disorder. With regard to central speech tests in particular, it is not clear whether the decrement in performance observed with increasing age of the subject (Bosatra and Russolo, 1982) is due to speech-specific central neural dysfunction or to deterioration of peripheral auditory coding that is known to occur with advancing age (e.g. Patterson *et al.*, 1982). Nevertheless, similar criticisms can be levelled at electrophysiological tests of central auditory neural function which have enjoyed a rapid and not wholly justifiable ascendancy in the audiological armamentarium over the last decade.

Future Developments

Lyregaard *et al.* (1976) concluded, for both theoretical and practical reasons, that the efficient diagnostic application of speech audiometry is limited to CANS disorders, requiring reduced-redundancy test materials. A decade later, audiological and medical professionals in the UK continue to rely heavily on monosyllabic word lists for the differential assessment of peripheral sensorineural hearing loss. In part, this is due to excessive concern with the identification of peripheral neural lesions, particularly acoustic neuromata, which undoubtedly often exhibit disproportionately poor speech recognition. This, combined with the clinical acceptability of simple speech-based tests, makes it unlikely that the use of monosyllabic word lists will diminish rapidly.

However, with the considerable advances that have been made in auditory physiology and psychoacoustics over the last 10 years, the opportunity now exists for the development of a more analytical and functional approach to diagnostic assessment, investigating basic auditory processing. Psychoacoustic tests are becoming clinically more acceptable with the use of adaptive procedures, but speech-based tests such as the FAAF procedure (Foster and Haggard, 1979) offer the additional advantage of stimulus familiarity. Synthesized speech features (Fourcin, 1979) allow precise control of parameters of the speech signal and investigation of specific aspects of auditory processing. Recent dramatic improvements in neuro-radiological procedures should help to overcome some of the specificity problems involved in the assessment of central auditory nervous system disorders, so that speech-based CANS tests should undergo a deserved revival in the UK. Control of the linguistic redundancy of the speech signal, while maintaining its acoustical structure (as in the SSI test), along with the use of competing speech rather than noise masking, should enable higher auditory processing to be investigated more accurately.

Appendix I

Method of Performing Speech Audiometry with Monosyllabic Word Lists

(a) The first word list should be presented at a level which is comfortable to the patient and is likely to give rise to a high identification score. Estimate the level at which the patient is likely to score 50% correct (the *half-peak level* or HPL). This can be calculated by adding the HPL for normals to the average of the patient's *best two* pure-tone thresholds for the test ear (over the frequency range 250 Hz–4 kHz). The presentation level of the first word list should be at the estimated HPL + 10 dB.

(b) Calculate the contralateral masking level required for the first speech level, using the formula in Appendix II.

(c) Test at estimated HPL + 10 dB
estimated HPL + 0 dB
estimated HPL − 10 dB
and at 10 dB lower levels until the discrimination score drops below 10%. The contralateral masking level should be adjusted in line with the speech presentation level.

(d) Test at HPL + 30 dB and in increasing 20 dB steps to complete the speech audiogram curve (up to the maximum output of the audiometer or the loudness discomfort level of the patient).

(e) Sketch by eye the 'best fit' sigmoid speech identification function, as judged from the identification scores plotted on the chart.

(f) Except where the identification score, averaged over three adjacent test levels, is 95% or more measure this maximum or optimum discrimination score separately. To do this, present three word lists at the level which is judged by eye to be most likely to give the maximum speech identification score.

Appendix II

Masking for Speech Audiometry

For accuracy of masking, the effective masking level of the audiometer should be known (see Fuller, this volume). Coles and Priede (1975) published formulae for the masking of the non-test ear in speech audiometry and their derivation is outlined in Coles and Priede (1974).

The formula to determine the masking noise dial setting when the effective masking level is known is:

$$D_m = D_s + E_m + maxABG_{nt} - 40$$

where D_m = masking noise dial setting
where D_s = speech dial setting
where E_m = effective masking level
maxABG$_{nt}$ = maximum difference between air-conduction and bone-conduction pure-tone thresholds in the non-test ear for any frequency in the range 250 Hz–4 kHz.

   Where the effective masking level is not known, the formula derived by Coles and Priede is:

$$D_m = M_w + D_s - C_s - BBC_{nt}$$

where D_m = masking noise dial setting
where M_w = the threshold, in the non-test ear, for the wide-band masking noise
where D_s = speech dial setting
where C_s = speech dial setting at which an average of 50% speech recognition is obtained by a group of normally-hearing listeners (i.e. the normal half-peak level)
BBC$_{nt}$ = best bone-conduction threshold in the non-test ear in the range 250 Hz–4 kHz.

Appendix III

Instructing the Patient

The following instructions are suggested for use in speech audiometry using monosyllabic word lists with phoneme scoring. It is not important that the exact wording be adhered to, as long as the main points are covered:

   'You are going to hear someone speaking single words through the earphones, one ear at a time. The words are spoken slowly like this . . . BUS . . . FUN . . . SHOP . . . TOY. . . At the beginning the words will be at a comfortable level but they will gradually become quieter and then later they will be much louder. Please listen carefully and repeat after each word whatever you think you heard. Even if you hear only part of the word or a word that doesn't seem to make sense, or even a single sound like /a/, /o/ or /ch/, please repeat it because it adds to your score. From time to time you may hear a rushing noise in the opposite ear to the speech. Ignore the noise and concentrate on repeating the words that you hear. It is important to go to quite loud levels, but if the words or the rushing noise get uncomfortably loud, let me know. Do you have any questions?'

Chapter 7

The Uses and Misuses of Speech Audiometry in Rehabilitation

R. Green

Rehabilitation is a wide area of audiology, and speech audiometry has been used extensively within it. However its uses can be summarized into two main categories. Firstly it is used to measure a patient's ability to understand speech and so to predict the degree of handicap they are likely to suffer. Secondly it is used to evaluate treatments, such as the fitting of a hearing aid or the introduction of an auditory training programme.

It would be useful to be able to write a chapter outlining practical details of tests appropriate for each of these roles and the procedures which would yield the best results with such tests. However in reality speech audiometry is not yet sufficiently well developed for such recommendations to be made. Furthermore it has considerable potential for abuse. All that can really be achieved here is to make the reader aware of its limitations as well as its strengths.

This chapter will begin by looking at the meaning of rehabilitation. It will go on to discuss how speech audiometry has been used to measure disability and evaluate treatments. It will focus in particular on hearing aid intervention as this is both a common treatment and one with which speech audiometry is often linked. The use which has been made of speech audiometry in making inferences both about handicap and treatment benefit will be discussed. It will be necessary to look at some theoretical issues (in particular test sensitivity and reliability) in order to achieve a clearer understanding of the need for choosing appropriate test conditions, and of the importance of making critical interpretations of the test results. Finally some practical suggestions will be made though these will refer more to the qualitative than the quantitative uses of speech audiometry.

Auditory Rehabilitation

The aim of auditory rehabilitation will vary from clinic to clinic. In some institutions it is considered sufficient simply to fit a hearing aid on the

129

assumption that self induced rehabilitation will automatically follow. At the other extreme, considerable effort may be expended in quantifying the extent of the patient's auditory disability, and then fitting aids and conducting auditory training programmes which focus on bringing about as much reduction in that disability as possible, in order to alleviate the resulting handicap.

A clear, if modest, definition of the aim of auditory rehabilitation is necessary if the place of speech audiometry within a rehabilitation programme is to be understood. A possible definition of rehabilitation then is as follows:

> rehabilitation is the process by which patients are enabled to come to terms with the disabilities which result from their hearing impairment, and to reduce as far as possible the impact of those disabilities on their daily life.

It is also worthwhile, in the context of this definition, to differentiate between the terms impairment, disability and handicap. Hearing *impairment* describes the extent of the underlying dysfunction of the patient's auditory system. This impairment is commonly (though not exclusively or exhaustively) 'measured' by the pure tone audiogram. A hearing impairment will in turn give rise to *disabilities* in performing various more complex processing tasks such as discriminating speech. The relationship between such disabilities and the underlying impairment which gives rise to them is not straightforward. For example, two patients with the same pure tone audiogram may not have the same ability to discriminate speech. Finally the patient's degree of *handicap* will be governed by the extent to which their disabilities interfere with their way of life. Thus a mild high frequency hearing loss may provide a serious handicap to a young teacher coping with speech at different distances and in a sometimes noisy classroom. The same loss may go almost unnoticed in a retired person whose life is mainly centred around the home.

Disability Measurement

It is often thought useful to measure the effect of the patient's hearing loss on their ability to discriminate speech. There is as expected some relationship between the speech discrimination scores and the pure tone audiogram, with typically correlations of around 0.6–0.7 being found between the pure tone average and the maximum speech discrimination score (see Figure 1). The degree of correspondence of this relationship suggests that some idea of a patient's difficulties in coping with speech discrimination can be obtained from the pure tone audiogram alone. Poorer audiometric thresholds are associated with poorer speech discrimination. However it seems to be also true, for reasons discussed elsewhere in this book, that the pure tone audiogram does not tell the whole story. Patients with identical audiograms will not

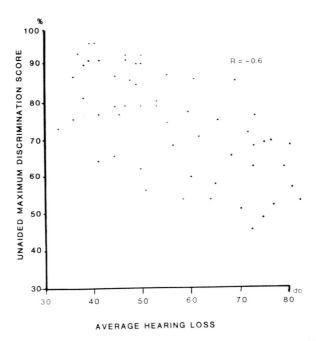

Figure 1.   Relationship between hearing loss (averaged across frequency) and unaided maximum discrimination score (FAAF Test).

always give similar speech discrimination scores. Most clinicians will be familiar with the patient who seems to be having a lot more difficulty coping than his pure tone audiogram would have lead them to expect, or the patient who appears to be doing surprisingly well despite his impairment.

If measures of speech discrimination are to be useful in rehabilitation then they must tell us something about the patient's ability to cope in the world outside the audiology clinic. In other words we should be able to make predictions about the degree of handicap from such disability measures. Unfortunately a close relationship between disability and handicap does not exist though it is often assumed, with the result that many unfounded inferences are made from one or two brief speech discrimination measures. This practice underlies the all too familiar situation in which the general medical practitioner conducts his own version of speech audiometry (by interview in a one-to-one situation in a quiet consulting room) and makes unjustified predictions based on the 'test result' ('I had no trouble making myself understood, therefore you do not have a hearing handicap in any situation').

In the audiology clinic more precise, quantitative measures of speech discrimination are possible, such as maximum discrimination score, speech reception threshold and so on. However such increase in precision is in a sense only useful if it allows us to predict the extent of the patient's handicap.

131

If a patient has a maximum discrimination score of 82% what can we say about her ability to cope as a secretary in a noisy open plan office, or as a nurse needing to understand patients on an intermittently noisy ward?

Some light is shed on this issue by examining studies in which Hearing Handicap Questionnaire scores have been compared with speech discrimination scores in order to see how closely related they turn out to be. Several such questionnaires have been developed. (Ewertsen *et al.*, 1973; Noble *et al.*, 1970; Berkowitz *et al.*, 1971; High *et al.*, 1964). Usually they contain questions relating to typical real life situations and require the patient to circle the category of answer that best fits his experience. Extracts from the Hearing Measurement Scale are shown in Figure 2. Several studies have compared such measures and some of these are summarized in Figure 3. Thus Jupiter (1982) showed a correlation of 0.57 between speech recognition measured under headphones and handicap. (A higher correlation was found between the handicap score and free field speech measures, implying perhaps that more 'realism' in the clinic does enable better prediction of real-life handicap, at least for some tests and conditions.)

Findings such as these seem to emphasize three points. Firstly there is some relationship between discrimination scores and handicap. Secondly the relationship depends on the test conditions under which speech discrimination was carried out. In the Jupiter study, free field test scores using voice levels typical of normal speech intensities were more closely related to handicap than scores measured under headphones and at higher signal levels than are typical in everyday life.

All ·· All the time   **Mo** — Most of the time   **Half** — About half the time
Occ ·· Occasionally   **Ne** — Never

Against each relevant question put a circle round the short form of the phrase that most closely describes your experience.

1. Do you have difficulty hearing in a conversation with **one** other person when you're at home?

           All   Mo   Half   Occ   Ne

2. Do you have difficulty hearing in **group** conversation at home?

           All   Mo   Half   Occ   Ne

3. Do you have difficulty hearing in a conversation when you're with **one** other person **outside**? (by 'outside' is meant some place outside the house where you would be talking to others)

           All   Mo   Half   Occ   Ne

4. Do you have difficulty hearing in **group** conversation outside?

           All   Mo   Half   Occ   Ne

Figure 2. Extract from the Hearing Measurement Scale (Noble and Atherley 1970).

Study	Speech Recognition (40dBSL)	Sound-field Speech Recognition (50dBHL)
Jupiter (1982)	-.57	-.74
Bernstein (1981)	-.63	-.65
Weinstein & Ventry (1983)	-.50	-.54
Berstein (1981)	-.50	-.74

Figure 3.   Correlations between speech recogination ability and self-assessed hearing handicap.

Thirdly the relationship between the two measures is at best only loose which implies, hardly surprisingly, that there is more to handicap than can be encompassed in a single measure of disability. Handicap is a multidimensional entity, affected by all the different situations that a person comes across in their daily life. In order to tighten up the relationship between what goes on in the clinic and in real life it would be necessary to measure speech discrimination in a variety of situations similar to those encountered by the patient. Thus it would be necessary to measure speech in quiet and in a variety of different background noises, in conditions with various degrees of reverberation, using a variety of different voices, both live and amplified, with and without lipreading. Clearly this is not a practical proposition in most clinics.

It seems then that we cannot hope for a close relationship between disability and handicap. However it is worth considering just how close we can make the relationship. In other words which test or clinically feasible combination of tests *best* allows us to predict hearing handicap? This is currently a question to which research has not supplied a complete answer, but some insight is obtained from studies in which the correlation between handicap and both disability (e.g. speech discrimination) and impairment (e.g. pure tone average) measures have been compared.

Figure 4 shows the results of a number of studies in which handicap scores were related to both speech discrimination scores and the pure tone average. (The former correlations are negative because as speech discrimination scores get smaller, i.e., worse, handicap scores get larger.) The correlations are better for the pure tone results than for the speech results. These studies suggest that handicap is in fact better predicted from the pure tone audiogram than from speech measures. The fact that speech audiometry is a relative rarity in rehabilitation may then be due to more than just lack of

133

equipment or time. It may also be that pure tone audiometry gives in practice a better 'feel' for the degree of handicap than speech discrimination measures even though the latter seem at first sight more valid.

We have discussed so far the possibility of predicting a patient's handicap from speech discrimination scores. We have seen that the relationship appears to be only a loose one. Therefore if we are to use speech tests what use can such scores be put to in helping each individual? What can we say to them as a result of their discrimination scores? Perhaps the most useful concept we can get across is that of 'distortion'. It is important for patients to understand that there is more to their hearing impairment than simply a loss of sensitivity, that the 'distortion' introduced by their damaged ear can make it difficult to unscramble even loud speech. The extent of this difficulty is well demonstrated by measures of maximum discrimination. The fact that many will score less than 100% at any level provides a good starting point for discussing the difference between clarity and loudness that puzzles so many patients.

It also provides a starting point for discussing the likely benefit that a hearing aid will provide, as the degree of cochlear distortion which underlies less than perfect discrimination scores must limit the potential success of an aid. However this takes us into a further area of rehabilitative speech audiometry.

Study	Age	X PTA	Scale	Pure Tone Average Loss & Hearing Handicap	Speech Discrimination Score & Hearing Handicap
High *et al.* (1964)	21–73	38dBHL	HHS	·65	−·46
Berkowitz & Hochberg (1971)	60–87	36dBHL	HHS	·57	−·30
Noble & Atherly (1970)	35–65	37dBHL	HMS	.60	−.58
Rosen (1978)	16–65	?	SHHI	·58	−·33
Weinstein & Ventry (1983)	65–92	37dBHL	HHIE	·62	−·42

(from Weinstein 1984)

HHS = Hearing Handicap Scale
HMS = Hearing Measurement Scale
SHHI = Social Hearing Handicap Index
HHIE = Hearing Handicap Inventory for the Elderly

Figure 4. Correlations among pure-tone sensitivity, suprathreshold speech recognition ability, and hearing handicap in selected studies.

Treatment Evaluation

Rehabilitation involves more than simply predicting and assessing handicap. Indeed its primary function is to provide treatment aimed at alleviating that handicap as much as possible. Various forms of rehabilitative intervention exist, for example the fitting of a hearing aid, or the use of an auditory training programme. The success of such a treatment is sometimes monitored with the help of speech audiometry. Thus a patient may be given speech discrimination tests before and after undertaking an auditory training programme and the difference between scores used as a measure of the effect of the programme. Comparison of aided and unaided speech scores is a frequently suggested method for measuring the effect of a hearing aid. Indeed the latter idea is so common that even if many clinics do not practice it, it probably lingers close to the top of many a list of priorities intended for implementation just as soon as time and finances permit. It is therefore worthwhile focussing on the potential of speech discrimination as a means of hearing aid evaluation.

In practice discrimination scores are obtained with and without a hearing aid. Let us for example take a situation in which a patient's discrimination score unaided is 70% and aided is 90% with a fixed input level typical of normal conversational speech. Is such information useful? What can we do with it? Firstly it may seem to indicate that the aid is definitely helping. However most hearing aids, unless grossly misfitted, will provide some benefit. In that sense we have achieved a result which is so highly predictable anyway as to not really warrant the time taken to do the test.

A more useful comparison may be between the unaided maximum discrimination score (rather than the score at normal speech intensities) and the aided maximum discrimination score. Suppose we do this and find that the patient's unaided maximum score is 80% and his aided score 90%. This result suggests that the aid is indeed doing more than simply making speech louder. It is also clarifying it to some extent, as the maximum discrimination score has improved by some 10%.

Such a comparison suggests that the hearing aid is providing some benefit (though we will have cause to question this inference shortly). However a further question arises here. Is the aid fitted the *best possible* aid for that patient, or would a different aid demonstrate an even greater improvement? This question takes us into the area of predicting optimum benefit, in which an attempt is made to predict the best possible improvement in speech discrimination score we can expect, given certain background information about the patient. If such a prediction can be made with any certainty then it should be possible to compare the predicted discrimination score with the measured discrimination score and so decide whether a particular hearing aid is providing optimum benefit. Currently this is still a research question, which is being investigated by the author. As an illustration of the problem taken from our current work, Figure 5 shows the relationship between the unaided maximum discrimination score and the 'benefit' provided by a hearing aid (difference between aided and unaided score). The relationship between the two is approximately defined by the following equation:

PREDICTED AIDED SCORE = (UNAIDED SCORE)/2 + 50

Thus if his unaided score was 80%, the predicted aided score would be 90%. In this study (Green and Bamford, 1986) aids were carefully fitted according to the configuration of the individual audiograms. However it is still not possible to state with certainty that each represents the *best* aid for each patient. (Indeed strictly speaking we can never be sure we have the *best* of all possible aids). Furthermore there is still a considerable 'spread' of scores, so that it is difficult to predict with any certainty the aided score for each patient. The correlation between the aided and unaided scores is not high (R = 0.5). A patient with an unaided score of 80% could have an aided score anywhere between 85% and 100%.

It is possible to predict aided scores with more certainty if we take into account more background information about the patient. Thus in the same study a closer relationship (r = 0.9) was obtained when a different speech test was used and certain other background information was taken into account, such as the patient's age, audiometric configuration and unaided most comfortable level (MCL).

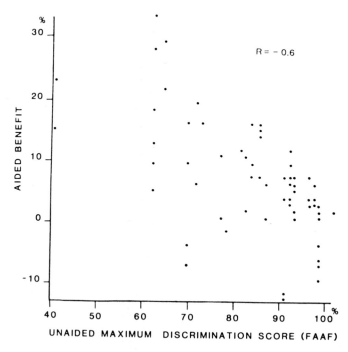

Figure 5.   Relationship between unaided maximum discrimination score and aided benefit.
The relationship demonstrates the extent to which benefit (aided-unaided score) experienced by patients is predictable from their unaided discrimination score.
Patients with lower unaided scores tend to show more measurable benefit than patients with higher unaided scores.

The interesting thing about this result is that it was obtained by choosing from a considerable amount of background information (such as age, degree, slope and configuration of hearing loss, measures of cochlear distortion, hearing aid frequency response slope) those features of the situation which contributed most to predicting the aided score. Thus prediction of the 'benefit' provided by a hearing aid was possible to some extent from the patient's unaided score for the same test. Prediction was considerably improved by allowing for the age of the patient, the unaided MCL and the configuration of the audiogram. However one feature included which made very little difference to prediction of the aided score was the slope of the hearing aid frequency response. Changing the slope does not appear to significantly influence the aided score. Thus we can to some extent predict this score, we can measure it, but in many cases we can do very little to influence it. Again this calls into question the usefulness of performing speech audiometry as a means of measuring the success of a hearing aid fitting other than for detecting an aid which is grossly misfitted.

Treatment Comparisons

Speech testing has also been used as a tool for differentiating between treatments. For example we may wish to compare the benefit provided by several different hearing aids, in order that the most successful can be selected for the patient.

Various procedures for performing such a comparison have been suggested. The most straightforward is simply to compare the aided discrimination scores for the various hearing aids under identical conditions. This form of speech testing formed part of a procedure for comparative evaluation of hearing aids first described by Carhart (1946). Because of its face validity and subsequent influence on comparative evaluation, it is worth describing the Carhart procedures in some detail.

Carhart's original procedure consisted essentially of 5 steps:

STEP 1 Measure the subject's unaided soundfield speech reception threshold, threshold of discomfort and discrimination score at a fixed sensation level (25 dB SL).

STEP 2 Fit the first hearing aid for evaluation. Set the gain so that the subject reports a speech signal 40 dB above normal speech threshold as being comfortably loud. Measure the aided speech reception threshold and threshold of discomfort.

STEP 3 Set the aid on maximum gain and repeat the aided speech reception threshold and threshold of discomfort.

STEP 4 Set the gain so that the subject reports a speech signal 50 dB above normal speech threshold as being comfortably loud. Measure the speech reception threshold in noise. (Carhart advocated two types of noise, white noise and saw tooth noise).

STEP 5 Reset the aid as in STEP 2 and remeasure the aided speech reception threshold (as a check for reliability). Measure the speech discrimination score at a 25 dB sensation level.

Steps 2 to 5 were repeated for each hearing aid to be evaluated.

The method enables a number of dimensions of hearing aid performance to be examined, in particular the discrimination in quiet and background noise, and the aided dynamic range. Experience with the procedure has led to a number of modifications. For example the full procedure proved time consuming and so not practical for comparing more than a few hearing aids. The signal and noise levels, as well as types of noise have also been varied to suit the tastes of the clinician performing the procedure. However, in its modified form the Carhart method still finds favour.

The status of hearing aid selection and evaluation has changed substantially since Carhart's day as a result of thorough and critical examination of the issues. The background to this area is well covered in many audiology texts (Byrne 1983; Schmitz 1980; Ross 1978) and it is not the author's intention to review that material in any detail here. Briefly the usefulness of comparative evaluation was brought into question following a number of studies which seemed to show that differences between hearing aids were simply not detectable (e.g. Shore *et al.*, 1960; Resnick *et al.*, 1963) unless aid parameters were manipulated so as to be grossly inappropriate (e.g. Jerger *et al.*, 1966). It was not clear whether this failure to differentiate between aids was due to the fact that the aids used really were equivalent or simply because the speech tests used were just not sensitive enough to reveal any differences.

More recently interest in comparative evaluation has been revived. There are two main reasons for this. Firstly, with the developments in microelectronics and consequent versatility in hearing aid design, the debate about individual selection has reopened, particulary in the form of a plethora of hearing aid selection procedures (e.g. Berger *et al.*, 1977; Byrne *et al.*, 1976; Shapiro, 1978; Pascoe, 1975). Often the claims of such procedures are backed by their apparent success as measured by speech discrimination scores. Secondly speech tests themselves have developed to the point where they are now more likely to be sensitive to differences between hearing aids.

Quality Judgement

One development in this area is in the introduction of more qualitative comparisons between hearing aids. In this type of test patients are asked to listen to speech through each of a number of different instruments and to decide on the basis of this listening test which aid they prefer. Various versions of this test occur. For example one rather elaborate procedure has been developed by Studebaker *et al.* (1982). In their procedure speech signals from a large number of aids are prerecorded on two channels of a tape recorder. Each possible pairing of the hearing aids is recorded and comparison between pairs is performed by the patient switching between channels on the tape recorder. In Studebaker's method the pairs 'compete' against each other rather like soccer teams aiming for a place in the World Cup. This method enables a fast switching between pairs so that subtle differences between aids can be more readily identified than may be the case in more conventional speech audiometry. It also enables each patient to sample in one session all the aids held in a clinic's stock, or at least all those recorded. However the difficulties associated with making such recordings make it clinically rather a formidable undertaking.

In its simplest form, quality judgement is probably the method used most often to differentiate between aids. It is common practice for the patient to try a number of aids in the clinicians office and each time to be asked 'How does that one sound?'. Indeed this situation is so common that a note of caution must be introduced concerning the validity of its underlying assumption. This assumption is that when a patient makes a judgement about a particular aid this judgement says something meaningful about that aid. In other words if the patient states that he prefers aid A to aid B, there is some essential difference between aids A and B which is causing him to say this. In a recent study (Green and Bamford, 1986) different hearing aids were compared using this quality judgement type of task. Each time a patient, listening to speech in various types of background noise, was asked which of two hearing aids they preferred. The results showed a marked order effect, suggesting that regardless of the type of aid fitted, the more frequently preferred aid was the one fitted second. This preference for the second aid persisted even when the 'two' aids tried were (unbeknown to the patient) actually the same aid. The implication here is that a patient's quality judgements, or more casual comments, about different hearing aids do not necessarily reflect important differences between aids. It may have more to do simply with the patient becoming more accustomed to the environment (acoustic and otherwise) in which the aid is being fitted.

Speech Discrimination and Benefit

In an earlier section we examined the relationship between speech discrimination measures of disability and a patient's degree of handicap. It was demonstrated there that the two measures are only loosely related. Inferences about handicap are also implicit in taking speech discrimination measures of the effect of a hearing aid. Such tests are performed partly on the assumption that differences between unaided and aided scores will reflect the degree of benefit, or reduction in handicap, experienced by the patient in real life. Furthermore differences between hearing aids measured in the clinic are assumed to reveal which hearing aid is most likely to provide the greatest benefit for the patient outside the clinic. Does this prove to be the case?

Benefit is a difficult thing to measure. Like handicap it comprises many dimensions, such as how well the patient copes with the aid in quiet conditions, noisy conditions, at home, at work and so on.

Often benefit is encapsulated in overall measures such as patient satisfaction or hours for which the hearing aid is worn. Figure 6 is taken from a study (Gerber *et al.*, 1979) in which different test conditions were used to measure discrimination scores and these differences were then correlated with the patient's average use (hours per day) of their hearing aid. As much as 50% of variability in the patient's aid use was predictable from their discrimination scores, though this depended on the particular test and conditions used.

In particular the study reveals that a test becomes most sensitive as a predictor of hours of use in a restricted range of signal to noise ratios. Discrimination scores in quiet seem to bear little relationship to hours of use. Discrimination scores in high levels of background noise are also poor predictors. However across a range of intermediate conditions some relationship does exist between speech discrimination and hours of use.

This relationship is apparently tightened up considerably if further background information is also taken into account. Foster *et al.* (1981) looked at how well the amount of use of a hearing aid (hours per day) could be predicted, and found that if allowance was made for the patient's discrimination score, tolerance thresholds, age and some other easily obtained background information, almost 80% of the variability in use time could be accounted for.

The relationship between speech discrimination and patient satisfaction is more complex. It might be expected for example that if patients do show better speech discrimination with one hearing aid rather than another, then they would also tend to prefer it. A number of studies have given results which suggest that this is not in fact the case. Thompson and Lassman (1969) for example showed that although a frequency response which provided more high frequency emphasis gave better speech discrimination scores, patients tended to prefer aids with less high frequency emphasis. Haggard *et al.* (1981) found a slight tendency for more favourable responses about the benefit of a hearing aid from subjects whose speech results show less rather than more improvement.

The reasons for this somewhat paradoxical finding must presumably lie in overriding importance of the 'tone colour' of a hearing aid. Punch (1980) for example has shown that the amount of low frequency in a hearing aid strongly influences patient judgement about it. The more low frequency, the more

	Signal to noise ratio	Correlation (R^2) between test score and aid use
Carhart	−10 dB MCR	(50·8%)
SSI	−10 dB MCR	(48·1%)
SSI	−20 dB MCR	(47·8%)
SSI	0 dB MCR	(41·6%)
Carhart	−20 dB MCR	(36·1%)
Carhart	0 dB MCR	(34·6%)
Carhart	+20 dB MCR	(13·8%)
Carhart	+10 dB MCR	(11·8%)
SSI	+10 dB MCR	(8·4%)
SSI	+20 dB MCR	(0·4%)

Figure 6.   Rank order for predicting the subject's use of a hearing aid.
The figures show the correlation between aid use and scores from the Synthetic Sentence
Identification Test (SSI) and W22 Word Lists (Carhart) with various levels of competing signal.
SSI = Synthetic Sentence Identification Test
Carhart = W22 Word Lists
MCR = Message to Competition Ratio

they like it. Whatever the reasons it puts the clinician in something of a spot.
Speech audiometry is performed as a means of evaluating hearing aids.
Common sense suggests that the aid with the best discrimination score is best
for the patient. Unfortunately it is also more likely to be received by the
patient with less than optimal enthusiasm. The way out of this impasse is not
clear. However it seems likely that any relationship between speech discrimination and satisfaction is likely to change over time. Indeed such an influence
presumably is implied in the often heard comment that 'I didn't like the aid at
first but now that I am used to it I think it is much better'.

Treatment Evaluation Over Time

If treatment evaluation by using speech discrimination is to be useful in
rehabilitating patients then it must, as has already been stated, tell us something useful about the patient. In the light of the discussion of the previous

141

section what it actually tells us is in some sense paradoxical, in that the aid the patient performs best with will not necessarily be the aid they prefer. However rehabilitation is not instantaneous and very little work has been done on the way changes occur over time in measures such as speech discrimination, patient satisfaction, hours of use and so on. It may well be that patients will grow to like the aid which gives them better discrimination, once they have had time to adjust to it. Alternatively it may be (though intuitively this is less likely) that an aid which initially demonstrates poorer discrimination, shows a marked improvement as the patient becomes accustomed to it. The point is that we do not really know yet what kind of predictions we can make about the long term rehabilitative prospects of a particular aid, simply based on speech discrimination scores, which again throws their quantitative application into doubt.

So far in this chapter we have concerned ourselves with looking at the rehabilitative uses to which speech audiometry has been put. We have stressed the need for looking not simply at the test scores but further at what those scores tell us about a patient's handicap and likely benefit from a hearing aid. Indeed such considerations suggest that speech audiometry has a rather limited potential in one particular but common area of rehabilitation, namely the fitting of hearing aids. However, given that limitation it is necessary to look at some important underlying concepts that will enable us to be more effective in selecting tests and conditions which are most likely to be of use.

Sensitivity

Much misuse of speech audiometry results from a lack of understanding of how speech tests work. In particular tests are often used in situations and under conditions which render them insensitive to the process under examination, or in which they become so unreliable that the scores derived from them are meaningless. Thus a clinician trying to assess a patient's speech discrimination using live voice in free field may well obtain different scores in different conditions simply because of uncontrolled changes in the level of the clinician's voice. We have already seen the effect of background noise on the sensitivity of speech tests as predictors of aid use.

If we wish to differentiate between two hearing aids we need a speech test which is sensitive to differences between hearing aids. For example if two aids differ in terms of their frequency response a speech test will only successfully differentiate between them if it contains items which are made easier with one frequency response than with the other. This may appear obvious but tests are frequently employed in the hope that they will be sensitive to these differences, rather than because such sensitivity has been proven. This practice has largely stemmed from the idea that because speech can partly be defined in terms of frequency, changes in frequency response will therefore elicit changes in the ability to perform tests containing speech items. Although this has a grain of truth it misses two important points. Firstly speech is very redundant, so that changes in frequency/gain characteristic of the hearing aid or impaired ear or both, through which the speech is being perceived need to be rather extreme if differences are to be detectable. Secondly the time domain is also important in defining the speech signal. Indeed the transient quality of many speech sounds suggests that it is likely to be at least as important as the frequency domain.

The clinician theoretically has some control over test sensitivity by choosing a test which is known to be sensitive to differences he wishes to examine. Unfortunately the day is not yet with us when he can decide what he wishes to use speech audiometry for and then consult a 'catalogue' of tests and procedures in order to find a test known to be particularly effective for that use.

Some progress has been made in specifying target sensitivity. There now exist tests specifically for hearing impaired children and comprising items taken from the language typical of such a population such as BKB sentences (Bench and Bamford, 1979), or modelled after tests for adults but incorporating items suitable for children (Jerger and Jerger, 1982). The FAAF test (Foster and Haggard, 1979) claims sensitivity to high frequencies and should therefore be useful for both hearing aid work and assessing disability in milder high frequency impairments, though this is as yet only beginning to be tested rigorously in practice.

Further control can be exercised by selection of the conditions under which the test is performed. If for example two hearing aids are to be compared on a patient with a mild hearing loss there may be little point in measuring maximum discrimination in quiet, as scores are likely to be close to 100% with both hearing aids. Alternatively if the test is performed using a considerable amount of background noise the patient may score 0% with both aids. In neither of these conditions is the test proving 'sensitive' to hearing aid differences. Somewhere between these two extremes the test is likely to reach its greatest sensitivity (assuming, as we have already discussed, that it has any sensitivity at all to differences between aids).

Unfortunately this point of maximum sensitivity is seldom known. It is likely to depend on the test itself, the nature of the background noise and the type and degree of hearing loss of the patient being tested. However experience suggests that tests are likely to be most sensitive when the patient is scoring in the region of 50–90% and Dillon (1982) has shown that theoretically at least the best point to aim at is a score between 70% and 90%.

Reliability

Perhaps the greatest misuse of speech tests arises from a poor understanding of the idea of test reliability. Scores on an ideal speech test will be exactly repeatable. However in practice if a patient performs a speech test and scores say 70% it would be unrealistic to hope that everytime he performed the test under those conditions he scores exactly 70%. If this were the case and if with another aid he scored 72%, we could be confident in asserting that this difference represented a small but significant improvement for the second aid. In practice the test score will show some random variation from test to test. Furthermore this variability will depend on the test itself and on the conditions under which it was performed. There is in fact a trade off to be made between the sensitivity of a test and its reliability. It is possible to make a test perfectly reliable. To do this it is simply necessary to make the test very easy, so that the patient always scores 100%, or very difficult so that they always score 0%. Unfortunately at these points we have a test which is perfectly reliable but, as discussed above, completely insensitive. As the level of difficulty increases and the patient's score falls below 100%, so the sensitivity is likely to increase and the reliability decrease. Technically the rate at which they change is not quite the same for sensitivity as reliability. Thus sensitivity is greatest between 50% and 100%, and variability at 50%. The region of test difficulty which maximizes this sensitivity/reliability trade off is the region of maximum efficiency.

Minimal Differences

A critical concept is that of minimal differences. We have stated that if the test is not ridiculously easy or hopelessly difficult then the test score will have associated with it a degree of variability. Given a test score of 70% on one occasion, repeating that test on a separate occasion will give a score which is not necessarily or even probably the same. The problem arises when the two scores are obtained from two different treatments,for example two hearing aids. How large a difference would there need to be between scores before we could say with any certainty that the difference really was due to a difference between hearing aids and not simply due to the expected variability associated with the test.

It turns out that we can calculate the variability associated with a particular speech test. This variability depends almost entirely on the number of items in the test and the test score itself. Figure 7 represents the 95% confidence limits for establishing significant difference between two test scores for a typical speech test containing 30 items, such as the AB word lists (Boothroyd, 1968) when scored phonemically, i.e., 10 words in each list with

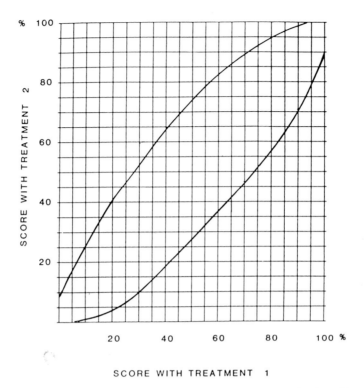

Figure 7.   Minimal differences between treatment scores for significance (95% confidence limits).
If the score for treatment 2 falls within the boundary of the curves at the points of intersection with the score for treatment 1, then the difference between scores cannot be attributed with any certainty to a difference between treatments.

3 phonemes per word making 30 phonemes per test. The area bounded by the curves represents the amount of uncertainty associated with any particular test score. If we use the horizontal axis to represent patient test scores for a particular condition, we can determine for any score how much smaller or greater a second score (e.g. with a different hearing aid) needs to be before we can say with any certainty that the difference between scores really is due to a difference between hearing aids. Assume that a patient scores 70% with hearing aid A and 85% with hearing aid B. Follow the 70% grid from the horizontal axis to the points where it is crossed by the curves. Reading these points off the vertical axis establishes that the second aid must score 47% to be regarded as significantly worse than the first aid and 90% to be regarded as significantly better.

The striking point here is that the differences do need to be quite large before any importance can be attached to them. It would have been tempting to see the second aid as being better than the first as the difference in

145

discrimination score was 15%. Examination of the 95% confidence limits shows that the size of this difference could simply be due to chance. Note also that the size of difference which can be regarded as significant depends on the scores themselves. For scores in the 50% region, differences need to be larger than for scores close to either extreme (100% or 0%) before significance can be attached to them.

The only steps that can be taken to improve the reliability of the test scores without sacrificing sensitivity involve increasing the number of items on a test. This can be done by repeating the test more than once for each condition or by using a test which intrinsically contains more items. Figure 8 shows reliability plots for a number of typical test situations, and in the Appendix the same data are presented in tabular form. From these figures a number of comparisons can be made. For example if in the above situation

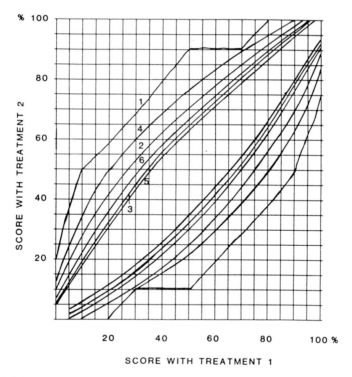

Figure 8.   Minimal differences (95% confidence limits) for:
1) AB Words (% of Words Correct; 1 List)
2) AB Words (% Phonemes Correct; 1 List)
3) AB Words (% Phonemes Correct; 2 Lists)
4) FAAF (% Correct; 1 Page)
5) FAAF (% Correct; 1 Complete List)
6) BKB Sentences (% Correct; 1 List)

the test had been performed twice for each hearing aid and scores obtained were those averaged over two lists, then we could regard the test scores as suggesting a significant difference between aids. Given a score of 70% the second score need only be 83% to be regarded as significantly better. If the scores had been obtained with the FAAF test where the minimal score is also 83% significance could again be accredited to the differences.

These concepts should be valid whatever rehabilitative situations are being compared, whether it is aided versus unaided scores, comparison between aids, comparison of auditory training programmes or discrimination in quiet at different distances from the speaker. They serve again to emphasize the limitations of current speech audiometry in individual rehabilitation. Speech tests are useful in research as they can be performed a lot of times on different subjects. However speech audiometry is not a very precise instrument for use with individual patients, and its quantitative uses in that role are not therefore particularly great when only one or two test scores are considered.

It is possible with shorter speech tests to take several measurements of discrimination at different intensities and so plot aided discrimination functions. This has the advantages of testing across a range of performance levels for the subject (and so including regions of greater sensitivity) and comparing the plotted performance/intensity curves. The variability associated with such curves will be less than that associated with a single test score. Figure 9 demonstrates the use of this procedure in comparing performance at different

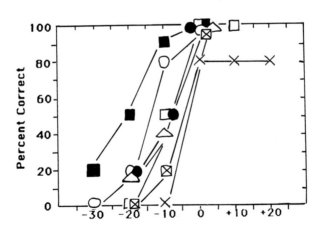

Figure 9.   Unaided and aided paediatric speech intelligibility scores as a function of the message-to-competition ratio (MCR). The SPL of the test sentences was 50 dB. The SPL of the competing sentence messages was varied to produce MCRs from +20 to −30 dB. Test conditions are listed in the order of administration.
(X), unaided – pretest; (□), Aid A – Binaural; (■), Aid B – Binaural; (○), Aid B – Left Ear; (●), Aid B – Right Ear; (△), Aid C – binaural; (⊠), Unaided – Post-Test.

signal to noise ratios using monaural and binaural combinations of different aids (Jerger and Jerger, 1985).

Test Types

If speech audiometry is to be performed in a rehabilitative setting then the test chosen should be governed by the use to which it is intended to be put. Much previous discussion has centred around work with hearing aids, but speech audiometry does have its wider uses. For example Watts *et al.* (1977) used speech discrimination scores to assess the effects of an auditory training régime. By comparing a group of subjects who were given lip reading and auditory training with a group of subjects who were given only lip reading, they were able to show that discrimination scores did indeed improve with auditory training.

A useful test to incorporate into an auditory training programme would be the FAAF test. Although it requires a small microcomputer for scoring to obtain a full feature analysis, the resulting breakdown of scores into particular feature errors should enable those areas of difficulty to be targeted and monitored with serial repetitions of the test. An audio visual version of the test, FADAST (Summerfield and Foster, 1983), is also available so that lip reading skills can be explored.

The problem with longer tests such as the FAAF test (which takes about seven minutes to run) is that for optimal sensitivity some idea of response rate is necessary so that conditions can be suitably adjusted (either by increasing the noise level or decreasing the speech level). A test procedure currently under development is an 'adaptive procedure' in which, rather than running the test in fixed conditions, test conditions are continually adjusted until a target rate of response is achieved. Such a procedure has the advantage that the scoring region likely to be most sensitive can be selected. However in practice the procedure is not straightforward (again being best handled by on line computing techniques) and in the case of FAAF will not produce feature error scores.

The time taken to perform FAAF (other than as an adaptive procedure) tends to prohibit its use for plotting discrimination functions and test lists such as the AB word lists or Jerger's Paediatric Speech Intelligibility test (Jerger and Jerger, 1982) would be more useful here.

Many tests even in the most favourable conditions are not easy enough for the profoundly deaf and tests such as the Connected Discourse Tracking test (De Filipo *et al.*, 1978) may provide help here. This test is run by a patient trying to follow and repeat continuous discourse, either with or without lipreading. The number of words correctly repeated per minute can be used as the score. Such a test has been used for example in monitoring the effectiveness of cochlear implants. It does however require good language skills on the part of the patient.

Test Conditions

The conditions under which the test is performed can be manipulated to be more or less representative of 'real life'. Thus speech testing has been performed with a variety of different background noises. Continuous white, pink or speech shaped noise are typical. If more 'realistic' noises are introduced such as canteen noise, traffic noise or whatever then the reliability of the test score tends to deteriorate owing to the intermittencies present in such noise.

Another approach to realism has been through using different amounts of reverberation on the assumption that many important living environments will be considerably more reverberant than the clinic in which tests are usually performed. The range of reverberation times commonly encountered is considerable. Results from a study by Wills (1985) for example suggested that a hearing impaired child moving between a normal classroom and a partial hearing unit classroom, could experience reverberation times varying between 0.36 and 1.42 secs, depending both on the classroom itself and the number of people in the room at any one time. Moncur and Dirks (1967) were able to show that speech discrimination deteriorated in reverberant conditions when background noise was present.

Directional effects can also be explored. Optional directional microphones are becoming more and more a feature of modern hearing aids, and studies using directional versus non directional microphones have demonstrated their effectiveness. However placement of speakers in a test room can be critically important in such studies, both for the speech signal and the background noise. Owing to head shadow effects signals tend to be louder to each ear from its respective side and softest from the rear. Using rear speakers for the noise and optimally placed speakers for the speech does tend to produce scores favouring directional microphones. However it is likely that factors such as the amount of reverberation present in a room will have some influence on directional advantage, and it is unclear to what extent laboratory demonstrations of such advantage carry over into the patient's normal environment.

The problem with any manipulation of test conditions is the same problem we have come across repeatedly in this chapter. We can perform tests and obtain scores under more or less any condition we choose, however inferences from such scores about individual rehabilitation cannot be more than very general. Furthermore equally valid inferences can often be made with information already obtained. We have seen for example that handicap is better predicted from pure tone thresholds than from speech discrimination scores, and that only gross differences between hearing aids will be apparent unless considerable time and effort are devoted to obtaining scores in a variety of conditions.

Qualitative Uses of Speech Audiometry

If the reader detects a note of scepticism concerning the strictly quantitative uses of speech audiometry in rehabilitation with individual patients, let me redress that somewhat by pointing to its qualitative value.

Patients are often impressed by the improvement which an aid can provide in their discrimination score if both are performed with stimulus levels appropriate for normal speech. It is not difficult in this situation to get a significant improvement and this improvement can be a powerful tool for 'selling' the idea of a hearing aid. AB word lists are useful here due to their speed of administration and provision of a number of equivalent lists. Speech tests performed with and without lip reading give a sometimes dramatic demonstration of the extent to which a patient relies on lip reading skills. This can be done live voice (with care) using AB words or BKB sentences, or by using lipreading tests such as FADAST or the audiovisual version of BKB (Rosen and Corcoran, 1982).

A speech test such as FAAF serves to focus a patient's attention on particular areas of difficulty and as such serves as a useful catalyst to patient counselling and as a guide to auditory training needs.

With children it is very often useful to 'score' tests not so much by the number right or wrong as by the way in which their behaviour changes as they go from certain to uncertain responses. It is an attribute of tests such as BKB that their steep performance/intensity functions can cause rapid changes in behaviour from confidence to hesitation and faltering with small changes in intensity. Again this can be a telling demonstration to parents of both the extent of a child's loss and, if aided tests are also performed, the benefit provided by the hearing aid.

In summary, if time and effort are to be expended in performing speech audiometry on individuals as an aid to rehabilitation, its limitations must be understood. Only a loose relationship between speech scores and handicap exists. Current speech tests are not particularly sensitive to differences between hearing aids. Furthermore speech test scores show considerable variability. On the positive side rehabilitation will be helped if patients and their families understand what is happening to them. Speech discrimination scores often provide a meaningful demonstration of the patient's difficulties, and so can be used to lead them to a better understanding of the nature of the problems for which they have sought our help.

Appendix

Critical Differences

These tables show the lower and upper limits beyond which two treatments can be said to be significantly different at the 95% level of confidence.

For example assume that a patient performs one AB word list with hearing aid A (scored as phonemes correct) and scores 60%. For hearing aid B to be significantly better he would need to score 80% with it (37% for it to be significantly worse).

CRITICAL DIFFERENCES FOR:
FAAF

% correct 1 page			% correct 1 complete list		
SCORE	LOWER	UPPER	SCORE	LOWER	UPPER
0	0	10	25	14	39
5	0	25	26	15	40
10	0	35	28	15	41
15	5	40	29	16	43
20	5	50	30	18	45
25	5	55	31	19	46
30	10	60	33	20	48
35	10	65	34	20	49
40	15	70	35	21	50
45	20	75	36	23	51
50	20	80	38	24	52
55	25	80	39	25	54
60	30	85	40	26	55
65	35	90	41	28	56
70	40	90	43	29	58
75	45	95	44	30	59
80	50	95	45	30	60
85	60	95	46	31	61
90	65	100	48	33	63
95	75	100	49	34	64
100	90	100	50	35	65
			51	36	66
			52	38	68
			54	39	69
			55	40	70

CRITICAL DIFFERENCES FOR:
AB WORDS

% of words correct
1 list

SCORE	LOWER	UPPER
0	0	20
10	0	50
20	0	60
30	10	70
40	16	80
50	10	90
60	20	90
70	30	90
80	40	100
90	50	100
100	80	100

% phonemes correct 1 list			% phonemes correct 2 lists			% phonemes correct 2 lists		
SCORE	LOWER	UPPER	SCORE	LOWER	UPPER	SCORE	LOWER	UPPER
0	0	7	0	0	5	52	35	68
3	0	17	2	0	10	53	37	70
7	0	23	3	0	12	55	38	72
10	3	30	5	0	15	57	40	73
13	3	33	7	2	18	58	42	75
17	3	37	8	2	20	60	43	77
20	7	43	10	2	23	62	45	77
23	7	47	12	3	25	63	47	78
27	10	50	13	5	27	65	48	80
30	10	53	15	5	28	67	50	82
33	13	57	17	7	32	68	52	83
37	17	60	18	7	33	70	53	83
40	20	63	20	8	35	72	55	85
43	20	67	22	10	37	73	57	87
47	23	70	23	10	40	75	58	88
50	27	73	25	12	42	77	60	90
53	30	77	27	13	43	78	63	90
57	33	80	28	15	45	80	65	92
60	37	80	30	17	47	82	67	93
63	40	83	32	17	48	83	68	93
67	43	87	33	18	50	85	72	95
70	47	90	35	20	52	87	73	95
73	50	90	37	22	53	88	75	97
77	53	93	38	23	55	90	77	98
80	57	93	40	23	57	92	80	98
83	63	97	42	25	58	93	82	98
87	67	97	43	27	60	95	85	100
90	70	97	45	28	62	97	88	100
93	77	100	47	30	63	98	90	100
97	83	100	48	32	65	100	95	100
100	93	100	50	33	67			

CRITICAL DIFFERENCES
FOR:
BKB SENTENCES

SCORE	% correct 1 list LOWER	UPPER	SCORE	% correct 1 list LOWER	UPPER
0	0	4	56	41	70
2	0	10	58	43	71
4	0	14	59	44	73
6	2	18	60	45	74
8	2	22	61	46	75
10	2	24	63	48	76
12	4	26	64	49	78
14	4	30	65	50	79
16	6	32	66	51	80
18	6	34	68	52	80
20	8	36	69	54	81
22	8	40	70	55	83
24	10	42	71	58	84
26	12	44	73	59	85
28	14	46	74	60	85
30	14	48	75	61	86
32	16	50	76	63	88
34	18	52	78	64	89
36	20	54	79	65	90
38	22	56	80	66	90
40	22	58	81	69	91
42	24	60	83	70	93
44	26	62	84	71	93
46	28	64	85	73	94
48	30	66	86	75	95
50	32	68	88	76	95
52	34	70	89	78	96
54	36	72	90	79	96
56	38	74	91	81	98
58	40	76	93	83	99
60	42	78	94	85	99
62	44	78	95	86	99
64	46	80	96	89	100
66	48	82	98	91	100
68	50	84	99	93	100
70	52	86	100	96	100
72	54	86			
74	56	88			
76	58	90			
78	60	92			
82	66	94			
84	68	94			
86	70	96			
88	74	96			
90	76	98			
92	78	98			
94	82	98			
96	86	100			
98	90	100			
100	96	100			

Chapter 8

Speech Tests of Hearing for Children

A. Markides

All tests of hearing using speech as stimulus are conveniently grouped under the heading of speech audiometry. Such tests are used for a multiplicity of purposes. In addition to their function as valuable checks on pure tone audiometry, they also contribute in differentiating between sensory and neural dysfunctions, in evaluating a patient's every day difficulties in hearing, in assessing the practical significance of therapeutic, educational, (re)habilitative and compensatory procedures and in studying various factors affecting speech perception.

The main concern here is with those speech tests of hearing, specially designed for English speaking children, that evaluate a child's ability to make correct phonemic classification mainly on the basis of acoustical information. Such tests are commonly referred to as speech articulation, speech inteligibility, speech discrimination or speech recognition tests. In this chapter the latter term will be adopted and used throughout mainly because it describes more accurately the process involved (Olsen and Matkin, 1979).

This chapter begins with a brief description of the historical developments of speech audiometry and it goes on to consider the wide variety of speech materials used in the construction of speech recognition tests. The major criteria for the construction of speech tests of hearing for children are then presented and discussed. This is followed by a description of the main speech tests of hearing for children in current use in the United States of America and in the United Kingdom, with the latter ones being discussed in more detail. The chapter concludes with two major recommendations for developments in this area. The main speech recognition tests for children currently used in the UK are given in the Appendix.

Historical Developments

Specially designed speech recognition tests have been in regular use for just over 40 years. It is of interest to note, however, that speech was used as test

155

material for hearing assessment as far back as two centuries ago when Ernaud and Pereire in the middle of the eighteenth century and Itard at the beginning of the nineteenth century used speech to evaluate the effects of auditory training on their patients' speech perceptual abilities (Urbantschitsch, 1895).

It is true that these early attempts in the measurement of hearing for speech have very little in common with what we now refer to as speech tests of hearing. They did, however, stimulate discussion especially among otologists towards the end of the nineteenth century (Gruber, 1891). This debate was also facilitated by a series of timely scientific inventions that had a considerable influence on the development of speech audiometry. In 1876 Alexander Graham Bell invented a transducer that converted sound energy to electrical energy and vice versa. In 1877 Thomas Edison patented the phonograph which was later on suggested for use in the measurement of hearing for speech (Bryant, 1904).

At the beginning of this century these and other inventions brought about rapid developments in electro acoustic communication systems. These systems called for precise and quantifiable measurement of their speech reproducing capabilities and the first person to respond to this need was Campbell in 1910. Campbell was involved with telphone transmitting equipment at the Bell Telephone Laboratories in the USA. His evaluative method, referred to as 'articulation testing', involved a speaker reading out a list of nonsense syllables at one end of the telephone and a listener trying to identify these syllables at the other end. The percentage of correctly identified syllables was taken as a measure of relative intelligibility (Levitt and Resnick, 1978). Many of the materials and methods used by Campbell were later found to be relevant for evaluating hearing (Fletcher and Steinberg, 1929). The major development in this direction came from the Psycho Acoustic Laboratory of Harvard University and from the Central Institute for the Deaf (CID), in the USA. It was just after the Second World War that Egan (1948) developed the now well known PAL 20 PB-50 Lists. It soon became evident, however, that many patients had difficulties with the vocabulary used in these lists as they contained a number of generally unfamiliar words. In 1952 Hirsh and his associates at the CID devised a modification of Egan's word lists referred to as the CID W-22. According to Martin and Pennington (1971), and more recently, Martin and Forbis (1978), this is the most extensively used monosyllabic (open set response) test in the United States.

These tests and subsequent ones were comprehensively dealt with by a number of authors especially Davis and Silverman (1978) and Bess (1982). In view of this, and the contents of Chapter 11, it is not intended to repeat the same information here. Only a selection of the most widely used tests will be mentioned in a historical context.

In the last twenty years a large number of speech tests of hearing using a variety of speech materials were developed in the United States. Using nonsense syllables Resnick and his associates (Levitt and Resnick, 1978;

Resnick *et al.*, 1976) developed the well known Nonsense Syllable Test (NST). Using monosyllabic words (open set response) Tillman, Carhart and Wilber (1963) developed a new test of the consonant-vowel-consonant (CVC) variety based on the criteria of phonemic balancing. Similar tests using monosyllabic words but of a closed set response type (multiple choice) were also developed, the most popular being the Modified Rhyme Hearing Test (MRHT) by Kruel and his associates (1968). Using sentences as stimulus materials Silverman and Hirsh (1955) introduced their Everyday Speech Sentence Test which was developed and recorded at CID. The most commonly used sentence test in the USA at present, according to Bess (1983) is the Synthetic Sentence Identification (SSI) test which was developed by Speaks and Jerger in 1965.

Similar developments were also evident in the UK. Lists of words were constructed by Fry and Kerridge (1939) as part of a study sponsored by the Medical Research Council which led to the development of the MedResCo hearing aid used in the UK National Health Service. A later study, Fry (1961) at University College, London, developed phonetically balanced word lists for use with adults. The same author also designed a speech test of hearing based on sentences again with deafened adults in mind. There were also developments in speech audiometry for children which will be dealt with later in this chapter.

Speech Materials

Since the early report of Fletcher and Steinberg (1929), a wide variety of speech materials has been employed in the construction of speech recognition tests. They have included individual sounds, nonsense syllables, PB monosyllabic words, disyllabic words, sentences and continuous discourse. Darbyshire (1970) and Ling (1978) for example recommended the use of isolated sounds as stimulus material for evaluating the hearing potential of very deaf children. In 1929 Fletcher and Steinberg devised several lists of nonsense syllables. It has been claimed on numerous occasions that speech tests of hearing consisting of nonsense syllables have certain advantages (Edgerton and Danhauer, 1979). It is true that they lack meaning and therefore their auditory recognition is not dependant on the vocabulary of the listener. It must not be forgotten, however, that this lack of meaning in turn can also be a disadvantage since the listener does not commonly need to identify meaningless speech material. Also the composition of such syllables by definition does not follow the normally allowed sequence of the language and thus the combination of the sounds uttered are not necessarily the appropriate representations of the phonemic sequence in the language. Moreover, nonsense syllables are so abstract that they baffle many listeners and their auditory recognition is also greatly affected by previous experience (Berger, 1971). It was mainly because of these reasons that Fletcher (1929) recommended the use of monosyllabic words for speech tests of hearing.

The use of monosyllabic word lists in speech recognition tests has been widely accepted. This is mainly due to the fact that such tests must consist of relatively non-redundant items, otherwise the multiplicity of clues available to the listener can obscure some of the inabilities to differentiate speech sounds by their acoustical properties. Such tests, however, do not eliminate contextual clues and it is not always clear to what extent they are true measures of the ability of the listener to make phonemic classifications based solely on auditory clues (Hirsh, 1964).

In principle tests using sentences are preferable because they are nearer to the speech material which the listener is exposed to in every day life. It is well known, however, that the meaning of a sentence and word sequence can easily be conveyed by one or two key words and therefore, speech recognition scores derived from sentences are highly influenced by guessing. It is mainly because of this factor that the same hearing ability under similar listening conditions gives a higher score for sentences than for isolated words. As it has been repeatedly shown that there is a close correlation between the results of sentence and word recognition tests the use of the latter can be justified in view of the great saving of time which they afford. Sentence tests have a useful rôle to play, especially when used with people who are so deaf that they cannot understand amplified speech without having a great deal of help from context. In view of the linguistic redundancy inherent in sentences and also the fact that it is exceedingly difficult to construct equivalent sets of 'real' sentences in terms of vocabulary, word familiarity, word length, sentence length and syntactic structure, Fry (1964) departing from conditional procedures suggested the use of 'artificial' sentences based on the traditional probabilities of word sequence. This suggestion was immediately taken up by Speaks and Jerger for experimentation and in 1965 they reported in favour of the test, but cautioned on the high learning effect associated with such material.

The most logical speech message to use for speech recognition testing is continuous discourse (Hirsh, 1952). One major deterrent to the use of such materials is the difficulty of quantification. Ulrich (1957) devised such a test based on a fifteen minute lecture on 'The Food Resources of Africa' which can be administered to a group of listeners and scored in terms of information retained. Its use has been very limited indeed.

In all routine uses of speech recognition tests the responses of the listener must be recognized and quantified by the tester. The tester is therefore placed in a listener's position, thus creating an unwanted variable. Moreover, many subjects, especially children, have accompanying defects of speech so that scoring can become extremely difficult and prone to errors since the examiner tends to be uncertain as to whether the imperfect spoken response is due to faulty hearing or faulty speech or both. To remove, or at least to lessen, the examiner's involvement in the recognition score tests of multiple choice (Watson, 1957) or of the word completion type (House *et al.* and Kryter, 1963, 1965) have been compiled. This approach has three important advantages over classical speech recognition techniques. First the message set is always closed and of controllable size. Secondly the testing procedures can be easily automated thus minimizing experimental error and finally, the learning or practice effect can be determined with relative ease. Such tests have serious drawbacks in that the final score is contaminated by a chance factor and when word completion is involved by the spelling, handwriting legibility and reading ability of the subject. It must be remembered that speech tests of hearing should investigate the listeners' hearing function not their speech production or their mental, physical, linguistic or educational abilities.

Speech Tests of Hearing Specially Designed for Children

Before presenting and discussing the various speech tests of hearing which have been specially developed for hearing-impaired children in the UK it seems appropriate to consider the major criteria upon which such tests are based.

When using speech tests of hearing with children our primary concern is threefold. First we would wish to establish the intensity level at which the child can just detect the presence of speech — the Speech Detection Threshold (SDT). Secondly, we want to establish the intensity level above which the child is not prepared to tolerate speech — the Uncomfortable Loudness Level (ULL) and thirdly, we want to find out how well the child recognizes speech at several suprathreshold levels with a view to maximizing residual hearing. Tests and procedures for the first two items are simple and have been presented and discussed by Markides (1980). Tests of speech recognition, our present concern, are more complicated.

Major Criteria

According to Watson (1957) the major criteria for valid speech recognition tests for children are the following:

(a) They should be constructed of monosyllables.
(b) The words should be within the vocabulary range of the child.
(c) The lists should be phonetically balanced.
(d) The lists should be equal in difficulty.
(e) The responses required must not involve a skill which will cause the subject any difficulty or the tester any uncertainty.

The use of monosyllabic words, preferably of the consonant-vowel-consonant type, is recommended because contextual clues are relatively absent with such materials. It is true that the same can be said for nonsense syllables. Watson (1957) however found that nonsense syllables make too difficult a test for children. He observed that the tendency among children when presented with nonsense materials was to try and perceive them as real monosyllables.

The monosyllabic words used must be within the vocabulary of the children for which the test is intended. If they are not the most likely happening is for the children either to make no response at all or to respond with the nearest known word in their vocabulary. In speech recognition tests the listener is comparing the words heard with a large portion of the vocabulary contained in their memory. Therefore, word familiarity (Broadbent, 1967) together with the number of alternatives with which each word may be confused (Miller *et al.*, 1951; Rosenenzweig and Postman, 1958) have been found to influence speech recognition scores. Ideally the monosyllabic word lists developed for speech recognition testing should be phonemically balanced. In other words the frequency of occurrence of the phonemes in each word list should reflect the frequency of the occurrence of the phonemes as found in the English language. According to Egan (1948) the minimum number of monosyllabic words required in each list to achieve such a phonemic balance is fifty.

Since it is necessary to assess speech recognition ability at several suprathreshold levels or in a variety of acoustic conditions it is essential to have a number of word lists. These word lists should be of equal difficulty (not more than 8% variability) so that the differences in scores obtained reflect the relative ability of the listener to recognize speech and are not due to inequalities in difficulty between lists.

Finally, the type of response required must reflect the child's ability to hear and this must not be contaminated by any other factors. For example, an oral response is inappropriate for those children with severe articulatory problems because the tester cannot be sure whether such a response is due to faulty hearing or faulty articulation, or both. Similarly, it is inappropriate to accept a written response because this may reflect the child's ability to write correctly rather than his ability to hear. In this context it also needs to be mentioned that the tester's hearing should be near normal otherwise difficulty will obviously occur in assessing the oral responses of the child.

Tests

This section will be divided into two parts. The first part will present in summary the most commonly used speech recognition tests for children used in the USA. The second part will present and discuss in more detail the speech recognition tests for children in current use in the UK. This emphasis is deliberate. The former tests have been well documented by previous writers (Bess, 1983) whilst the latter have been existing in relative obscurity.

160

United States of America

One of the first workers to design and develop a speech recognition test for children was Hudgins. He introduced his test, consisting of four monosyllabic word lists based on familiar words in 1944 and referred to it as the Phonetically Balanced Familiar (PBF) lists. A similar test was also developed by Haskins in 1949. It consisted of four lists, fifty words in each list, and was called the Phonetically Balanced Kindergarten 50s (PBK-50s) test. These two tests were based on an open response design and as such they proved rather difficult for young children below the age of 6 years. This difficulty led to the development of speech recognition tests based on the closed set or multiple choice format (Sortini and Flake, 1953; Pronovost and Dumbleton, 1954; Myatt and Landes, 1963).

The test devised by the latter authors was later on revised and improved by Ross and Lerman (1970) and it soon became known as the Word Intelligibility by Picture Identification (WIPI) test. It is suitable for three to six year olds and consists of four lists of monosyllabic words arranged into twenty five plates with each plate having a 6 picture matrix.

A similar test was also developed by Katz and Elliott in 1978. Their test referred to as the Northwestern University — Children's Perception of Speech (NU — CHIPS) test, was specially designed for very young (3 year old) inner-city children. It consists of four monosyllabic word lists with fifty items in each list.

Erber (1974, 1977, 1980) developed a series of tests, the most widely known being the last one. This is a simple test specially designed for children with severe to profound hearing loss and who, owing to severe linguistic retardation are unable to respond to traditional word recognition tests. This test is known as the Auditory Numbers Test (ANT). It requires that the child can count from 1 to 5 and it is suitable for children in the age range of 3 to 8 years.

In 1976 Weber and Redell were of the opinion that tests for children based on single words underestimate the speech recognition abilities of hearing-impaired children. Because of this, they constructed sentences using the stimulus words of the WIPI test developed by Ross and Lerman (1970). This test referred to as the WIPI Sentences, consists of 4 twenty five sentence lists. The child's task is to identify and point to the picture on the WIPI six picture matrix plate that best represents the spoken sentence.

Bess (1983) reported that a number of authors were in favour of using adult monosyllabic material of the open set response type with young children. It may be that certain adult lists can be used effectively with some children, but the consensus of opinion on this matter is that the selection of speech materials for children should be within the children's speech and language competence. There is no doubt that some hearing impaired-children, mainly because of severe linguistic retardation, are unable to take part in conventional speech recognition tests. In order to assess the speech perceptual abilities of such children, Ling (1978) put forward a rather simple speech recognition test referred to as the Five Sound Test using three vowels /u/, /a/ and /i/ and two consonants /ʃ/ and /s/. According to Ling, these sounds cover the frequency range of all phonemes and the vowels contain sufficient harmonics to convey suprasegmental information.

Another test in this category which deserves special mention is that developed by Finitzo-Hieber and his associates (1980). They developed a non-linguistic test for very young children around 3 years old. Their test is based on 30 environmental sounds (plus 1 practice item) and is referred to as the Sound Effects Recognition Test (SERT). The 30 environmental sounds are divided into 3 lists with each list consisting of 10 items represented on 4 picture matrix plates.

United Kingdom

According to Watson (1957), one of the first workers to develop a speech recognition test specially designed for children in the UK was D. C. Kendall 1953, 1954) working in the University of Manchester under Professor Ewing.

THE KENDALL TOY TEST (KT TEST)

The KT Test was intended for very young children (3 to 5 years old) who had developed a moderate vocabulary. It consists of 3 lists, each list containing 10 monosyllabic words which are represented by small toy replicas. Each word list contains a range of the most common vowels, diphthongs and consonants. The test is administered in a free field situation using live voice which is monitored with a sound level meter situated close to the child's ear. First of all the child is presented with each toy replica and is encouraged to name it. This procedure is followed in order to make sure that the objects in the test are within the known vocabulary of the child being tested. All 10 toy replicas are then presented and arranged on the table in front of the child. The child is then required to point to the appropriate toy when he hears the instruction 'Show me the . . .'. In order to lessen the possibility of a chance response and also to give some practice before beginning the test, an additional 5 toys are placed with the 10 test items. This is a useful little test and provided the tester takes special care in monitoring the loudness of his speech, quite a lot of information can be gained not only regarding the speech detection level but also the child's speech recognition abilities at several suprathreshold levels. Since this test can only be administered in a free field situation (and masking is not practical for very young children) both the SDT measurement and the Speech Recognition scores obtained relate only to bilateral hearing. This test is widely used in paediatric audiology clinics throughout the country.

In order to meet the special needs of school aged hearing-impaired children, Watson (1957) working at Manchester University developed a series of speech tests comprising the Manchester Junior (MJ) lists, the Manchester Picture Vocabularly test (MP) and the Manchester Sentence (MS) lists.

The Manchester Junior (MJ) Lists

This test was specially designed for hearing-impaired children from about the age of six and upwards. It consists of 4 word lists with 25 monosyllables in each list. Each list is scrambled once thus giving a total of eight 25 word lists. Although a serious attempt was made to achieve phonemic balance, this, owing to the small number of words in each list and also to the restricted vocabularly used, proved very difficult to meet. The end result however reflects a reasonable compromise. The test was tape recorded and standardized on normal hearing children. The 8 word lists proved to be equal in difficulty giving a normal speech recognition curve based on whole word scoring which rises by 5% per dB. This test has proved to be satisfactory for children with minor linguistic retardation. It presents, however, difficulties to children with severe linguistic retardation and associated speech problems.

The Manchester Picture (MP) Vocabulary Test

This multiple choice test was developed for hearing-impaired children of six years and over who because of their handicap are unable to take part in an open set type of speech recognition task.

It consists of six lists of twenty monosyllables each. The vocabulary used is simple. An attempt was made to secure homogeneity and equality of difficulty between word lists but experience has shown that there exist significant differences in difficulty between the lists. The lists are not phonemically balanced but the words in each list are carefully chosen to give as wide a selection as possible of the phonemes from the English language.

The test is configured in the form of three sets of twenty cards each. At the initial stages of the development of this test each card contained six pictures. Later on the number of pictures drawn on each card was limited to four. One of the pictures on each card illustrates the stimulus word whilst the other three relate to words containing the same vowels or the same consonants as the stimulus word.

The administration and scoring of this test is carried out as follows: The child is presented with the practice card and is asked to name the pictures on the card. The tester then asks the child to 'show me the . . .'. When the child shows that he understands the procedure then the tester (or preferably a helper) introduces the other cards one by one giving the child sufficient time between each stimulus word to respond. Only one stimulus word is given for each card. If the child is uncertain or mistaken in his choice the word given must not be repeated — the tester should proceed to the next item.

This test is usually administered in a free field situation using monitored live voice. With cooperative children it can also be administered through a closed circuit system comprising of a tape recorder, speech audiometer attachment and earphones.

The responses of the children are scored on the number of words correctly identified, expressed as a percentage of the total number of words in each list. The test was standardized with normal hearing children listening through a closed circuit arrangement. The normal speech recognition curve obtained showed a slight curvilinear rise of 4% per dB covering the 10% to 90% recognition function. It must not be forgotten that this is a multiple choice type of test and as such chance cannot be entirely ruled out and guessing is certainly taking place. Watson (1957) suggested that when the highest score obtained by a subject at any level is less than 20% this should be ignored as it might have come about as result of chance.

THE MANCHESTER SENTENCE (MS) TEST

This test was developed to ascertain the speech recognition abilities of hearing-impaired children when presented with connected speech. It consists of five lists of ten sentences each. The sentences consist of familiar statements, commands and questions and they reflect a linguistic level within the abilities of hearing-impaired children of 10 years and over. The test was standardized with normal hearing pupils in the seven to nine year age range. The normal speech recognition curve obtained has a gradient at its linearly rising section of 5% per dB.

Each sentence consists of five key words and each word correctly repeated carries two percentage points. Although attempts have been made to standarize this test in terms of equality of difficulty between the sentence lists the end result is not satisfactory. Even a casual analysis of the use of this test reveals wide discrepancies in scores in the region of plus or minus 20% between the various lists. Furthermore, some of the sentences used are now out of date — this test has not really enjoyed any popularity but unfortunately is still in use in several paediatric audiology clinics in the UK.

THE AB ISOPHONEMIC WORD LISTS

At present the most widely used speech recognition test for children in the UK is the one developed by Arthur Boothroyd in 1968. This test is commonly referred to as the AB Isophonemic Word Lists and consists of fifteen ten word lists with each list containing the same thirty phonemes, ten vowels and twenty consonants. The monosyllabic words used in constructing the test were of the consonant-nucleus-consonant (CNC) type and were selected from the author's vocabulary — first names and obscenities excluded.

This test has several major advantages over the other tests so far mentioned in this section.

(a) It consists of short word lists thus allowing the exploration of a large number of listening conditions within a relatively short period of time (this factor is very important in busy audiology clinics).
(b) The considerable number of word lists employed ($N = 15$) reduces the possibility of repeating various word lists within a session thus diminishing the effects of learning factors.
(c) The recognition score is based on the number of phonemes correctly repeated and thus, according to Boothroyd, produces a high interlist equivalence and good reliability.

The test also has several shortcomings. A considerable number of the words used are not within the vocabularies of junior children and some of these words are emotionally biased. Boothroyd was of the opinion that the phonemic scoring employed in the test diminished the influences of linguistic factors but this is an opinion which is strongly contested. Furthermore the word lists because of their short nature, do not reflect the phonemic balance of the English language.

Three versions of this test are available on tape. The first version reflects a strong northern English accent whilst the second version recorded at the Institute of Sound and Vibration Research, University of Southampton, reflects a 'standard' BBC type of English accent. Using the first version, Boothroyd (1968) reported a maximum gradient of speech recognition of 4% per dB for children in the age group 5–9 years. Using the second version Markides (1978) reported varying gradients of speech recognition depending on the age of the normal hearing children. For 6 year olds, he reported a 4.2% rise per dB from 10–90% recognition score. For 7 and 8 year olds, this rise was 4.8% per dB and for 9, 10 and 11 year olds it was 5% per dB. A third version of the lists was produced by the Royal National Institute for the Deaf and is commercially available. This version contains all the lists and has two practice words at the beginning of each list.

THE BKB SENTENCE LISTS

The most recently developed speech recognition test for children in the UK is the BKB sentence lists (Bench, Koval and Bamford, 1979). This is an open set response test and according to the authors it better reflects the natural language usage of hearing-impaired children. The construction of this test was based on the responses of hearing-impaired children in the age range 8–15 years when asked to describe familiar pictures depicting everyday activities from home and play situations. It consists of 21 lists of 16 sentences (not more than 7 syllables in each sentence). Each list contains 50 stimulus words. The scoring is achieved by calculating the percentage of key words repeated correctly. A simplified version of this test referred to as the Picture-Related BKB Sentence Lists for Children (BKB-PR) was also developed. This simplified version consists of 11 lists of 16 sentences with 50 stimulus words in each list. This test has potential but has not yet been widely accepted or used in the UK.

The Reed Hearing Test (Reed, 1959) consists of a set of cards, each one containing four pictures. The pictures each depict a single object which on one card have a common vowel e.g., mouse, house, owl, cow but with differing consonants. There are eight cards in all. The child is required to point to the picture that is named e.g., 'Show me the cow'. After a practice with the tester in front of the child to ensure that the correct names are associated with the pictures and that the child understands the test, the test is repeated with the tester 6ft behind the child and speaking in a normal conversational voice. Three or four cards are used and if the child fails to select the correct picture more than once or twice it should be referred for a full audiometric examination. If the child is successful the test should be repeated with a whispered voice and should be referred if it fails on more than one or two pictures.

Reed revised the test and it was published by the Royal National Institute for the Deaf in 1970 as the RNID Hearing Test Cards.

OTHER TESTS

Several other attempts (Dodds, 1972; McCormick, 1977; Holsgrove and Halden, 1984) have been made in producing speech tests of hearing suitable for children in the UK. The tests developed have not been widely accepted.

Conclusion

Most of the speech recognition tests for children currently used in the UK were designed and developed more than 20 years ago. They are in need of updating and there is also an urgent need to construct and develop new tests for children of all ages especially for those children below the age of 5 years.

Administration and scoring procedures of speech recognition tests of hearing for children were considered to be beyond the scope of this chapter and have not been discussed fully here. One important point pertinent to this area however which needs to be made relates to the lack of standardization and calibration of the relevant equipment used for speech audiometry. This has created and continues to create serious problems in the use of speech audiometry as a diagnostic procedure in the assessment of hearing. This may in turn account for the restricted use of speech audiometry in the UK National Health Service (Fuller and Moss, 1985).

Appendix

Main Speech Tests of Hearing for Children in the United Kingdom

The Kendal Toy Test (K. T. Test)

Preliminary Practice List	*KT/1*	*KT/2*	*KT/3*
chair	knife	fork	house
church	bath	cat	spoon
nail	soap	tree	fish
ring	car	watch	duck
plane	bus	match	cow
	tin	dog	gate
	boat	horse	brick
	pig	bed	shoe
	brush	key	cup
	pipe	egg	plate

The following distractors should be used:

	pin	ball	mouse
	duck	sheep	book
	jar	hen	string
	comb	mat	glove
	wheel	doll	plane

The Manchester Junior (M.J.) Lists

MJ/1	*MJ/2*	*MJ/3*	*MJ/4*
farm	bad	ship	book
bird	dish	home	kind
school	keep	cup	train
but	milk	made	last
play	boy	egg	three
duck	some	day	pot
them	fall	fish	does
soon	house	took	field
pig	put	park	had
doll	time	shoe	poor
for	know	horse	give
shop	bed	night	ball
hand	five	just	mouse
have	with	seat	hair
from	yes	man	big
cat	sheep	hat	room
green	her	bus	saw
door	down	long	can
white	food	chair	stick
nice	car	boat	good
that	take	seen	when
come	red	black	wash
brown	dog	road	floor
get	has	girl	one
could	gun	cow	said

167

MJ/5	MJ/6	MJ/7	MJ/8
hand	with	took	good
white	put	seat	room
but	milk	chair	last
them	car	road	one
doll	down	egg	ball
farm	bad	ship	pot
nice	fall	horse	kind
from	dog	bus	big
door	know	seen	train
soon	keep	cow	wash
for	time	cup	had
bird	sheep	long	mouse
that	red	day	said
shop	food	girl	hair
play	gun	night	book
come	bed	hat	give
cat	some	home	can
school	yes	boat	when
get	has	fish	field
green	boy	shoe	stock
pig	five	black	poor
could	house	man	does
have	her	park	three
duck	take	made	saw
brown	dish	just	floor

The Manchester Picture (M.P.) Vocabulary Test (Modified Version)

List 1	List 2	List 3	List 4
pin	ship	pig	sea
well	leg	fire	tie
boot	bus	cup	duck
coat	dog	saw	cake
star	cat	house	bird
dish	drum	bed	doll
tie	three	cake	plate
stair	fish	sock	spoon
fly	three	chair	ring
man	wall	mouse	light

List 5	List 6	List 7	List 8
key	hill	brick	sheep
bell	pen	pipe	kite
moon	book	sun	foot
boat	shop	wall	spade
car	cap	cow	man
ball	gate	dog	bat
tap	teeth	car	cup
house	star	bus	feet
snake	foot	seat	brush
bun	mat	leg	moon

168

The Manchester Sentence (M.S.) Test

LIST *A*
1. The *girl's mother* has a *new red hat*.
2. *Some people send cards* at Easter.
3. The *tits built* a *nest* in the *apple tree*.
4. *Mother* will *bake* a *cake* for *my birthday*.
5. *Indians make birch bark canoes*.
6. *Some countries have summer* in *December*.
7. *Is* a *twopenny stamp blue* or *brown*?
8. *Leave* the *door* key *under* the *mat*.
9. *Put*, a *tight bandage round* his *thumb*.
10. *Very early houses* had *roofs* of *straw*.

LIST *B*
1. My *friend's father drives* a *blue car*.
2. *Would* you *like some water* with your *meal*?
3. *Swallows sometimes fly near* the *ground*.
4. *People squeeze lemons* to *get* the *juice*.
5. The *brown deer licked* its *baby fawn*.
6. *Stars seem brighter* on a *dark night*.
7. *Open* your *sum book* at *page fifty-two*.
8. *School ends* at *ten past four*.
9. *Put clean paper on top* of the *table*.
10. The *names* of *some towns end* in *-ham*.

LIST *C*
1. You *can't buy fish* in a *baker's shop*.
2. *New shoes* are *often tiring* to *wear*.
3. *Most mice* have *long thin tails*.
4. The *shops don't open before eight*.
5. *People sometimes cross* a *fence* by a *stile*.
6. *Many plants begin* to *flower* in *May*.
7. The *American flag* has *red* and *white stripes*.
8. *Buy some toothpaste* in the *Chemist's shop*.
9. *Most car engines* are *cooled* by *water*.
10. *Tigers* and *leopards* are *members* of the *cat family*.

LIST *D*
1. *Father comes home* from *work* at *six*.
2. *Please sew* a *button on* the *vest*.
3. The *man* had *chesse* and *dry biscuits* for *supper*.
4. *Fresh water fish are caught* with *flies*.
5. *We do not often have snow* in *September*.
6. *Many women use gas* for *cooking*.
7. *Bears often sleep* on the *branch* of a *tree*.
8. *Fetch some sticks* to *lay* the *fire*.
9. The *box* of *nails weighs half* a *pound*.
10. *Men used* to *hunt animals* with a *spear*.

LIST *E*
1. We *read* a *fairy story after tea*.
2. *Father carried* his *white shirt upstairs*.
3. *Frogs come out* of the *water* to *breathe*.
4. The *boy likes bread* and *jam* for *tea*.
5. *Trees* do *not grow* on *high mountains*.
6. *Farmers usually cut* their *hay* in *June*.
7. *Put* the *glass jar under* the *water*.
8. *Don't come home without* your *cap*.
9. *Six o'clock* is *too late* to *start*.
10. The *first wheels* were *made* from *slices* of *log*.

169

A.B. Isophonemic Short Word Lists

No. 1	No. 2	No. 3	No. 4	No. 5	No. 6
ship	fish	thud	fun	fib	fill
rug	duck	witch	will	thatch	catch
fan	gap	wrap	vat	sum	thumb
cheek	cheese	jail	shape	heel	heap
haze	rail	keys	wreath	wide	wise
dice	hive	vice	hide	rake	rave
both	bone	get	guess	goes	goat
well	wedge	shown	comb	shop	shone
jot	moss	hoof	choose	vet	bed
move	tooth	bomb	job	June	juice

No. 7	No. 8	No. 9	No. 10	No. 11	No. 12
badge	bath	hush	jug	man	have
hutch	hum	gas	match	hip	whizz
kill	dip	thin	whip	thug	buff
thighs	five	fake	faith	ride	mice
wave	ways	chime	sign	siege	teeth
reap	reach	weave	bees	veil	gauge
foam	joke	jet	hell	chose	poach
goose	noose	rob	rod	shoot	rule
not	got	dope	vote	web	den
shed	shell	lose	shook	cough	cosh

No. 13	No. 14.	No. 15
kiss	wish	hug
buzz	dutch	dish
hash	jam	ban
thieve	heath	rage
gate	laze	chief
wife	bike	pies
pole	rove	wet
wretch	pet	cove
dodge	fog	loose
moon	soon	moth

RNID Hearing Test Cards

1.	EGG	PEG	HEN	BED
2.	CUP	DUCK	JUG	BUS
3.	SHIP	DISH	PIG	FISH
4.	KNIFE	PIPE	PIE	KITE
5.	KEY	SHEEP	FEET	TREE
6.	HAT	CAT	LAMB	FAN
7.	DOG	COT	DOLL	SOCK
8.	OWL	HOUSE	MOUSE	COW

Chapter 9

Speech Perception Tests for the Profoundly Deaf

A. B. King

In conventional speech audiometry the test items are single words with a consonant-vowel-consonant structure, or words embedded in a fixed 'carrier phrase', or sentences. Standard lists of such items are presented auditorily at each of a number of different intensity levels and the patient is required to identify the word or sentence heard. What is measured is the percentage of words or individual speech-sounds (phonemes) correctly identified at each intensity level.

For many profoundly deaf listeners, even at an intensity level which yields the best result, the score is likely to be close to zero, or zero. But this does not mean that, with amplification, such people cannot make some sound-discriminations which are useful in the perception of speech. They may not be able to identify single words, but they may at least be able to distinguish speech from other kinds of sound. Secondly, any ability which they have to discriminate between simple sound-patterns may provide a helpful supplement to the information they obtain from lip reading, so that their lip reading ability with appropriately amplified acoustic input is greater than with visual information alone. Thirdly their auditory discrimination, though limited, may enable them better to monitor their own speech, particularly in its prosodic aspects such as timing, rhythm, pitch and intonation.

For these reasons, it makes sense to look for a method of assessing speech perception in profoundly deaf people, even though conventional speech audiometry is not appropriate. Speech audiometry was developed primarily as a diagnostic tool, as has been discussed in previous chapters. The development of speech perception tests for the profoundly deaf has a different focus: the aim has been to develop tests of either (a) ability in a realistic audio-visual speech reception task which relates to everyday function, or (b) ability to discriminate between the kind of simple acoustic patterns which give information that facilitates lip reading. A secondary aim in the development of some of these tests has been to enable an analysis of *which* features of speech the person fails to perceive.

Audio-Visual Speech Perception Tests

Profoundly deaf people rely heavily on lip reading in their perception of speech in everyday life. Furthermore, visual and auditory information complement each other linguistically. Distinguishing one word from another involves the perception of contrasts between different speech sounds. Sensorineural hearing impairment can make certain of these contrasts very difficult to perceive auditorily, even with amplification. Where vowels are concerned, some contrasts are more difficult than others: for example, the vowels in 'hard' and 'hid' may be much easier to distinguish between than those in 'hid' and 'hood'. This is partly because the vowel in 'hard' is relatively long and the other two are short, but also because the resonance which distinguishes the vowel in 'hid' from that in 'hood' is in a higher frequency area of the spectrum than that which distinguishes 'hard' from the other two. However, different vowels are reasonably easy to lip read and so visual information can be used to overcome auditory impairment.

Certain consonant contrasts also cause difficulty auditorily to those with sensorineural hearing loss. In phonetic terms, consonants differ in the *place* in the mouth where they are articulated, in the *manner* of articulation, and in whether they are *voiced* or not (i.e. whether the vocal folds of the larynx are vibrating throughout the articulation of the sound or not). To know whether the speaker has said 'by' or 'die' it is necessary to perceive the difference due to contrast in *place* of articulation of the two consonants (bilabial and alveolar respectively) but they are both voiced and both articulated in the same manner (plosive). To someone with hearing impairment this contrast may be difficult to perceive auditorily, because the relevant acoustic cue is a rapid change in the pattern of the higher part of the frequency spectrum. Fortunately, the difference between 'by' and 'die' is very easy to *see*. On the other hand, the differences between 'pie' and 'by' (contrast of voicing), and 'by' and 'my' (contrast of manner) are not easy to lip read as the consonants distinguishing these three words are articulated in the same place, by making a closure between the lips. Fortunately, the relevant acoustic differences in these cases are predominantly in the lower frequencies and so someone with hearing impairment may well be able to use auditory information to overcome the lack of visual cues.

There are other aspects of speech which are difficult to see, such as syllable rhythm and intonation. Although these aspects are prosodic, and have limited bearing on the contrasts between speech sounds, they do have important linguistic significance when it comes to perceiving word boundaries and appreciating the meaning of whole sentences. Fortunately it is again the case that these less visible aspects are conveyed by relatively low frequency acoustic patterns not requiring fine spectral resolution, and so the hearing impaired person is likely to be able to make use of this auditory information.

Two good examples of audio-visual speech perception tests which use videotaped presentation of the speaker's face to assess a person's ability to perceive speech-sound contrasts are the following: The FADAST — Four-alternative Auditory Disability and Speech-reading Test (Summerfield and Foster, 1983), and the Intervocalic Consonant Test (Rosen *et al.*, 1979; Rosen and Fourcin, 1983).

The FADAST uses audio-visual presentation of a set of single monosyllabic English words. Each word presented is accompanied by a subtitled group of four possible responses involving one vowel contrast and one consonant contrast, e.g. 'bull', 'wool', 'bell', 'well'. The whole test has a balanced distribution of contrasts which are relatively easy and relatively difficult to discriminate by vision alone.

The Intervocalic Consonant Test comprises 48 trials during which each of the 12 most commonly occurring English consonants is presented four times. In every spoken item the consonant is preceeded and followed by the same open vowel and each item is spoken with the same intonation contour. The response is to write down the consonant perceived.

Both the FADAST and the Intervocalic Consonant Test results can be analysed by confusion matrices to discover the distribution of errors over different types of consonant contrast (voice, place and manner). They therefore enable the person testing to gain a clearer idea of what kind of information a profoundly deaf person is using in speech-reading and where they are failing. Further information of remedial significance may be obtained by a comparison between aided and unaided performance, and between results when aided with different kinds of device.

A different kind of audio-visual test is Connected Discourse Tracking (De Filippo and Scott, 1978). This does not admit of the kind of analysis of utilized information made possible by the above two tests, but it does provide a very realistic speech perception task in which the person receiving is watching and listening to a complete spoken text. He or she can therefore make use of semantic and syntactic contextual clues in deciphering what is being said. The method employs live presentation of the test with the receiver being required to repeat back verbatim what is said, at manageable intervals. There are certain permissible types of interaction between speaker and receiver to clear up errors and the score is the number of words-per-minute correctly transmitted during a 5-minute period. As with the above tests, differences between aided and unaided scores provide a measure of benefit from hearing aids or other prosthetic devices. There is however, the disadvantage that because test/retest reliability is not very high, a number of sessions may be required under each condition to establish the statistical significance of any aided/unaided difference in score, and this is clearly time-consuming. The method is perhaps most appropriate when a patient's progress with a particular device is being monitored over a period of some weeks or months.

173

Sound Pattern Tests

A different approach is to concentrate on auditory ability alone, and to develop tests of whether the profoundly deaf person can discriminate between the kinds of simple acoustic pattern which give information that facilitates lipreading. Discrimination between such patterns is also likely to help in successful monitoring of his or her own speech, particularly in its prosodic aspects.

The History of Sound Pattern Tests

Distinguishing one word from another involves the perception of contrasts between different speech sounds (phonemes). The idea of examining specific acoustic patterns which are independent of speaker variability and which provide auditory cues for phoneme identification derives from speech science and, in particular, the acoustic theory of speech production and perception as expounded by Fant (1960, 1967), and Pickett (1980). A sound spectrum is a particular pattern relating intensity to frequency. Speech consists of a constantly changing spectral pattern in time, but it cannot be segmented strictly into individual phonemes. (For a detailed description see Richard Wright's chapter in this book on 'Basic Properties of Speech'.) The investigation of acoustic cues to contrasts between consonants has involved looking at what happens to the spectral pattern during vowels which come before and after the consonants in question. In addition to phoneme contrasts, there are the other linguistically significant contrasts of syllable rhythm and intonation to consider, and the relatively simple acoustic cues to these have also been studied.

The technology of speech synthesis has provided a vital tool in the study of acoustic speech cues, because it has enabled investigators to generate speech-like sounds, vary their spectral pattern over time in controlled ways, and then find out how people with normal hearing and language-development perceive them. In the case of phoneme cues, listeners have typically either been asked to 'label' the items by indicating for each item whether they heard this word/syllable or that word/syllable, or in some studies they have been presented with two items and simply been asked to indicate whether they heard them as 'the same' or 'different'. The relevant acoustic dimensions have been varied in graded steps to establish the critical boundaries for perception of one phoneme rather than another.

These studies of speech sound perception and the relative importance of different acoustic cues have been reviewed by Pickett (1980), and investigations of the development of speech sound perception in children are reviewed by Hazan (1986).

By the 1970s a substantial body of knowledge about acoustic cues had been built up, and investigators began to apply the same techniques to the study of difficulties in speech perception experienced by these with impaired hearing (Pickett *et al.*, 1983). Vowel contrasts are cued by differences in spacing between 'formants' (frequency bands of relatively high energy equivalent to vocal tract resonances). It has been found that the more severe the hearing loss, the more difficulty is likely to be experienced in discriminating formant differences particularly in the higher frequency region. Place of articulation of consonants is cued by relatively brief transitions in the frequency of the formants of adjacent vowel sounds. People with sensorineural hearing loss have been found to have poor discrimination of 2nd formant transitions, particularly in the presence of the lower frequency 1st formant (which is the condition obtaining in listening to natural speech). They also have shown very poor discrimination of the *rate* of transition, which for normally hearing listeners is the acoustic cue to whether a consonant is made in an obstruent (plosive) or approximant manner. Regarding perception of whether a final consonant is voiced or not, some hearing-impaired listeners have shown poor performance when the preceeding vowel-duration cue has been removed, but others have apparently been able to make use of the remaining spectral cues, and this latter group were those with relatively good hearing for frequencies below 1 kHz. The cue to voicing of initial obstruent consonants is the voice onset time (VOT), which is the interval between the transient burst (associated with release of the obstruent closure) and the onset of the strong periodic voicing excitation associated with the vowel. Moderately hearing-impaired listeners have generally been found to have little difficulty in discriminating and identifying voiced and unvoiced obstruents as a function of VOT, but among the more severely impaired, the ability is highly variable.

In fact, in all these acoustic cue investigations with hearing-impaired people, although the group results are as reported above, variability between individuals is high and it can in no way be predicted accurately from the pure tone audiogram how good discrimination will be for a particular acoustic cue to speech sound contrasts. Among children the variability is even higher. However, some studies report findings parallel to the results with adults. Fourcin (1976) presented synthesized two-formant vowels corresponding to /i/, /ɑ/ and /u/ (/i/ and /u/ had identical 1st formant values). Those hearing impaired children with more severe losses were able to identify /ɑ/ correctly but showed confusion in their identification of /i/ and /u/ which are distinguished by height of the 2nd formant. Children with less severe losses had little difficulty in the task. A second test was concerned with the syllable-initial voicing contrast cued by VOT as described above. A further cue, that of whether the 1st formant transition is cut back or not, was artificially manipulated so that on some trials the 1st formant cue did not coincide with the VOT cue as it would in natural speech. The conclusion from the results was that the children seemed to require both cues to identify the phonemes correctly and that those with more severe losses could not perceive the contrast at all.

175

Application of Sound Pattern Tests to Profoundly Deaf Listeners

The techniques of speech synthesis and acoustic cue studies can also be applied in the case of those with profound losses. However, for these people it makes sense to limit the sound patterns used to those which are the most basic in speech perception, since it is already established that their auditory perception of acoustic cues to consonant contrasts is very poor indeed and in many cases non-existent. What is proposed is a simple battery of tests employing sound patterns related to the prosodic aspects of speech: syllable rhythm and intonation. It would also seem to be worthwhile including a vowel contrast test, at least using vowels which differ in 1st formant position, and a test of whether they can identify periodic and aperiodic sound (the cue to whether a sound is voiced).

It is possible to generate suitable sound patterns using commonly available microcomputers and speech synthesis chips, but a certain amount of phonetic expertise is necessary on the part of the programmer to ensure that while the patterns are simplified to test perception of a particular acoustic feature, the parameters are kept appropriately speech-like.

The use of a microcomputer gives further advantages: automatic control of the randomized presentation of stimuli and automatic recording of responses and reaction-times. In addition, the procedure can be made adaptive so that progress to different levels of difficulty is based on a statistical criterion of success, and the hardest level of discrimination at which a particular listener can still succeed is pinpointed rapidly without the need for a tedious number of stimulus presentations or the discouraging effects of repeated failures.

One such battery of tests has been employed at the RNID in the past few years to assess the auditory discrimination ability of profoundly deaf patients using appropriate amplification. The task is a single-interval binary choice identification, i.e. the patient hears one of two possible sounds and is required to identify it by pressing one of two labelled buttons. Each test is preceeded by a practice session with immediate knowledge of success or failure on each item. The five tests are:

1. Gap detection: the sound is identified as 'broken' or 'smooth'. Duration of the gap is varied.
2. Detection of amplitude dip: the sound is again identified as 'broken' or 'smooth'. Duration of the dip is held constant but amplitude of the dip is varied.
3. Identification of aperiodic and periodic sound: the sound is identified as 'crackle' or 'hum'.
4. Identification of vowel-like sounds: the sound is identified as /i/ ('EEEE') or /ɑ/ (AAAH). The difference is in the pattern of formant spacing.
5. Perception of pitch contour: the sound is identified as 'falling' or 'flat'. The range of fundamental frequency over which the fall occurs is varied.

For all test items except 'crackle' the synthesized sound has a vowel-like spectrum with periodic excitation of resonances (formants). Apart from test 4, the formant spacing is that of neutral vowel-quality. The duration of each stimulus is approximately 1 second.

	Pass	Fail
1. Gap detection: 80ms or less	16	7
: 95–125ms	19	4
2. Detection of amplitude-dip: 3–6 dB	14	9
: 9–12 dB	19	4
3. Aperiodic/periodic sound	13	10
4. Vowel identification (/i/ vs /ɑ/)	8	15
5. Falling/flat pitch contour	2	21

Table I Sound Pattern Test Results from 23 Profoundly Deaf Listeners

Table I shows results on the Sound Pattern Tests given by 23 profoundly deaf listeners (with auditory thresholds in excess of 90 dBHL in the frequency range 500 Hz to 4 kHz), using appropriate amplication. Most of those tested could make some discrimination between sound patterns which could give useful information to supplement lip reading, even though in most cases this appears to be limited to the temporal pattern of amplitude changes rather than contrasts which involve frequency analysis.

To discover how well these listeners can in practice integrate such auditory discriminations with lip reading, it would be necessary to carry out audio-visual tests of the kind described earlier in this chapter. Sound Pattern Tests, as well as being a research tool, provide information useful to those carrying out auditory training programmes with profoundly deaf patients, enabling them to plan realistic programmes and monitor progress. But it can be argued that if a test of ability is required which relates to everyday function in speech perception, then audio-visual tests which incorporate the lip reading dimension are the most appropriate choice.

Chapter 10

Testing Visual and Auditory Visual Speech Perception

G. Plant and J. Macrae

The testing of a hearing-impaired person's speech perception skills usually concentrates on assessing his/her ability to understand speech via audition alone. Materials adopted for such testing usually consist of lists of monosyllabic words (Egan, 1948; Hirsh *et al.*, 1952; Fry, 1961) although testing materials utilizing nonsense syllables (Levitt and Resnick, 1978; Edgerton and Danhauer, 1979) and sentences (Davis and Silverman, 1970; Kalikow, Stevens and Elliott, 1977) have been developed. Although much useful information can be obtained through auditory testing alone, such an approach cannot adequately assess an individual subject's overall communication ability in everyday situations. Most conversations are typically conducted face-to-face. In such situations the receiver has access not only to the acoustic speech signal but also to the visible movements of the speaker's articulators. The importance of these visible movements for hearing-impaired persons should not be underestimated. Lip reading 'the correct identification of thoughts transmitted via the visual components of oral discourse' (O'Neill and Oyer, 1981) represents the primary mode of speech perception for many severely and profoundly hearing impaired persons. There are also many situations where hearing impaired persons with less severe losses also need to use lip reading to supplement the auditory signal. Speech perception via audition alone may be impossible for many hearing-impaired persons in noisy and/or reverberant conditions. Even in quiet surroundings hearing-impaired persons typically report that they can understand speech more easily if they can both hear and see the speaker. Comments such as 'I hear a lot better with my glasses on' and 'I don't hear so well in the dark' are familiar to clinicians working with hearing-impaired adults. Given the great potential value of lip reading for hearing-impaired persons it is perhaps surprising that standard audiological procedures do not routinely include visual and auditory-visual testing. Such testing would appear to offer a more comprehensive picture of an individual subject's overall communication competence.

Testing via vision alone can be criticized on the grounds that it represents a highly artificial situation, as almost all hearing-impaired persons potentially

179

have at least some auditory information available to them via hearing aids. Although such a criticism is perfectly valid, lip reading testing does enable the clinician to determine the limits of speech perception via vision alone. If this baseline can be determined a number of rehabilitative measures may then be evaluated. The relative value of auditory or tactual supplements to lip reading can then be measured by comparing the unaided (lip reading alone) and aided (lip reading plus the supplement) scores. Such testing may also assist the clinician in the planning and provision of appropriate rehabilitative strategies. Scores obtained in testing may also help the clinician to determine the sensory modality to be stressed in the training procedures. The effectiveness of various training procedures can also be evaluated by comparing the scores obtained pre- and post-training. Visual alone and auditory-visual testing may also serve as a valuable demonstration for those hearing-impaired persons who doubt the value of lip reading. The response made by many hearing-impaired persons to the suggestion that they should attend to visual as well as auditory cues is 'It's no use, I can't lip read'. Questioning usually reveals that this judgement is based on an unrealistic experience such as turning off the television sound and being unable to understand what is being said. A comparison of scores obtained auditory alone and auditory-visually usually results in superior performance in the bisensory condition especially if the test materials are presented in noise. This improvement can be used to highlight the value of lip reading as a supplement rather than a substitute for audition.

This chapter presents an overview of visual and auditory-visual research conducted at the National Acoustic Laboratories (NAL) over the past decade. Although the tests described were developed specifically for use in Australia they could be adapted quite easily for other dialects as this would involve only minor changes in idiomatic expression. Obviously, the filmed version of the tests described would be unsuitable for use in countries other than Australia as the speaker used is a native speaker of Australian English. This problem can be easily overcome, however, by recording the adapted materials using a speaker with an appropriate dialect.

Another factor which should be noted is that the tests described in this chapter were designed for use with adventitiously hearing-impaired adults. Although some of the materials may be suitable for use with congenitally hearing-impaired children and adults, care should be taken in using the tests with this group. A number of tests have been specifically developed for use with congenitally hearing-impaired children. These include the Monash Diagnostic Test of Lip Reading Ability (Perry, 1979) and the Craig Lip Reading Inventory (Craig, 1964). Rosen and Corcoran (1982) have also reported on the use of the BKB Sentence Lists (Bench and Bamford, 1979) as a lip reading test. These materials were based on a language sample taken from 263 hearing-impaired children aged from 8 to 15 years. It is suggested that these materials may be more suitable for testing congenitally hearing-impaired subjects than the tests described in the chapter.

Review of Visual and Auditory-Visual Tests

The first filmed test of lip reading ability was developed by the pioneering lip reading teacher Edward B. Nitchie in 1913. The test consisted of 3 proverbs — 'Tis love that makes the world go round', 'Spare the rod and spoil the child' and 'Fine feathers make fine birds' (O'Neill and Oyer, 1981). Unfortunately, it is not known if the test was ever used to assess the lip reading skills of hearing-impaired subjects. This test does appear, however, to have had a number of obvious deficiencies. The use of such highly predictable and familiar material means that subjects would only have to detect one or two words in order to guess the rest of the sentence. The sentences used do not reflect normal conversational speech. A final criticism which can be made is that the test consisted of an excessively small number of items. Conklin (1917) attempted to devise a test which provided a detailed analysis of lip reading abilities. The test, which was presented face-to-face, assessed the subject's ability to perceive consonant, word and sentence materials (O'Neill and Oyer, 1981).

Day, Fusfeld and Pintner (1928) administered two lip reading tests consisting of 4 lists of 10 sentences to 8,300 deaf children. The test materials were presented to the children by both an outside examiner and their class teachers. The results obtained provide an interesting insight into the abilities of hearing-impaired persons to lip read familiar speakers. The scores obtained when the children's teachers read the sentence were 50%–60% better than those obtained when the materials were presented by an outside examiner.

The 1940s saw the development of a number of lip reading tests designed specifically to assess the abilities of deaf children. Heider and Heider (1940) developed three filmed tests of lip reading consisting of words, nonsense syllables, sentences and stories. The test results obtained indicated that visual vowel recognition was related to overall lip reading skill and practice in vowel discrimination may lead to improvements in lip reading ability.

Mason (1943) described a test consisting of commonly occurring nouns which was designed for use with young hearing-impaired children. The final form of the test consisted of a closed-set response with the child asked to indicate which one of five possible alternatives had been presented as the stimuli. The best known and still most widely used lip reading test is that developed by Utley (1946). The test in its original form consisted of two equivalent forms each containing a word subtest, a sentence subtest and a story subtest. The test was standardized using 761 hearing-impaired persons ranging in age from 8 to 21 years and has become generally accepted as the most valid test of lip reading abilities. This is despite detailed criticism of the test made by DiCarlo and Kataja (1951) who claimed that the test was excessively difficult. They found that 50% of the material contributed only 3% to the scores obtained and was therefore non-functional. Jeffers (1967) believed that this excessive difficulty was, to a large part, related to the filmed version of the test. The speaker, 'an attractive, vivacious university co-ed, unaccustomed to speaking to the deaf or hard-of-hearing' (Utley, 1946) was criticized by DiCarlo and Kataja's (1951) subjects as being excessively difficult to lip read. As a result the test is now usually presented live-voice or via a filmed version using a more acceptable speaker. It should also be noted that only the sentence subtests are generally used.

Morkovin (1947) produced a series of films based on real life situations which were designed specifically for lip reading training. Despite this, one of the films 'The Family Dinner' has been used as a lip reading test. The film, which portrays 'a typical American family at dinner' (Lowell, 1974) was used by DiCarlo and Kataja (1951) in their analysis of the Utley Test. They asked their subjects 20 questions relating to the film's content and found a high correlation (0.77) between scores obtained for the Utley Test and the life situation film. 'The Family Dinner' was also used by Lowell (1957) to evaluate the Film Test of Lip Reading developed at the John Tracey Clinic in Los Angeles. This test consisted of two equivalent lists each containing 30 simple, unrelated sentences which were designed to reflect everyday usage. The scores obtained for the two tests resulted in a correlation coefficient of 0.89 (Lowell, 1974).

In all of the studies thus far described the test stimuli consisted, at least in part, of meaningful materials. The 1970s, however, saw a number of studies which concentrated on the visual perception of consonants. Binnie, Montgomery and Jackson (1974) developed a test consisting of 20 English consonants combined with the vowel /a/ to form CV syllables. The test consisted of 100 items with each consonant presented 5 times in a random order. The test was administered without sound to 36 normally hearing subjects. Analysis of the subjects' responses revealed that they were able to identify 5 visemic (visually distinctive) categories based on consonant place of articulation. Binnie *et al.* (1974) suggested that the test could be used to identify those individuals who were unable to detect the different visemic categories. These persons, they suggested, might derive benefit from lip reading training at the syllable level. Walden, Prosek, Montgomery, Scherr and Jones (1977) used a 400 item version of Binnie *et al.*'s (1974) test to evaluate the effects of training on visual consonant recognition. They found that the number of visemic categories their subjects could identify rose from 7 pre-training to 9 post-training.

Skamris (1974) developed a simple film test to assess the lip reading skills of deafened adults. The test consisted of Danish numerals, place names and a series of sentences about eating or meals. One major advantage of this test was the short time taken to administer it (3 minutes) and there appeared to be a good correlation between the subjects' scores obtained on the test and a rating made of their lip reading skills by therapists, family members and the subjects themselves.

The Manchester Speechreading Test (Markides, 1980) consists of two lists, each containing a word (33 CVC words) and a sentence subtest (25 unrelated sentences ranging in length from 2–6 words). Initial testing was conducted face-to-face and involved 340 subjects aged from 6–74 years. The results showed a rapid increase in scores from age 6 years to age 13–14 years at which point a performance plateau was reached. The scores for the adult subjects remained consistent across all age groups although there was a fall in scores for the oldest group (70+ years). The fall, however, was not statistically significant. A later study (Elphick, 1984) involved administering an expanded version of the test to a group of twenty 9-year old children using both live and recorded presentations. The study found no statistical difference between the two presentation modes with good test/retest reliability. The 1970s and 1980s have seen the development of a number of auditory-visual tests. The HELEN Test (Ludvigsen, 1974) was developed by an interdisciplinary group of Danish researchers in the early 1970s to test 'hearing handicapped persons' perception of speech in a manner which corresponds to the situation in everyday life' (Ludvigsen, 1974). It consists of 8 lists of 25 questions which were presented in a noise background. Each list involves a series of questions which may be divided into 5 broad categories:

1. Sentences with 'before/after' involving numbers, days or months e.g. 'What day comes before Friday?' 'What number comes after 24?'
2. Sentences with colours. e.g. 'What colour is red wine?'
3. Sentences with simple arithmetic computations e.g. 'What is 4 plus 2?', 'What is half of 2?'
4. Sentences with opposites. e.g. 'What is the opposite of hot?'
5. Miscellaneous question. e.g. 'What language is spoken in Sweden?', 'Which is bigger an elephant or a mouse?'

The sentences were designed to be relatively simple, require only a one-word answer and have only one possible correct response. Each of the 8 lists is identical in form with only the key words changed. In a pilot study conducted with the test, the materials were presented auditory alone and auditory-visually. Prior to administration of the test the signal-to-noise ratio (S/N) which resulted in a discrimination score of 50% or worse for the auditory alone condition was determined. The test was then presented auditory alone and auditory-visually with the signal-to-noise ratio held constant at the predetermined 50% point. The aim of the study was to try to specify the gain which resulted when vision supplemented audition. A pilot study (Ewertsen, 1974) conducted with 18 hard-of-hearing subjects resulted in improvements in scores ranging from 6–38% (mean = 23.4%) when the materials were presented auditory-visually. Ewertsen also reported that younger congenitally hard-of-hearing subjects evidenced more improvement in the auditory-visual condition than did older presbycusic subjects.

The QUAH Test (Jerger and Jerger, 1979) also represents an attempt to test subjects using 'a series of real-life listening situations'. The test consists of '25 questions or commands that require a specific motor response'. An answer sheet is provided for each question and this serves to provide some cues as to the task required of the subject. For example, one of the answer sheets has a circle drawn on it and the subject is asked to 'Draw another circle'. The sentences are presented in blocks of five auditory alone with a competing speech message and then the same questions are presented visually-alone but in a different order. The aim of the testing was to determine the subject's ability to understand speech in noise (normal hearers scored 90% at 0dBS/N) and to 'evaluate the possibility of performance deficits due to non-auditory variables'. An experimental study using these materials with 55 normally hearing subjects has been published (Jerger and Jerger, 1979) but unfortunately results obtained with hearing-impaired subjects have not been reported.

Walden, Schwartz, Montgomery and Prosek (1981) in a study investigating the effects of training on speech recognition reported on the use of a sentence test which was presented auditory-visually in noise. The test consisted of 38 sentences (100 key words) relating to a common theme — 'The United States Army's drill sergeant program' (Walden *et al.*, 1981). As the subjects of this study were either serving or had served in the US Army the topic was a familiar one. The subjects were required to repeat each sentence as it was presented and were scored on the percentage of key words correctly perceived. The intensity of the competing noise was individually set for each subject and was at the level where the subjects scored 40–50% correct for practice sentences presented auditory-visually.

A final set of test materials which are often used for auditory, visual and auditory-visual speech perception testing are the CID Everyday Sentence Lists (Davis and Silverman, 1970). Johnson (1976) for example, has reported on the use of the lists to measure the receptive communication abilities of students entering the National Technical Institute for the Deaf in Rochester, New York. Each list consists of 10 unrelated sentences containing 50 key words with the subject required to repeat each sentence as it is presented. Some care needs to be exercised in using these lists as a means of assessing auditory, visual and auditory-visual speech perception. Hinkle and Binnie (1979) in a study of test equivalence of 10 lists of the CID Sentences, found that although 'several groups of sentence tests were not statistically different on the basis of mean data. . . . standard deviations and correlations were not equal (and) equivalency was rejected'.

The NAL Lipreading Test

The NAL Lipreading Test (Plant and Macrae, 1981) was designed to assist therapists responsible for the rehabilitation of adults with acquired hearing losses to determine the basic lip reading skills of individual cases. It consists of two subtests which evaluate consonant recognition and sentence identification respectively. The consonant test enables the therapist to determine whether the hearing impaired person is able to group consonants into the appropriate visemic categories. Inspection of the results of this test will assist the therapist in deciding 'which particular visemic groups should be emphasized during training' (Shoop and Binnie, 1979). Although training in the recognition of individual phonemes is often dismissed as being inappropriate (see for example McCormick, 1979a), research by Walden and his associates (1981) indicates that training in consonant recognition can result in substantial improvements in the ability to recognize sentence materials. The sentence subtest presents materials which more closely replicate the realities of everyday communication. This subtest is designed to give the therapist a measure of an individual subject's ability to lip read in everyday life.

Factors Influencing Test Design

Presentation Means

An important consideration in the development of any speech perception is whether it should be presented 'live' or whether a recorded version should be used to ensure consistency of presentation. The use of live-voice testing does appear to have a number of advantages, the most obvious of which is that it does not require the use of play-back equipment. This is a potentially important factor as many clinics do not have access to video equipment. A second advantage of live-voice presentation is 'its greater fidelity to a three-dimensional real-life situation' (Elphick, 1984). This factor, however, does not appear to be of critical importance. A study by McCormick (1979b) comparing live and videotaped presentations of the same test materials concluded 'that there was strong evidence to support the hypothesis that the loss of the third dimension does not degrade lip reading scores if all other variables are carefully controlled'. The most important advantage of a filmed test is that it eliminates the problem of speaker differences. Martony (1974) found rather large variation between speakers presenting non-labial Swedish consonants and vowels as a lip reading test. The scores for individual speakers ranged from 19.8% to 33.3% with a mean score of 27.4%. A second study involving both vowel and consonant tests revealed significant differences between the speakers who had been found hardest and easiest to lip read in the first study. A second factor favouring recorded tests is that speakers cannot reasonably be expected to replicate their articulatory patterns across numerous present-ations of the same test. As Elphick (1984) has noted, 'rate of utterance, facial expression and movement of lips are but some of the variables which defeat exact repetition'. An additional problem is posed in attempting to present materials face-to-face without voice. This usually results in exaggerated, non-normal articulatory patterns. The possibility also exists that some auditory cues may be unintentionally provided. These problems are overcome by the use of a recorded test. The speaker can be encouraged to use normal voice and articulatory patterns and the audio signal removed during testing ses-sions. The factors outlined above prompted the decision to use a recorded version of the NAL Lipreading Test.

The Speaker

The problem of speaker variability has already been discussed and it was this fact that determined the use of the same speaker in all visual and auditory-visual studies conducted. The speaker chosen was a female audiologist in her late twenties who uses the General variety of Australian English. This repre-sents 'the form of English most characteristic of the Australian people . . . its use is widespread and to be found among all occupational groups' (Mitchell and Delbridge, 1965). There is some limited evidence available which indi-cates that one variety of Australian English — Cultivated — may be easier to lip read. Bernard (1970) in a cine-X-ray study of the vowels and diphthongs of Australian English found that speakers of Broad Australian English 'show smaller average maximum lip and teeth apertures than the General subjects and these show smaller average maximum lip and teeth apertures than Cultivated subjects'. The Cultivated variety of Australian English, however, is used by a relatively small number of speakers. Mitchell and Delbridge (1965) for example analysed the speech of 9,000 secondary students aged from 16–18 years and found that only 11% used Cultivated Australian English compared to 34% for the Broad variety and 55% for General Australian English.

A second major consideration in the selection of the speaker was that the person chosen should not be involved in any of the rehabilitative activities being undertaken at NAL at the time the test was developed. This was extremely important as it was intended to use the lip reading test as a means of evaluating training procedures adopted with adventitiously hearing-impaired adults. The previously cited study of Day, Fusfeld and Pintner (1928) found that familiar speakers are easier to lip read than unfamiliar speakers. A common concern of persons working with hearing-impaired adults is that the skills being developed may be specific to a particular speaker — the therapist — rather than generalizable to all speakers. The use of an unfamiliar speaker offers the opportunity to determine whether the skills acquired during training are being transferred to other communication situations and speakers.

Test Materials

The major aim in the design of the test was to develop a means of assessing hearing-impaired adults to determine whether individual cases need rehabilitative services and if so the type and extent of the programme provided. This aim motivated the development of a test which included a consonant identification test and a sentence test.

Consonant Subtest

The consonant subtest consists of the 20 English consonants /p, b, m, t, d, n, k, g, f, v, θ, ð, s, ʃ, dʒ, tʃ, w, r, j, l, / combined with the vowel /a/ to form 20 CV syllables, for example /pa/, /ba/ and /ma/. The syllables are presented in 5 lists which are identical in all but order of presentation of the individual consonants. Each syllable is preceded by the carrier phrase 'Please say . . .', with the subject's task being to repeat the syllable presented.

Sentence Subtest

Although a number of lip reading tests utilizing sentence materials were available at the time the test was developed, it was felt necessary to design a new list. Several factors determined the form of the test sentences eventually adopted. The use of the Utley Test sentences was considered but eventually rejected for a number of reasons. The criticisms of Di Carlo and Kataja (1951) have been cited but there are other factors which make the test unsuitable for use in Australian conditions.

Firstly the test was designed in the mid-1940s and consequently contains many idiomatic expressions which are outmoded and/or American in origin. Another major problem with the Utley Test and almost all others considered is that the sentences in the test lists are not related to each other. Thus for example the sentence 'I don't know if I can' in the Utley Test is followed by 'How tall are you?' This is a highly artificial situation which in no way reflects the reality of everyday speech which consists of related materials with a high degree of contextual redundancy. A further problem with the majority of available tests was the form of response expected from the subject — to repeat what had just been said. This is very rare in everyday conversation unless the receiver is attempting to verify what was said — 'Did you say . . . ?' The HELEN Test offers a solution to this problem through the use of questions while the QUAH test requires the subject to perform a motor task. These represent far more realistic responses but both tests suffer the disadvantage of using unrelated sentences. A final factor was the need to determine the scoring method to be adopted. The Utley Test, for example, utilizes a system whereby the subject receives credit for every word correctly perceived. This scoring method has one serious disadvantage in that it can lead to scores which in no way reflect understanding. An extreme example of this is that a subject responding to the test sentence 'We drove to the country' with 'We . . . to the . . .' receives as much credit as one who responds with 'We drove . . . country'.

A second, perhaps preferable means of scoring the Utley Test was developed by Northwestern University Audiology Clinic. 'In this method the number of sentences correct is recorded. A sentence is scored correct if the content is perceived with reasonable accuracy' (Jeffers and Barley, 1971). This is obviously a more realistic form of scoring but it does not overcome the previously stated objections to the Utley Test — idiom, non-related materials and the response expected from the subject.

The scoring methods for the HELEN and QUAH Test appear to be the most acceptable. In both cases there is only one possible correct response. This eliminates the need for the clinician to make any judgement as to whether the response meets criterion.

These factors determined to a large extent the form of the sentence subtest of the NAL Lipreading Test. The test consists of 50 questions (see Appendix) most of which can be answered with one word. The questions are divided into the following five categories:

1. Some questions about you. (What's your name?)
2. Questions about your relatives. (What was your mother's maiden name?)
3. Questions about where you live. (What's the name of your street?)
4. Questions about things you like. (Who's your favourite author?)
5. Questions with easy answers. (What is the opposite of happy?)

The questions within each category are related and the subject is informed of the category of each group of questions prior to presentation. The sentences were designed to reflect normal colloquial usage and range in length from 3 to 11 syllables with a mean length of 6.6 syllables. It was initially intended that the test subjects would answer the test questions, but this would have created difficulties in determining the correct response without biasing future present-tations of the test. For this reason the test subjects were asked to repeat each sentence as it was presented and their responses were recorded by the experimenter. Responses were scored as correct if they contained sufficient information to ensure that the subject could have answered the questions correctly. For example the response 'What was my mother's name before she was married?' for the test sentence 'What was your mother's maiden name?' would be scored correct. One point was given for each sentence correctly understood.

The recorded sentences were transcribed by two experienced users of the International Phonetic Association symbols. The frequency of occurrence of individual phonemes was calculated and the results are presented in Table I.

Consonants account for 59% of phoneme occurrences with vowels and diphthongs contributing 41% (vowels 35%, diphthongs 6%). The ten most frequently used phonemes were /ɔ, t, w, j, n, ɒ, s, u, l. z, m/. Mines, Hanson and Shoup (1978) in a study of conversational American English found that /ɔ, n. t, l, s, r, i, k, d, ɛ/ were the ten most frequently occurring phonemes and accounted for 47% of the data. The major differences between the sentence test results and those of Mines *et al.*, is the relatively high occurrence of /w, j, d/ in the sentence test. This can be accounted for by the type of sentence used in the test. Interrogative sentences (questions) are used and as a consequence there is a high occurrence of the words 'what', 'when', 'where' and 'which'. The personal nature of the questions accounts for the large number of /j/ occurrences. 'You' occurs 19 times and 'your' occurs 16 times and these two words account for all the occurrences of /j/.

Consonants (initial & final)		Consonantal blends	
Stops		/tr/	1
/p/	5	/dr/	—
/b/	18	/pl/	2
/t/	49	/kr/	2
/d/	30	/br/	1
/k/	20	/st/	2
/g/	5	/str/	1
		/fl/	1
Nasals		/pr/	3
/m/	31	/gr/	1
/n/	35	/tw/	1
/ŋ/	3	/fr/	1
		Vowels & Diphthongs	
Fricatives		/i/	19
/f/	13	/I/	32
/v/	22	/ɛ/	13
/θ/	4	/æ/	15
/ð/	10	/ɒ/	34
/s/	33	/ɔ/	29
/z/	31	/u/	32
/h/	23	/ʊ/	—
/ʃ/	3	/ʌ/	22
		/ɜ/	8
Affricatives		/ə/	63
/tʃ/	5	/a/	8
/dʒ/	4	/eI/	19
		/oʊ/	8
Semi-Vowels		/aI/	5
/r/	11	/aʊ/	11
/y/	35	/ɔI/	2
/w/	37	/Iə/	—
		/ɛə/	1
Lateral			
/l/	19		

Table I Frequency of occurrence of consonants, vowels and diphthongs for the sentence test

Further analysis of the data revealed strong similarities with that reported by Mines *et al.* (1978). Of the 463 consonant occurrences in the sentence test 34% were unvoiced and 66% were voiced. Mines *et al.* found that 65% of consonants in their study were voiced. Further analysis of the consonants revealed that stops accounted for 27% of all occurrences in the sentence test consonant 22% and nasals 15%. Mines *et al.* report 29%, 19% and 18% respectively. They further report that the vast majority of consonants are articulated at the front of the mouth with dental and alveolar sounds (61%) and labial and labiodental sounds (22%) contributing over 80% of consonant occurrences. The frequency of occurrence for these places of articulation in the sentence test are 56% (dentals and alveolars) and 19% (labials and labiodentals). Mines, *et al.* (1978) found that almost three-quarters (72%) of the vowels were articulated near the front of the mouth. In the current study 56% of the vowels were fronted or centred. The phonemic analysis of the test would seem to indicate that it is fairly representative of conversational English. The major difference in the relative occurrence of phonemes in the sentences and that reported by Mines *et al.* (1978) can be attributed to the use of interrogative sentences.

Test Standardization

The two subtests which make up the NAL Lipreading Test were developed and tested over a period of 5 years. Work on the consonant subtest was conducted during 1976–77 (Plant and Macrae, 1977) while the development and standardization of the sentence subtest occupied the period 1978–80 (Plant and Macrae, 1981; Plant, Macrae and Pearce, 1980).

Administration

The two subtests were administered without sound with the subject seated 1.8 metres (6 feet) from the television monitor. In the case of the consonant test the subjects were told that they would see 20 consonants combined with the vowel /a/ and they were asked to repeat what they thought had been said. To ensure subject familiarity with the material, a practice test containing all 20 consonants was presented auditory-visually prior to administration of the test. The five tests were then presented without sound and the subject's responses were recorded by one of the experimenters who was seated in the test room with the subject. The subjects were instructed that they must give a response for every item presented.

Prior to administration of the sentence test the subjects were given the following instructions:

> You are about to see a lip reading test. The test consists of a number of
> questions about you, your family, where you live, things that you like

plus a number of questions with easy answers. Don't answer the questions but tell me what you think the speaker said. Do you understand?

The subjects were encouraged to attempt to repeat every question even if their response appeared nonsensical. The subjects' responses were recorded by one of the experimenters who was seated in the test room with the subject.

Subjects

The five lists of the consonant subtest were presented to 30 subjects ranging in age from 18 to 50 years. No attempt was made to determine the audiometeric thresholds of this group although it was known that some of the older subjects had marked high frequency hearing losses. The sentence subtest was administered to 100 adult subjects (49 males, 51 females) all of whom spoke English as their first language. Of these 70 had normal or near normal hearing and 30 were hearing-impaired. The test was also administered to 24 normal-hearing subjects (12 males, 12 females) who spoke Engish as a second language and had learned it after the age of 8 years.

Recordings

The consonant test was recorded on black and white videotape and the sentence test was recorded in both black and white, and colour. The monochrome versions of the test were designed for use in situations necessitating the use of portable equipment as the colour equipment used at this time could not be easily or safely transported. McCormick (1979b) has reported that 'a life-sized black and white television picture does not degrade the visibility of speech movements compared to a colour picture of the same dimensions'. The monochrome version was made with a Sony Video Tape Recorder (Model AV3670CE) using a Sony Camera (Model AVC3250CI). The colour recording was made using a Sony Videocassette Recorder (Model VD2850P) with a Sony Television Camera (Model DXC1200P). In both recordings the speaker's image was approximately life-size on the television monitor. Frontal lighting was used during the recordings to ensure maximum illumination of the speaker's face and articulators.

Results

Consonant Subtest

The subjects' responses for the consonant subtest were analyzed using a Wang 2200 B computer which produced a detailed confusion matrix showing the percentage correct for each consonant and the direction of error responses. Examination of the confusion matrix revealed 7 distinct confusion clusters which can be classified as:

1. Bilabials /p.b.m/
2. Labiodentals /f.v./
3. Interdentals /ɵ, ð/
4. Rounded labials /w, r/
5. Alveolar continuants and velar stops /l, n, j, g, k/
6. Post alveolars /dʒ, tʃ, ʃ/
7. Alveolar fricative and stops /s, d, t/

These results indicate that the subjects were able to differentiate between the various places of articulation. With the notable exception of the alveolar consonants, however, the subjects were unable to differentiate manner of articulation within the various place of articulation categories. The subjects were also unable to differentiate between voiced and voiceless consonants sharing the same place of articulation. The mean percentage correct for the experimental subjects was 37.3 (range 30–46) and it would appear that this is near the upper limits of performance. When it is considered that such features as nasality and voicing are not visible, it is unreasonable to expect much improvement through lip reading alone. The exception to this is found with the rounded labials /w, r/. It appears that with training, these two consonants may be discriminable.

An interesting feature of the results was that within each confusion cluster there was a distinct preference for one of the consonants. For example, within the bilabial group /p, b, m/ there was a tendency to respond /ba/ for presentations of /pa/, /ba/ and /ma/. Within each category there was a similar trend. For the labio-dentals, 88% of reponses were for /f/; for the alveolars and palatals 85% of responses were for /l/; for the alveolars 54% for /s/; for the post alveolars 45% for /dʒ/; and for the rounded labials 85% of responses were for /w/. Only within the interdental group was such a trend not found.

Explanations for this phenomenon are difficult to find. At first it was assumed that it was related to the relative frequency of occurrence of the phonemes in the language, but Mines *et al.* (1978) found that the most commonly occurring consonants are /n, t, s, r, l. d/. Although there was preference for /s/ and /l/ in the test results, the other consonants were not identified to the degree expected if frequency of occurrence was the determining factor. A similar trend has been found in Danish (Skamris, 1977).

Sentence Subtest

The sentence subtest was initially administered to thirty normal-hearing subjects who spoke English as their first language. The mean score for this group was 39.7% (S.D. = 17.5%) with scores ranging from 2–76%. The test was then administered to twenty hearing-impaired persons attending lip reading lessons at the Australian Association for Better Hearing. The mean score for this group was 39.1% (S.D. = 25.6%) with scores ranging from 0–88%. The difference between the scores obtained by the two groups was not statistically significant.

In an attempt to validate the sentence test, the lip reading teachers at the Australian Association for Better Hearing were asked to rate their pupils on a 5-point scale devised by Skamris (1974). At the time of this rating, the teachers were not aware of the scores obtained by their pupils on the sentence test. In order to compare the scores with the rating the scores were ranked on a 5-point scale as follows: 0–20% = Rank 1, 21–40% = Rank 2, 41–60% = Rank 3, 61–80% = Rank 4 and 81–100% = Rank 5. The rank difference correlation coefficient between the score ranks and the ratings was then calculated and found to be 0.865, which indicates that level of performance on the test is a valid measure of a person's lipreading ability.

The sentence subtest has been presented to 100 persons — both normal-hearing and hearing-impaired — who speak English as a first language. The mean score for this group is 38.9% (S.D. = 20.8%) with a range of scores of 0–88%. Means were also calculated separately for the male and female subjects and were found to be 33.6% and 43.9% respectively. When a t-test was used, the differences between the means for the male and female subjects was found to be significant at about the 0.02 level. The mean score for the group of 24 normal-hearing persons who had learned English as a second language was 15% with scores ranging from 2–38%. The difference between the mean score of this group and that of the subjects who spoke English as a first language was statistically significant. It was hypothesized that this poor performance resulted from the lip readers' relatively poor knowledge of the English language. Much of the lip read signal is ambiguous or invisible and the lipreader has to use his/her language knowledge to supply the missing elements in the lip read pattern. Persons lacking an intimate knowledge of the rules and structure of the language find it difficult to insert the elements necessary to ensure understanding.

Practice Effects on the Sentence Subtest

In order to investigate any possible practice effects which might arise with repeated presentations of the sentence materials, the sentence subtest was administered to 30 normal-hearing subjects and readministered approximately one month later. The mean scores of the group were 39.8% for the first presentation and 46.5% for the second. Using a t-test, the difference between the means was found to be significant at the 0.01 level. If the test is repeated, for example when presented before and after lip reading training in order to evaluate any improvement due to the training, it must be realized that an improvement of about 7% is to be expected purely as a result of the retesting

193

of the subject. For an improvement to be significantly greater than that expected on the basis of practice, a score on the retest 25% or more better than the score on the first test would have to be obtained.

It is possible however, to avoid the influence of the practice effect. In order to discover how many presentations were required before no further improvements occurred in performance, the test was presented three times, at weekly intervals, to 25 additional subjects. The mean scores for the three presentations were 33·2%, 44·0% and 45·9%. An analysis of variance was carried out and it was found that a difference of 3% would be required between the means in order to be significant at the 0·01 level. The performance on the third presentation was therefore not significantly better than that on the second. This indicates that no further improvement can be expected after the second presentation purely on the basis of practice. If the test is used as a measure of improvement due to training it should be administered twice before training commences and readministered at the completion of the training period. If this procedure is followed then improvements equal to or greater than those given in Table II are required in order to be significant.

Score	Sig. change	Score	Sig. change
0	2	50	12
2	4	52	12
4	6	54	12
6	6	56	12
8	8	58	12
10	8	60	12
12	8	62	12
14	10	64	12
16	10	66	12
18	10	68	12
20	10	70	12
22	10	72	12
24	12	74	12
26	12	76	12
28	12	78	10
30	12	80	10
32	12	82	10
34	12	84	10
36	12	86	10
38	12	88	8
40	12	90	8
42	12	92	8
44	12	94	6
46	12	96	6
48	12	98	4
50	12	100	2

Table II Significant change in score on the third presentation of the sentence test, as a function of the score on the second presentation of the sentence test.

Distribution of Scores on the Sentence Subtest

In order to provide a means of assessing an individual's performance on the sentence test the centile distribution of the scores of the 100 subjects in the reference group was calculated. This is presented in Table III. A subject's score for the test can be compared with this Table to give an idea of the individual's performance level. Fifty percent of the reference group obtained a score of 40% or better; it therefore follows that an individual who obtains a score of 40% has obtained an average score. On the other hand, an individual who scores 90% has done better than anyone in the reference group and has performed outstandingly.

Score	Centile	Score	Centile
0	100	46	39
2	98	48	36
4	97	50	32
6	95	52	29
8	93	54	26
10	91	56	23
12	88	58	20
14	86	60	17
16	83	62	15
18	81	64	13
20	78	66	11
22	76	68	9
24	73	70	7
26	71	72	6
28	68	74	5
30	65	76	4
32	63	78	3
34	60	80	3
36	56	82	2
38	53	84	1
40	50	86	1
42	47	88	1
44	43	90	0

Table III Centile distribution of scores on the sentence test.
(Centile = percentage of group obtaining given score or better)

Use of the NAL Lipreading Test in a Rehabilitative Programme

The results obtained from the two subtests of the NAL Lipreading Test can be invaluable in planning rehabilitative strategies for individual subjects. The consonant subtest provides a means of determining whether the subject is able to group consonants into the appropriate visemic categories. Some care needs to be exercised at this point. The 7 visemic categories found in our study should be regarded as being speaker-specific unless proven otherwise.

This view is also supported by the results of Martony's (1974) study. If a new recording of the subtest is made using a different speaker, a preliminary study would need to be conducted to determine the consonant visemic groups for that particular speaker. It is probable that the labial groups will be constant across almost all speakers. Differences may be found, however, in the visibility of the non-labial consonants. Once the groups have been determined for the speaker the test can be used as a means of assessing subjects prior to training. Most subjects are able to categorize the consonants correctly without training but there will be some persons who will experience difficulty at this level. For these it may be necessary to provide training at the level of consonant recognition. Such an approach is supported by the results obtained by Walden *et al.* (1977, 1981).

Performance with the sentence subtest also offers interesting insights into subject performance. If the standardized recording of the test is used, the subjects' overall score can be used to provide an estimate of performance relative to the results obtained with the 100 reference subjects. If a new recording is made with another speaker, however, testing would again be necessary to determine the range of performance. Additional information can also be obtained by examination of a subject's performance for the various categories of the sentence test. The categories have been ordered so that they become progressively more difficult as the test proceeds. The initial 27 sentences are related to 3 specific topics and are as a result, more predictable than the final 23 'questions about things you like' and 'questions with easy answers'. The subject's ability to use contextual cues can be assessed to an extent by comparing performance for the more predictable categories 1–3 with the scores obtained for categories 4 and 5. The sentences in category 5 represent the most difficult task as they are unrelated questions. Many subjects will find the first 3 categories relatively easy but will experience difficulty with categories 4 and 5. Such subjects would appear to be able to use contextual cues to assist lip reading performance and training procedures which provide practice in the recognition of less predictable materials may be of greatest assistance. Conversely the subject who scores poorly on all sections of the test should be provided initially with materials with a high degree of predictability and as performance improves more difficult materials should be introduced.

Auditory–Visual Testing

Auditory–visual testing offers the clinician the opportunity to evaluate a hearing-impaired person's speech perception skills in a manner which most closely replicates everyday communication situations. A comparison of the person's performance when materials are presented visual alone, auditory alone and combined auditory–visual can help determine the relative contribution to speech perception of the various sensory modalities and assist in planning training procedures. Materials used in auditory–visual research at NAL have included nonsense syllables, an English translation of 4 lists of the Helen Test and Kallikow *et al.*'s (1977) SPIN Test. Subjects in these studies have included totally deaf young adults using vibrotactile supplements to lipreading, normal-hearing adults and a group of elderly mild-to-moderately hearing impaired persons.

Consonant Perception

Nonsense syllable tests presenting consonants in fixed vowel environments have been used extensively in research studies to determine the relative contribution of the various sensory modalities and their combinations. Erber (1972), for example, presented the consonants /p, t, k, b, d, g, m, n/ in an /a–a/ frame to groups of normal-hearing, severely hearing-impaired and deaf children. In the visual alone condition the normal-hearing, severely hearing-impaired and profoundly deaf groups scored 31·61%, 49·17% and 45·17% respectively. In all cases the subjects were able to recognize consonant place of articulation but were unable to determine whether the consonants were voiced or voiceless or stops or nasals.

Scores for auditory-alone. recognition for the 3 groups were 99·67%, 50·38% and 21·11% respectively. The severely hearing-impaired group were able to accurately identify voicing and nasality but were unable to detect place of articulation. The responses of the profoundly deaf group were essentially random. In the auditory–visual condition the subject groups scored 99·78%, 88% and 60·5% respectively. The severely hearing-impaired group were able to fuse the information available via audition and vision resulting in a very high performance level. The deaf subjects also evidenced improved performance, albeit to a lesser extent, in the auditory–visual mode. Examinations of the subjects' responses indicated that they were able to perceive some voicing and nasality cues.

Research projects conducted at NAL utilizing consonant recognition tasks have been concerned with evaluating the effectiveness of vibrotactile lipreading supplements. Plant (1986) presented the consonants /p, b, m, t, d, n, k, g, f, v, s, z, ʃ, h, dʒ, tʃ, w, r, l. j/ in an /a–a/ frame via lip reading alone and lip reading supplemented by a vibrotactile aid presenting voicing information and a cue to signal the presence of high frequency consonants. The consonants were administered in lists consisting of 40 test items with each of the consonants presented twice in a random order. Eight testing sessions were conducted using these materials. In each session one list was presented for lip reading alone and one list for lip reading plus the tactile aid. The materials were presented live-voice with the order of presentation and lists used varied from session-to-session. The results obtained by 4 deaf subjects for this task showed that aided performance exceeded that obtained when the materials were presented via lip reading alone. Confusion matrices were drawn up and used to gain a detailed description of the subject's ability to perceive consonantal features. The results of this analysis are presented in Table IV. It can be seen that the vibrotactile aid provides information assisting in the recognition of consonant voicing and manner of articulation especially in the identification of stops, sibilants and nasals. For 3 of the 4 subjects there were also improvements in the aided condition in the perception of the affricates and semi-vowels. The results obtained here highlight the value of analyzing the direction of error responses in consonant recognition tasks. Such analysis allows the clinicians to determine which consonant features have their recognition enhanced by the aid used and can assist greatly in planning remediation programmes and in the selection of appropriate aids.

Sentence Materials. Auditory–Visual Presentation in Quiet

The first auditory–visual test programme conducted at NAL used an English translation of the HELEN Test as the test material (Plant, Phillips and Tsembis, 1982). The aim of the project was to evaluate the communication skills of elderly hearing-impaired persons to determine how much benefit was gained when vision supplemented aided hearing. The use of such testing with the elderly was seen as being of great importance as a large number of studies have shown that the elderly experience more difficulty in auditory (Pestalozza and Shore, 1955; Jerger, 1973; Hayes and Jerger, 1979) and visual (Farrimond, 1959; Shoop, 1978; Shoop and Binnie, 1979) speech perception than younger subjects with comparable hearing losses. Little research has been conducted, however, into auditory–visual speech perception by the elderly. As a high percentage of NAL's case load consists of elderly persons with mild–moderate noise induced and/or age related sensorineural hearing losses, research into this area was needed to help determine the direction and content of future rehabilitative programmes.

Materials

An English translation of the first 4 lists of the HELEN Test was prepared and recorded on colour videotape using a Sony Video Tape Recorder (Model AV3670CE) with a Sony Camera (Model AVC3250CI). The recorded image approximated life size on a 48 cm video monitor and frontal illumination was used to ensure a well-lit picture of the speaker's face. The audio signal was recorded so that the most intense components of the speech signal peaked at 0 dB on the VU meter.

	1 L	1 LV	2 L	2 LV	3 L	3 LV	4 L	4 LV	Overall L	Overall LV
Overall	47.2%	60.9%	49.1%	66.7%	48.75%	74.7%	43.75%	69.7%	47.2%	68.0%
Voicing	67.5%	80.9%	71.9%	82.8%	72.2%	91.9%	68.4%	83.75%	70.0%	84.8%
Manner (overall)	65%	76.9%	68.75%	86.25%	71.6%	80.6%	66.6%	83.75%	68.0%	81.9%
Stops	63.5%	77.1%	58.3%	92.7%	80.2%	80.2%	74%	95.8%	69.01%	86.5%
Affricatives	50%	53.1%	28.1%	25%	40.6%	59.4%	9.4%	40.6%	32.0%	44.5%
Fricatives	100%	100%	100%	100%	100%	100%	100%	100%	100%	100%
Sibilants	29.2%	83.3%	79.2%	85.4%	66.7%	85.4%	52.1%	66.7%	56.8%	80.2%
Nasals	46.9%	53.1%	43.75%	84.4%	46.9%	53.1%	59.4%	81.25%	49.2%	68.0%
Semi-vowels	84.4%	78.1%	85.9%	98.4%	68.75%	87.5%	73.4%	89.1%	78.1%	88.3%
Place (overall)	90.6%	91.9%	90%	89.4%	95.6%	95.3%	82.5%	85.3%	89.7%	90.5%
Bilabials	100%	100%	100%	100%	100%	100%	100%	100%	100%	100%
Labio-dentals	100%	100%	100%	100%	100%	100%	100%	100%	100%	100%
Rounded labials	100%	100%	100%	100%	100%	100%	100%	100%	100%	100%
Alveolars	86.5%	92.7%	88.5%	92.7%	90.6%	95.8%	77.1%	82.3%	85.7%	90.9%
Post-alveolars	66.7%	62.5%	56.25%	43.75%	89.6%	79.2%	37.5%	52.1%	62.5%	59.4%
Palatal velars	97.9%	97.9%	100%	100%	100%	97.9%	91.7%	85.4%	97.4%	95.3%
Glottal	100%	100%	100%	100%	100%	100%	100%	100%	100%	100%

Table IV Scores obtained by 4 profoundly deaf subjects for a task involving discrimination of 20 consonants in an /a c a/ frame with lipreading alone (LA) and lipreading supplemented by a vibrotactile aid (LV)

Subjects

The test was presented to 48 subjects (27 males, 21 females) who had been fitted with hearing aids and were attending for follow-up appointments. The subjects ranged in age from 58–89 years with a mean age of 75.4 years. The average pure tone thresholds (500 Hz, 1 kHz and 2 kHz in the better ear) ranged from 8.5 to 81.5 dB HTL with a mean of 46.5 dB HTL.

Procedures

The test materials were presented with the subject seated 2 metres from the video monitor. The audio signal was presented at a level which was considered appropriate for the test room. This was arrived at by consultation among 3 normal-hearing audiologists.

The subjects were initially presented with one of the tests auditory-visually as a practice list. They were instructed to adjust their hearing aid/s to their preferred level and were given the option of either answering the questions or repeating what was said. The subjects were then presented with the remaining 3 lists auditory alone, visual alone and combined auditory-visual. The list order and method of presentation were varied for each of the subjects in an attempt to minimize possible test differences and/or order effects. The subject's responses were recorded by the examiner who was seated in the test room.

Results

The group means for the three methods of presentations were calculated and found to be: vision alone 17.1%, auditory alone 82.3%, and auditory–visual 90.8%. Two-way analysis of variance was used with replications across subjects and this indicated that the effect of method of presentation was significant at better than the 1% level while order effects were not significant. A contrast (F ratio for presentation effect variance and error variance) was performed between the auditory alone and the auditory-visual conditions and there were significant differences at better than the 1% significance level. Clearly the difference between the visual alone condition and the other two methods of presentations was also highly significant. Means were also calculated for each list for each method of presentation. Two-way analysis of variance revealed no significant differences between lists but again highly significant differences between conditions. Group means were calculated for the 3 presentation conditions with subjects divided into 5 year age categories. These showed a gradual decline in score for both the auditory and auditory–visual condition as a function of increasing age, but such a trend was not discernible for the visual alone condition. A Spearman's Rho correlation was performed comparing the subjects' ages and scores obtained for each of the three conditions. This showed an insignificant correlation of -0.1 for the visual alone condition but a significant correlation -0.3 (at better than the 5% confidence level) for both the auditory and auditory–visual conditions, i.e. the scores tended to worsen slightly as the subject's age increased.

The results obtained showed the value of auditory–visual speech perception for the elderly hearing impaired. In only 3 cases was the auditory–visual score lower than that obtained by audition alone and in all 3 instances the decline was of only one test item (5%). Of the remaining subjects, 14 had identical scores in both conditions and 31 had auditory–visual scores which were higher than those obtained through audition alone. The overall improvement for auditory–visual over auditory alone of 8.5% appeared however to be an overly pessimistic indicator of the value of vision supplementing audition. This was due to the high auditory alone score obtained by almost all of the subjects. In cases where the subjects scored less than 80% for the auditory alone condition there was a mean improvement of 18% in the auditory–visual mode. This indicated that where the auditory alone score was low enough to allow substantial improvement the auditory–visual gains over audition alone closely approximated the visual alone score.

This should not be taken as implying that audition and vision provide two independent channels of information, even though there are some speech features which the hearing impaired find easier to see than hear and vice versa. For example, it is impossible to discriminate between voiced and voiceless cognates by lip reading alone (Plant and Macrae, 1977), whereas the ability to recognize consonant place of articulation, which is an extremely difficult task for the hearing-impaired via audition alone is easily accomplished through vision. Rather, it is assumed that much of the same information is provided by the two sensory inputs, and that the resultant redundancy makes the perceptual task comparatively easier.

Auditory–Visual Presentation in Noise

In order to provide a more accurate measure of the communication skills of the elderly, it was necessary to modify the test procedure. This involved the addition of competing speech noise in the auditory and auditory–visual conditions.

Materials

The four sentence lists were re-recorded on black and white videotape using a Sony Video Recorder (AV3670CE) with a Sony Camera (AV3250CE). The lighting and image size were the same as those used in the first study. The speech signal was recorded on one of the audio tracks with the most intense components peaking at 0 dB Vu. Four speaker babble at −3 dB VU was recorded as the second audio channel.

Subjects

The revised test was administered to 12 subjects (6 males, 6 females) attending for follow-up after hearing aid fitting. The subjects ranged in age from 67–81 years with a mean age of 72.1 years. The mean average hearing loss for the subjects was 48.9 dB HTL with a range from 37–74 dB HTL.

Procedure

The materials were presented using the equipment described for the first study with the audio signal again at a level which was considered appropriate for the test room. The subjects were divided into two groups each of whom was presented with one list auditory–visually as a practice list and then the remaining three lists as one of the two following orders: auditory alone, visual alone, auditory–visually or auditory–visually, visual alone, auditory alone.

Results

The group means for the three presentation conditions were: auditory alone 31.25%, visual alone 39.2% and auditory–visual 81.7%. Two-way analysis of variance revealed no significant differences between the auditory alone and the visual alone conditions. The score for the auditory–visual condition, however, was significantly better than those obtained for the other two conditions.

The mean improvement of 50.45% (range 10–95%) for the auditory–visual condition over audition alone indicates that, although the auditory skills of the elderly may decline with increasing age this may be overcome to a large extent by auditory–visual speech perception. When the results obtained in the two studies are compared, it appears that presentation of the test in quiet may not be the most appropriate measure of receptive communication skills. The addition of an adverse signal-to-noise ratio probably represents a more realistic measure of an individual subject's speech perception skills. Many elderly hearing aid users report great benefit in quiet, but extreme difficulty when noise is present. It is interesting to note that the amount of benefit gained from auditory–visual perception rose as the average hearing loss of the subjects increased. Subjects with average hearing losses greater than 45 dB HTL had improvements in scores ranging from 40–95% over those obtained auditory alone, while those with average losses less than 45 dB HTL had improvements ranging from 10–55%. It could be argued, however, that this represents a ceiling effect and that the latter group would show greater improvements if their auditory-alone scores were lowered by a more difficult signal presentation condition.

Use of Auditory–Visual Test Results in a Rehabilitative Programme

Clinicians providing aural rehabilitation for hearing-impaired adults should find that an auditory–visual test procedure such as the HELEN Tests serves as a useful addition to the diagnostic battery administered prior to training. The administration of test lists in the three sensory conditions auditory alone, visual alone and combined auditory–visual enables the clinician to evaluate the relative contribution of the different sensory modalities. The results may also enable the clinician to make realistic predictions about the individual subject's future performance with a hearing aid. Those clients who score poorly in noise may benefit from a training programme and can also be counselled as to possible 'Hearing Tactics' which may alleviate the problem, at least to some extent. Realistic advice can also be given as to what to expect from the aid in adverse conditions. The results of testing can also help determine the complexity of materials initially adopted with those subjects who require training and the mode of presentations to be used. For example, subjects with poor auditory alone scores in noise may benefit initially from auditory training in quiet and gradually have noise introduced as they become more competent and confident at the task. Subjects with good auditory alone scores but only a small gain in the auditory–visual mode may benefit from bisensory training with a distorted auditory signal forcing them to attend more closely to the visual signal. This can be achieved through the use of auditory masking, low pass filtering (Plant, Macrae, Dillon and Pentecost, 1984), intensity gating (Montgomery, Walden, Schwartz, and Prosak, 1984) or by the extraction and presentation of one speech feature such as funda-mental frequency (Rosen, Fourcin and Moore, 1981; Plant *et al.*, 1984).

In administering testing in noise, consideration also needs to be given to the level of the competing signal. Wherever possible this should be adjusted individually for each subject. The use of a fixed S/N may result in conditions which are excessively difficult or easy for individual subjects. Walden *et al.* (1981) adjusted the level of speaker babble until their subjects scored 40–50% recognition of key words in sentences. A similar approach was adopted by the HELEN Test group (Ewertsen, 1974). If such an approach is not feasible and a fixed level is used, an S/N of +3 dB appears adequate for most elderly subjects. The use of this S/N with many younger subjects, however, would probably result in very high auditory alone scores. Testing would need to be carried out to specify a fixed level resulting in an acceptable auditory alone score for most young subjects. Finally, with many profoundly deaf subjects it may be unrealistic and unwise to attempt auditory and auditory–visual testing in noise. For such subjects the task may prove excessively difficult and result in extremely low scores. With these subjects, testing in quiet should be attempted initially with masking added if the scores obtained in quiet indicate that the subject is able to make good use of auditory information.

Conclusion

The tests and procedures outlined in this chapter have been developed as part of an attempt by NAL to introduce comprehensive aural rehabilitation programmes for hearing-impaired adults. The tests can be used to assess the communication skills of individual subjects, help determine whether training programmes should be initiated, provide useful information as to the appropriate level of complexity of training and help determine the effectiveness of the training provided. The tests presented represent one approach to the problem of effectively assessing the communication skills of the hearing-impaired and can form part of a comprehensive test battery for use in audiological clinics. Further tests and procedures need to be developed and implemented. A special problem which needs to be confronted is the development of tests which can more effectively and accurately provide information as to rehabilitative procedures to be adopted with individual hearing-impaired persons. Such tests would assist greatly in the provision of individualized appropriate training procedures.

Appendix

Questions About You
 1. What's your surname?
 2. What are your Christian names?
 3. How old are you?
 4. What's your date of birth?
 5. Where were you born?
 6. Are you married or single?
 7. When were you married?
 8. What's your job?
 9. How much do you weigh?
10. How tall are you?
11. What's the colour of your eyes?
12. What's your doctor's name?

Questions About Relatives
13. What is your father's Christian name?
14. What was your mother's maiden name?
15. How many brothers do you have?
16. How many sisters do you have?
17. How many children do you have?

Questions About Your Home
18. Which suburb do you live in?
19. What's the name of your street?
20. Do you live in a house or a flat?
21. What's the number of your house?
22. What's your telephone number?
23. How many bedrooms does your house have?
24. Do you have a gas or an electric stove?
25. Where do you go shopping?
26. How do you get to the shops?
27. Do you have milk delivered?

Questions About Things That You Like
28. What's your favourite colour?
29. Do you prefer tea or coffee?
30. Which TV programme do you like the best?
31. Who's your favourite author?
32. Do you prefer butter or margarine?
33. What sort of pet do you have?
34. What's your favourite hobby?

Some Questions with Easy Answers
35. What's the time?
36. What day is it?
37. What colour are your shoes?
38. What month comes after August?
39. What colour is coal?
40. What month is it now?
41. What is four plus six?
42. What number comes before 26?
43. Is Peter a boy's name or a girl's name?
44. What is half of six?
45. What day comes before Friday?
46. What language is spoken in France?
47. Is Jane a boy's name or a girl's name?
48. What is five plus three?
49. What colour is milk?
50. What is the opposite of happy?

Chapter 11

Speech Audiometry in the USA

B. Kruger and R. M. Mazor

The purpose of this chapter is to review the present status of speech audiometry in the United States of America. Current clinical practices are discussed and some limitations of these practices are suggested. Both the application of speech audiometry techniques to rehabilitation, and some research trends are summarized.

Speech audiometry provides a means of assessing communication ability: the ability to understand speech. A primary use of speech audiometry in the USA is as an integral component of the differential diagnosis of hearing impairment. Speech audiometry, as it is commonly practiced, refers to obtaining a 'speech reception threshold' and a 'speech discrimination score'. As part of the basic audiologic evaluation it plays an important part in distinguishing conductive hearing losses from sensorineural or mixed losses. These and other speech tests are also used for differential diagnosis of retrocochlear involvement, central auditory nervous system involvement, and functional hearing loss or pseudohypacusis. A secondary use has been in the selection and fitting of hearing aids. More recent applications of speech audiometry are in the prognostic and rehabilitative evaluation of communication ability and handicap, and in communication training.

Terminology

The terminology used in speech audiometry is imprecise and is often quite confusing. For example, the term 'speech threshold' has different meanings to different clinicians and researchers. Is it a speech reception threshold, a spondee threshold, a word detection threshold or a word recognition threshold? For the purposes of clarity in this chapter, we will define the following terms: psychometric function, performance-intensity function, articulation, articulation index, threshold, detection, recognition, intelligibility, and discrimination. These definitions are discussed in order to clarify the terminology currently used in speech audiometry.

A *psychometric function* describes the relation between some measure of performance and a stimulus dimension. For example, a psychometric function might describe the detection of a pure tone in noise. In the case of speech audiometry, a psychometric function might display the percent correct identification of the speech stimulus as a function of its intensity. This is sometimes called a *performance-intensity function*. Figure 1 illustrates the psychometric functions for recognition of 36 spondees (a); 50 monosyllables (b, c, d, f); and synthetic sentences (e). The average slope of the function for CID W-1 spondees is 10% per decibel (dB) over the range 20–80%. The average slope for CID W-22 monosyllables is 4% per decibel, not as steep as the slope for spondees. Generally, a steeper psychometric function results when the task is simpler, the stimuli are more familiar or more homogeneous, or the subject is more experienced. Although the average psychometric function should best predict the slope of an individual subject's psychometric function and, therefore, predict a subject's performance at a given level, it is important to remember that an individual's psychometric function differs from the average function.

The performance-intensity function is currently used to describe what was previously called the *articulation-gain function*. This function is simply a psychometric function which describes per cent correct word recognition or identification as a function of intensity. *Articulation*, as it is used today, refers

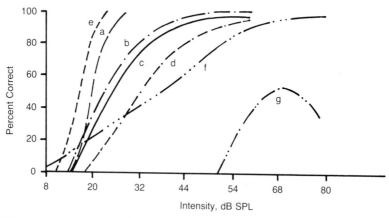

Figure 1.   Performance-Intensity functions for a variety of speech stimuli. Modified from Wilson and Margolis (1983) and Olsen and Matkin (1979).
a   CID W-1 36 spondees
b   CID W-22
c   NU 6
d   PAL PB-50
e   SSI (closed-set)
f   CCT (closed-set)
g   CID W-22 – Sensorineural Listeners

to speech production. The only exception is the *Articulation Index* where articulation refers to the relative prediction of intelligibility under a wide range of listening situations (French and Steinberg, 1947; Kryter, 1962a, b).

Threshold is that statistical point on a psychometric function which specifies the intensity level (in dB) at which a patient correctly identifies the stimulus a predetermined percentage of the time. This percentage (probability of responses) is between chance performance and perfect performance. For example, one might select 50%, or 75% correct stimulus identification to define the threshold.

Threshold performance clearly differs with the type of response required by a particular test. A threshold based on *detection* requires a judgement of stimulus presence or absence. This is called a *detection threshold*. The subject's familiarity with the stimulus often lowers (improves) the threshold. A threshold based on *recognition* requires a judgement made not only on stimulus presence or absence, but also on correct stimulus identification from a set (open or closed) of possible stimuli. This is called a *recognition threshold*. Recognition is a more difficult task than detection. Therefore, recognition thresholds are higher (poorer), that is, they require more energy than detection thresholds. Recognition is not only a threshold measure. A recognition judgement may be made at suprathreshold levels, e.g., 'speech discrimination testing' as well as at threshold, e.g., 'speech reception threshold'.

The American Speech-Language-Hearing Association (ASHA) *Guidelines for Determining the Threshold Level for Speech* (1979) define 'speech threshold audiometry' as 'a procedure for measuring an individual's intelligibility for speech material'. The *speech threshold* is the hearing level (dB HL) at which at least 50% of the test material is correctly identified. The recommended practice is to specify the speech material used, e.g. *spondee threshold* (ST) if the standard test materials — spondaic words (two-syllable equal-emphasis words) are used. However, the term still most often used to describe a spondee threshold is a *speech reception threshold* ('SRT'). The term speech reception threshold originally referred to the intelligibility of sentences (Hughson and Thompson, 1942), and has evolved to refer to threshold for a non-specified speech stimulus. Spondee threshold is more precise, but is not yet accepted as the most common usage.

More important, the problem with using the term speech reception threshold is that it does not accurately describe the performance required of the patient. The ST task requires that the speech stimulus (spondees) must be heard, *recognized* and repeated, although not necessarily understood. The more appropriate general term recommended for a speech threshold is *speech recognition threshold*, SRT (Feldmann, 1960; Bilger and Wang, 1976; Olsen and Matkin, 1979; Wilson and Margolis, 1983). Throughout this chapter *SRT* is used as the abbreviation for speech recognition threshold, and not for speech reception threshold.

A *speech detection threshold* (SDT) describes the level at which the presence of a speech signal is identified 50% of the time. Although the term *speech awareness threshold* (SAT) is used interchangeably with SDT, speech detection threshold is recommended, since speech awareness suggests the psychological preparedness of the listener while SDT is task specific.

Intelligibility is a term used to describe how well speech is understood. It originally referred to how well speech was transmitted over a communication system and thus was understood by an observer. It has also come to mean how well everyday-speech or other speech materials are understood by a listener whose hearing may or may not be impaired. Intelligibility is most often described by an individual's performance on a word recognition task, i.e. the percentage of words correctly recognized at a particular intensity level. Therefore, the terms intelligibility and recognition are used interchangeably. Recognition does not necessarily imply understanding. To make matters worse, *discrimination* has incorrectly been used as a synonym for both *intelligibility* and *recognition* to describe suprathreshold word recognition ability. Audiologists in the United States continue to refer to this recognition task as 'word discrimination' or 'speech discrimination' testing. For the purposes of clarity in this chapter, a suprathreshold intelligibility test is considered a recognition task and is described by the type of speech material used, e.g. word recognition test or sentence recognition test. The performance score on the word recognition test is abbreviated *WRS* for *word recognition scores*.

Discrimination is a judgement based on the comparison of two or more stimuli. The judgement can be made at threshold or at suprathreshold levels. Classical psychophysics distinguished between absolute or detection thresholds and discrimination or difference thresholds. Modern psychophysics does not make this distinction, since for both there is a background noise against which the stimulus must be differentiated.

Current Clinical Practices

Most audiologists in the USA currently obtain both a speech recognition threshold (SRT) and a word recognition score (WRS) for every patient undergoing a basic audiologic evaluation. Each are discussed separately below under the heading of *Speech Threshold*, and *Suprathreshold Speech Recognition Tests*. The information presented here on current practices in speech audiometry reflects the findings of a recent survey of audiometric practices (Martin and Sides, 1985), of two older surveys (Martin and Forbis, 1977; Martin and Pennington, 1971), and of recent literature in this area.

Speech Threshold

PURPOSE OF SPEECH RECOGNITION THRESHOLDS: The primary reason that a speech recognition threshold (SRT) or spondee threshold (ST) is considered a valuable part of a diagnostic audiologic evaluation is that it lends validity to pure-tone thresholds. There is generally good correspondence between speech and pure-tone thresholds both for normals (Fletcher, 1929) and those with hearing loss (Hughson and Thompson, 1942). The other very common reason for determining a speech threshold is its use as a reference level for suprathreshold recognition tests. Additional reasons include its reliability with the difficult-to-test patient, and the apparent face validity of using speech stimuli to assess sensitivity since communication depends upon listening to speech rather than pure tones.

| | Surveys on Audiometric Practice | | | | | |
| | Martin and Pennington 1971 | | Martin and Forbis 1978 | | Martin and Sides 1985 | |
Speech Material	Number	%	Number	%	Number	%
CID Auditory Test W-1	161	57.9	179	61.3	118	55.9
CID Auditory Test W-2	40	14.4	63	21.6	47	22.2
PAL Auditory Test No. 9	11	4.0	15	5.1	5	2.4
PAL Auditory Test No. 14	1	0.4	0	0.0	2	0.9
Children's Spondees	22	7.9	—	—	—	—
Connected Discourse	2	0.7	1	0.3	0	0.0
Other	15	5.4	26	9.0	40	18.9
More than one response	26	9.5	8	2.7	—	—
(Number of respondents)	(278)		(302)		(212)	

Table I Speech test materials used to obtain a Speech Recognition Threshold (SRT)

TEST MATERIALS: The commercially available speech threshold materials are listed in Table I. The most commonly used test material is the Central Institute for the Deaf (CID) Auditory Test W-1 (Hirsch, *et al.*, 1952). The CID Auditory Test W-2 is less commonly used. The 'other' stimuli used were primarily spondees selected from non-standard sources. Auditory Tests No. 9 and No. 14 (the original spondaic word lists developed at the Harvard Psycho-Acoustic Laboratory [PAL] by Hudgins *et al.*, 1947) are hardly used clinically any more. These two lists each consist of six randomizations of 42 words; there are 84 different spondees. In the former recording (PAL No. 9), each six words is attenuated 4 dB below the previous set for a total attenuation range of 24 dB. The latter recording (PAL No. 14), has a constant presentation level relative to the carrier phrase. The more widely used CID W-1 and W-2 lists (Hirsh, *et al.*, 1952) consist of the 36 more familiar spondaic

211

words: the W-1 recording attenuates the spondee 10 dB relative to the carrier phrase 'say the word'; and the W-2 recording is progressively attenuated 3 dB for each block of three words. The primary impetus to revise the PAL recordings was to achieve better homogeneity of audibility. The CID recordings were adjusted to be homogeneous within ±2 dB, for mean recognition thresholds of 20 dB SPL for experienced listeners and 21 dB SPL for inexperienced listeners. The variability in the physical characteristics of speech and the variability introduced by use of a VU meter to monitor the presentation of recorded spondee tests, make it impossible to achieve perfect homogeneity. Clinicians need to be aware of the expected sources of increased variability (Wilson and Margolis, 1983).

RECORDED VS MONITORED LIVE VOICE PRESENTATION: The clinician typically presents spondee test materials using monitored live voice (MLV) in preference to using recorded materials (Martin and Sides, 1985; ASHA, 1979; Martin and Pennington 1971). This mode is selected primarily because it offers greater flexibility. MLV permits modifications to suit the patient's ability and the available test time: it permits either faster or slower presentation, omission of the carrier phrase, and/or use of selected words. The use of monitored live-voice presentation of the test materials is often indicated by the clinical situation, e.g., testing very young children, difficult-to-test children or adults, or some elderly patients. It should be remembered, however, that a speech test is not a list, but an utterance that varies with the speaker or recording (Kruel *et al.*, 1969). Therefore, when MLV presentation is used and standardized stimulus materials must be sacrificed, the clinician should keep in mind that another source of variability is introduced. The use of the VU meter to monitor the presentation level is then very important in order to achieve maximal homogeneity of audibility for each talker.

For either recorded or monitored live voice presentation, the level, in dB SPL, at which the speech stimuli are equivalent to 0 dB HL is dependent upon the output transducer used. Typically spondees and other speech stimuli are presented through the standard audiometric earphone, TDH 39 or 49, mounted on an MX41/AR cushion. In this stimulus presentation mode (earphone), 20 dB SPL is the reference for speech stimuli. Current standards for audiometer calibration (ANSI S3.6, 1969) recommended calibration of speech by adjusting the rms SPL of a 1 kHz signal so that its VU meter deflection is equal to the average peak VU meter deflection produced by the speech. Sound field conditions are indicated when difficult-to-test children, or adults, will not accept earphones, or when aided and unaided SRTs are compared as a part of the hearing aid selection and fitting process. Calibration of loudspeakers must consider the orientation of the listener to the loudspeaker in the soundfield. In this stimulus presentation mode (sound field), the sound field should be calibrated to 16.5 dB SPL for 0 degrees azimuth and 12.5 dB SPL for 45 degrees azimuth (Dirks *et al.*, 1972). The complexity of specifying the sound pressure level of speech is emphasized by the fact that speech calibration techniques are still being researched. Although standards exist for earphone testing, sound field calibration standards are still in the development phase.

TEST METHODS: Although a number of clinical methods have evolved to obtain speech recognition thresholds, currently there is no preferred clinical method used. A concise summary of the differences in the various procedures can be found in Olsen and Matkin (1979). In spite of the lack of a standardized SRT procedure, Chaiklin and Ventry's (1964) protocol is commonly used and recommended. As with pure-tone threshold assessment, a modified method of limits is used to determine the SRT. However, the speech threshold is most commonly obtained using a descending method rather than an ascending method. Assessment begins at a level above suspected threshold to familiarize the listener with the words and the task. The level is then decreased in 5 dB steps, presenting 1 to 3 words at each level decrement until a word is missed. At this point the stimulus level is raised 10 dB and then lowered in 5 dB steps, presenting 3–6 spondees with each change in stimulus level. The level at which 50% of the spondees are correctly repeated is recorded as the speech recognition threshold (SRT) or spondee threshold (ST).

| | Surveys on Audiometric Practice | | | | | |
| | Martin and Pennington 1971 | | Martin and Forbis 1978 | | Martin and Sides 1985 | |
Step size in dB	Number	%	Number	%	Number	%
2	144	49.8	100	33.1	38	17.5
4	15	5.2	13	4.3	5	2.3
5	117	40.5	172	57.0	170	78.3
Other	8	2.8	8	2.6	5	1.7
More than one response	5	1.7	9	3.0	—	—
(Number of respondents)	(289)		(302)		(217)	

Table II Increment size used to obtain a Speech Recognition Threshold (SRT)

INCREMENT AND RESPONSE CRITERION: According to Martin and Sides (1985), most (78%) of the survey respondents use a 5 dB increment size to obtain the ST, although the second most common step size (17.5%) was 2 dB (Table II). There has been an increase in the use of the 5 dB step size since 1971 (Martin and Forbis, 1978; Martin and Pennington, 1971). The literature supports this practice in that there is little difference in spondee thresholds obtained with either step size (Chaiklin et al., 1964, 1967). The majority of the audiologists (43.4%) use a response criterion of two out of three correct responses to determine the ST (Table III), compared with the

213

previous two surveys where the response criteria were fairly equally distributed. Clearly, many other criteria are in use which highlights the fact that many different methods are still used to obtain an SRT.

| | Surveys on Audiometric Practice | | | | | |
| | Martin and Pennington 1971 | | Martin and Forbis 1978 | | Martin and Sides 1985 | |
Response Criteria	Number	%	Number	%	Number	%
2 out of 3	72	25.2	82	27.1	93	43.4
2 out of 4	77	26.9	68	22.4	50	23.4
3 out of 4	15	5.2	16	5.2	16	7.4
3 out of 5	26	9.1	21	7.0	12	5.6
3 out of 6	52	18.2	64	21.0	21	9.8
Lowest level with 3 Correct Responses	27	9.4	30	10.0	13	6.1
Other	17	5.9	17	6.0	9	4.2
More than one response	—	—	4	1.3	—	—
(Number of respondents)	(289)		(302)		(217)	

Table III Response criteria used to obtain a Speech Recognition Threshold (SRT)

PROPOSED METHODS: Two different procedures for obtaining an SRT and an ascending method (ASHA, 1979). Neither one has come into common usage yet, but the 5 dB decrement version of the descending method (Huff and Nerbonne, 1982; Wall *et al.*, 1984; Wilson and Margolis, 1983) holds promise. Both methods, however, are somewhat more time consuming than the method presented above.

The recent descending procedure recommended by Tillman and Olsen (1973) represents a methodological revival of the speech recognition threshold technique of Hudgins *et al.* (1947). The procedure requires familiarization of the patient with the spondees presented at a most comfortable listening level and elimination of any unfamiliar or incorrectly identified words. The initial presentation level is 30–40 dB above expected threshold. As the level is decreased in 10 dB steps, 1–2 words are presented at each level. When two words are missed, the presentation level is raised 10 dB, and the test descent is begun again in 2 dB steps. For every 2 dB decrement two words are presented. Threshold criterion is reached when five of six words are missed. The SRT is the number of correct words minus the starting level plus a correction factor (1 dB) of half the attenuation rate. A simplification of this method based on ease of administration on current clinical audiometers has been recommended by Wall *et al.* (1984) and Wilson and Margolis (198). This method calls for 5 dB decrements, five words per decrement, termination when all 5 words at an intensity level are missed, and use of a 2 dB correction factor.

The ascending method recommended by ASHA (1979) begins at the lowest audiometer attenuator setting and ascends in 10 dB steps presenting 1 word per level until a correct response is obtained. The stimulus level is then decreased 15 dB, and 4 words are presented for each 5 dB increment until three words are correctly repeated. The stimulus level is then decreased 10 dB, and the ascending procedure is repeated two more times. The SRT is the lowest level at which at least half of the words are correctly repeated in a minimum of two ascents. This procedure seems more awkward and time consuming than the simplified descending method (Wall *et al.*, 1984). A recent comparison (Wall *et al.*, 1984) of two descending methods (Chaiklin and Ventry, 1964) and two ascending methods (Chaiklin *et al.*, 1967; ASHA, 1979) suggests that: there are no significant differences among the SRTs using these four methods, the descending methods are the most sensitive (lowest thresholds) and are equivalent in time consumption and test-retest reliability, but the ascending methods agree best with a three frequency pure-tone average. The ASHA (1979) method is the most time consuming. Time will determine whether either of these more recently developed techniques is accepted for clinical use and whether more reliable determinations of the speech recognition threshold are even necessary.

FAMILIARIZATION: The importance of familiarity with the speech stimulus materials dates back to Hudgins (1949) and has been reinforced by Hirsh *et al.* (1952), by ASHA (1979), and by many more recent studies (for example, see Olsen and Matkin, 1979; Wilson and Margolis, 1983). In addition, most methods stress the importance of familiarizing the patient with the spondees face-to-face. Despite the fact that familiarization can improve threshold and reduce variability, few clinicians take the time to familiarize the patient with the stimuli prior to obtaining an SRT. Only 55% of the respondents reportedly familiarized their patients (Martin and Sides, 1985); this number is probably an over-estimate (ASHA, 1979).

CARRIER PHRASE: When obtaining an SRT in clinical practice, the carrier phrase is often omitted. According to Martin and Sides (1985), more than half of the audiologists disregard the carrier phrase; this practice has increased over the past 15 years (Martin and Pennington, 1971; Martin and Forbis, 1978). Of those who use a carrier phrase, 41% use 'say the word', and 81% present the carrier phrase and the stimulus word at the same hearing level. Although use of a carrier phrase helps the audiologist monitor the presentation level and helps the patient define the listening level, the contribution of a carrier phrase is probably negligible when the speech stimulus is as redundant as spondees.

RELATIONS BETWEEN PURE-TONE THRESHOLDS AND SPEECH THRESHOLDS: A clinical value often ascribed to the SRT is its correspondence with pure-tone thresholds. The SRT can be predicted with some precision from an average of selected pure-tone thresholds. For flat and gradually sloping losses, a three-frequency pure-tone average (PTA) of the thresholds obtained at 500 Hz, 1 kHz and 2 kHz optimally predicts the SRT (Fletcher, 1929; Carhart, 1946). Although the three-frequency pure-tone average is the most popular prediction method, it can overestimate the SRT, especially for patients with sloping high frequency losses. For steeply sloping losses, the average of the two best pure-tone thresholds is a better predictor of the SRT (Fletcher, 1950). More recently, Carhart and Porter (1971) have recommended that averaging the thresholds at 500 Hz and 1 kHz minus 2 dB since that average adequately predicts the SRT from most audiometric configurations (see also Carhart, 1971).

In clinical practice, the audiologist considers that agreement between the SRT and PTA of ±6 dB (to as much as ±10 dB) is within acceptable limits (Olsen and Matkin, 1979). If the SRT is significantly lower (better) than the PTA, results are most often considered pathognomonic of pseudohypacusis. It suggests that the pure-tone results are suspect and that additional testing is indicated. However, a discrepancy of 10 dB or greater can also be obtained from very young children or difficult-to-test adults (e.g., psychiatric or mentally retarded patients). This discrepancy is thought to result from the patient responding to the loudness of speech and does not reflect threshold for speech (Ventry, 1976). Although less common, a disparity of 10 dB or greater such that the PTA is lower (better) than the SRT can be obtained from patients with severe communication or word finding difficulties (e.g. retrocochlear lesions).

The relationship between the speech threshold and the PTA is dependent not only on the speech materials, the method, and the configuration of the loss, but also on the type of speech threshold obtained. A speech detection threshold requires less energy than a speech recognition threshold, thus the SDT is typically detected at levels 8–9 dB lower (better) than the SRT or the PTA (Chaiklin, 1959; Beattie et al., 1975a, b). Often, better agreement is found between the SDT and the 250 Hz pure-tone threshold. Either the SRT or the SDT may be used to indicate agreement with pure-tone thresholds.

MASKING: Often during speech audiometry acoustic signals presented to the test ear are sufficiently intense that they can be perceived in the non-test ear. In practice, most audiologists mask when cross-hearing is suspected but they do not apply a uniformly accepted masking criterion for determination of the speech recognition threshold. Rather, two masking criteria are quite widely used during SRT testing (Martin and Sides, 1985). Table IV indicates that most audiologists use a specific difference criterion to indicate the need for masking. The masking criterion used by almost half of the respondents (48%), according to Martin and Sides (1985), is a 40 dB or greater difference between the SRT of the test ear and the best bone-conduction threshold of the nontest ear. The other most popular criteria (41%) is a difference of 40 dB or greater between the SRTs from each ear. Acceptance of the former technique (SRT of the test ear re: the nontest ear's

	Surveys on Audiometric Practice					
	Martin and Pennington 1971		Martin and Forbis 1978		Martin and Sides 1985	
Masking Criteria	Number	%	Number	%	Number	%
Mask all SRTs	—	—	1	0.3	4	1.8
Patient hears speech in nontest ear or in middle of the head	11	43.7	5	1.6	50	1.8
40 dB or greater difference between SRTs of each ear	115	43.7	97	31.1	92	40.5
40 dB or greater difference between SRT of test ear and the best bone conduction threshold of the nontest ear	93	35.4	169	54.2	109	48.0
Never	—	—	17	5.4	6	2.6
Other	18	6.8	7	2.2	12	5.3
More than one response	26	9.9	16	5.2	—	—
(Number of respondents)	(263)		(312)		(227)	

Table IV Masking criteria used to obtain a Speech Recognition Threshold (SRT)

best bone-conduction threshold) seems to have increased somewhat since the earlier surveys (Martin and Forbis, 1978; Martin and Pennington, 1971). This division in approaches to masking criteria for SRT testing is consistent with the recommendations of the ASHA (1979) guidelines which specify two criteria: the SRT of the test ear is 40 dB or more greater than the SRT of the nontest ear; the SRT of the test ear is 40 dB or more greater than the pure-tone bone-conduction thresholds of the nontest ear at 500 Hz, 1 kHz, or 2 kHz. Fortunately, fewer than 5% never mask or always mask when obtaining an SRT. Masking practices are in agreement with the critical interaural differences for. air-conducted stimuli presented to the poorer ear (with a standard supra-aural earphone) and the better ear's bone conduction thresholds (Zwislocki, 1953; Liden, 1954). The amount of masking introduced into the nontest ear (Table V) is determined by the plateau method (Hood, 1957) by a majority of the audiologists (50%). Variants of the plateau method that are used by the rest of the respondents include an arbitrary starting level (29%) and a safety factor of 10–60 dB before beginning to plateau. This latter approach was reported by some of the 21% who indicated using an 'other' amount of masking (Martin and Sides, 1985).

BONE CONDUCTION: In the typical practice of audiology, an SRT or SDT is most often determined with air-conducted signals. However, at times it is clinically indicated to determine bone-conducted speech thresholds.

217

	Surveys on Audiometric Practice					
	Martin and Pennington 1971		Martin and Forbis 1978		Martin and Sides 1985	
Amount of Masking	Number	%	Number	%	Number	%
SRT of opposite ear then plateau	—	—	125	41.9	109	50.0
Arbitrary beginning then plateau	—	—	96	32.3	63	28.9
Other	—	—	77	25.8	46	21.1
(Number of respondents)			(298)		(218)	

Table V Amount of masking used to obtain a Speech Recognition Threshold (SRT)

Bone-conducted speech is used to assist in confirming the presence of an air-bone gap, as well as in estimating the size of the air-bone gap. This provides useful information for the medical management of the difficult-to-test patient. Bone-conducted speech thresholds correlate with either 500 Hz–1 kHz for an SRT or 250 Hz for an SRT.

RE-EVALUATION OF THE USE OF THE SRT: Most audiologists customarily obtain a speech recognition threshold for every patient. In fact, it is often clinical protocol to obtain a speech recognition threshold prior to assessing pure-tone air-conduction thresholds because the task of repeating spondees is easy for most patients. The speech recognition threshold is an admittedly helpful clinical check on the correctness of pure-tone thresholds, and appears to be assessing communication ability to the patient (and sometimes even to the audiologist). According to the procedures commonly used to obtain an SRT (discussed above), many short-cuts and compromises are introduced in a busy clinic practice with only minimal changes in the obtained level of the SRT. Thus, some re-evaluation of the rationale for the wide use of the SRT may be indicated. Wilson and Margolis (1983) correctly suggest that the routine use of the SRT for patients who have been tested before and who have reliable pure-tone thresholds is redundant and not cost effective. Perhaps the SRT should only be determined when there is a question of unreliable pure-tone thresholds (pseudohypacusis) and for the difficult to test.

Clinical resistance to selective use of the SRT rests with one of the primary reasons an audiologist gives for obtaining an SRT, that is to determine a reference level for suprathreshold speech recognition tests. The suprathreshold speech test is typically presented at some specified number of decibels in sensation level, relative to the SRT. This sensation level is based on the mean psychometric function or performance-intensity function for the test material thought to indicate the level at which maximum word recognition ability is attained. The inference that the mean level for maximum recognition is appropriate for the individual patient under test is questionable (see suprathreshold recognition testing below). More important, sensation level implies that the same stimulus is used for both the threshold and the suprathreshold test. This is not so in practice. Less variability is introduced when the presentation level for the suprathreshold test is referenced to a pure-tone detection threshold since the reference psychometric function is steeper. Wilson and Margolis (1983) suggest that an appropriate pure-tone average (e.g., Carhart and Porter, 1971) provides an adequate and efficient means of determining the reference level for suprathreshold speech recognition tests.

Further, comparison of two SRTs obtained under two different test situations (pre/post treatment) confounds the clinical conclusion. Each SRT represents a point on a psychometric function for the individual. The two points (levels) may differ if two different recordings were used and especially if MLV presentation of two different lists was administered by two different talkers. These differences may be exaggerated by the treatment (medication or amplification) thus changing the slope of the psychometric function.

Most clinicians recognize that the validity of the speech recognition threshold is questionable. Clinically, the use of speech stimuli to obtain an estimate of auditory sensitivity was considered an appealing and valid approach to understand communication disability. However, the speech recognition threshold has only an apparent face validity since neither the spondee nor the recognition task are directly related to the communication process. In addition, the specification of speech stimuli is difficult, and its resultant threshold is not frequency specific. Pure-tones thresholds, however, provide a valid estimate of auditory sensitivity.

DIFFICULT-TO-TEST PATIENTS: The SRT continues to be used clinically for testing children, psychiatric patients, and some limited-functioning geriatric patients. However, it is sometimes difficult to obtain an SRT from patients with limited or unintelligible speech (e.g., young children), those with mental retardation, profoundly hearing-impaired individuals, or deaf patients. Simple modification of test procedure may be sufficient. Typically, the audiologist changes the response mode by having the patient point to pictures or toys which illustrate the spoken spondee words rather than repeating the spondee heard. Flexibility of administration may include use of a modified carrier phrase (e.g., 'show me'), monitored-live-voice presentation, selected spondees, children's spondees (e.g. Newby, 1958), or monosyllables (TIP — Siegenthaler and Haspiel, 1966). When it is impossible to determine an SRT by any means, most difficult-to-test patients will perform an SDT test with spondees, or simple, more familiar words, such as 'go' or 'mama'. Modification of behavioural techniques used to obtain the SDT include visual reinforcement audiometry (VRA), conditioned orienting response audiometry (COR), and tangible reinforcement operant conditioning audiometry (TROCA) under earphones or in the sound field.

Suprathreshold Speech Recognition Testing

TEST MATERIALS AND THEIR PURPOSES: Some of the available speech recognition tests are listed in Table VI. The two word recognition tests used most often in the USA (Martin and Pennington, 1971; Martin and Forbis, 1978; Martin and Sides, 1985) are the CID Auditory Test W-22 (Hirsh, *et al.*, 1952) and the Northwestern University No. 6 (Tillman and Carhart, 1966). Much less frequently used are the CNC Word lists (Peterson and Lehiste, 1962) and the PAL PB-50 Word lists (Egan, 1948).

Each of these word lists consists of 50 open-set monosyllables. For each word correctly understood the patient receives a score of 2%. Normal-hearing patients and patients with conductive hearing loss generally score 90–100%, whereas patients with sensorineural or mixed hearing loss generally score less than 90%. Patients with central auditory problems usually have no difficulty with the word recognition test and score normally in the routine battery.

Thus, the word recognition test can be used for differential diagnosis by helping to determine the site of lesion of peripheral and central auditory pathologies. In addition, this measure is useful to the physician in determining surgical candidacy. The word recognition score (WRS) is also used by audiologists in hearing aid assessment and in planning aural rehabilitation programmes. Aural rehabilitation applications will be discussed later in this chapter.

Since the overwhelming majority of audiologists use open-set monosyllabic word lists (see Table VI), our summary of available clinical speech recognition tests begins with those types of stimulus materials. Some other types of speech materials used primarily in aural rehabilitation applications and in research are also presented below: nonsense syllables, open set as well as closed set monosyllables, and sentences.

| | Surveys on Audiometric Practice | | | | | |
| | Martin and Pennington 1971 | | Martin and Forbis 1978 | | Martin and Sides 1985 | |
Speech Material	Number	%	Number	%	Number	%
CID Auditory Test W-22	202	71.6	217	70.7	113	61.0
CNC Word Lists	9	3.2	37	12.0	10	4.6
PAL PB-50 Word Lists	25	8.9	22	7.2	4	1.8
Modification of Fairbanks Rhyme Test	2	0.7	0	0	0	0
Synthetic Sentences	0	0	0	0	0	0
Northwestern Univ. No. 6	—	—	—	—	51	23.4
Other	28	9.9	17	5.5	20	9.2
More than one response	16	5.7	14	4.6	—	—
(Number of respondents)	(282)		(307)		(218)	

Table VI Speech test materials used to obtain a Word Recognition Score (WRS)

Open-Set Monosyllables

PAL PB-50 MONOSYLLABLES: The PB-50 monosyllables were the first speech materials used in the evaluation of the hearing impaired. These speech tests were originally designed to assess the efficiency of communication systems. It was for this purpose that, during the Second World War, Egan developed the PB-50 monosyllables (1948). They were designed in order to meet the following criteria: all of the sounds of English speech should be represented with a relative frequency of occurrence which reflects their common usage, test items should have an equal average difficulty and equal range of difficulty. Twenty 50-word lists of familiar monosyllables were constructed. Unfortunately, these lists did not satisfy the criteria as well as expected. The phonetic balance was not exact, and words used were not all equally familiar. Eight of the original twenty lists were recorded at Central Institute for the Deaf (CID) by Rush Hughes and are currently referred to as the *Rush Hughes PB-50s*. Contrary to the original design-criteria, these recordings are noted for their low reliability and for their difficulty; an important variable was the speech production of the speaker. The resultant recordings are so poor that even a normal listener cannot achieve a perfect score. Although these lists are not commonly used for basic audiologic evaluation, audiologists do use these recordings when difficult material is needed, e.g. central auditory testing.

CID W-22 MONOSYLLABLES: In an effort to overcome the poor reliability and difficulty of the PB-50 word lists and to improve phonetic balance, Hirsh *et al.* (1952) developed the CID W-22 lists. Word difficulty was reduced and phonetic balance was improved (French *et al.*, 1930). Reliability was improved through the use of magnetic tape recording. The CID W-22 word lists are the most popular lists used by clinicians in the USA today. There are four 50-word lists with 6 randomizations of each list. These are commercially available on both records and tape from Auditec of St Louis (330 Selma Avenue, St Louis, MO 63119, USA).

CONSONANT-NUCLEUS-CONSONANT (CNC) MONOSYLL-ABLES: The CNC lists employ phonemic, rather than phonetic balance (Lehiste and Peterson, 1959). In order to achieve this phonemic balance Lehiste and Peterson used consonant-nucleus-consonant monosyllables in which each initial consonant, each vowel, and each final consonant appears with the same frequency of occurrence within each list. Lehiste and Peterson argue that phonetics is concerned with the physiological and acoustical pro-perties of speech, i.e. speech production, whereas phonemics is 'perceptual phonetics'. As the speech signal is not acoustically invariant, it would be impossible to achieve phonetic balance, therefore, intelligibility measures should use materials which are, instead, phonemically balanced. The original ten lists were revised (Peterson and Lehiste, 1962) in order to reduce the frequency of usage problem which occurred in the earlier lists. There are ten

50-word lists with 5 randomizations of each list in the commercially available CNC test.

NORTHWESTERN UNIVERSITY AUDITORY TEST NO. 4 and NO. 6 (NU-4, NU-6): The NU-4 test (Tillman, Carhart, and Wilber, 1963) was developed from the CNC lists (Peterson and Lehiste, 1962). The two NU-4 lists have high test-retest reliability and conform better to Lehiste and Peterson's plan for phonemic balance. The NU-6 lists (Tillman and Carhart, 1966) are an expansion of the NU-4 CNC lists; there are four, instead of two, lists available with four scramblings of each list. The NU-6 has achieved some popularity among clinicians here as can be seen in Table VI.

ISOPHONEMIC CNC WORD LISTS: Boothroyd (1968) published additional CNC lists which he described as isophonemic word lists. There are only 10 words per list, and each of 15 lists is phonemically balanced. Each of the 3 phonemes in a word is scored as correct or incorrect allowing for a phoneme-error score rather than a word-error score. In addition to allowing for phoneme error analysis, these short word lists have the advantage of being faster to administer. Nonetheless, they have not achieved clinical popularity in word recognition testing.

NONSENSE SYLLABLES: The primary advantage of using nonsense syllables for the speech recognition test is that they permit detailed analysis of the types of phonemic errors made by the listener. In addition, nonsense syllables insure that both word familiarity and memory effects are reduced. On the other hand, because of their inherent non-meaningfulness and resultant lack of intelligibility (Lehiste and Peterson, 1959) which increase the difficulty of the task for the listener, these stimuli are not usually used as part of the routine evaluation. A more appropriate use for these words is in hearing aid assessment and aural rehabilitation at which time phoneme error analysis may be important.

NONSENSE SYLLABLE TEST (NST): The *Nonsense Syllable Test* (NST) was developed for just this purpose (Resnick *et al.*, 1975; Levitt *et al.*, 1978). This test is a closed-set response test made up of consonant-vowel (CV) and vowel-consonant (VC) syllables. There are 7 test modules with 9 syllables in each module. There are three vowel contexts representing the extremes of the vowel triangle: /i/, /a/, and /u/. Consonants in each module are either voiced or unvoiced so that errors in voicing cannot be made. Levitt and his co-workers made no attempt at phonetic balance but were more concerned with the most frequent perceptual confusions made by both normal-hearing listeners (Miller and Nicely, 1955, and Wang and Bilger, 1973) and hearing-impaired listeners (Owens, Benedict and Schubert, 1972). The estimated reliability of the NST is 0.93 for 91 items (Dubno and Dirks, 1982). They suggest that the high reliability of these word lists make the NST a good choice when comparison scores are needed such as in hearing aid assessment and aural rehabilitation treatment programmes (Dubno, Dirks, and Langhofer, 1982).

CLOSED-SET MONOSYLLABLES: The traditional open-set testing paradigms have at least two disadvantages: 1. they do not control for the subject's previous linguistic experience and the extent to which that experience may affect his responses, and 2. subject response error scoring is difficult. Most closed-set tests are not commonly used in clinical practice.

RHYME TESTS: The *Rhyme Test* was developed by Fairbanks (1958) in order to reduce linguistic confounds and provide a test of 'phonemic differentiation'. This test is of the fill-in type in which the subject responds by filling in only the initial consonant from a set of 5 rhyming monosyllabic words. The Rhyme Test was later modified to include words in the forms consonant-vowel-consonant (CVC), vowel-consonant (VC), and consonant-vowel (CV), and called the *Modified Rhyme Test (MRT)* (House *et al.*, 1963). A multiple-choice type test, the subject chooses from 6 possible alternatives. The MRT has the advantage of assessing both initial and final consonants. Kreul *et al.* (1968) adapted the MRT to make it more clinically useful. Changes were made in recording technique, speaker control, carrier phrase, noise levels for masking the speech, instructions, test forms, and S/N levels for each of 3 individual speakers. However, this test is not often used clinically. The *Diagnostic Rhyme Test (DRT)* is a test developed for testing speech intelligibility over communication systems (Voiers, 1977), but is now beginning to find application for the hearing impaired and deaf (Milner and Flevaris-Phillips, 1985). The test consists of rhyming pairs. The consonants in each pair differ by a single distinctive feature of six possible features. It is designed for phonemic analysis of the initial consonant.

MULTIPLE CHOICE DISCRIMINATION TEST (MCDT): The MCDT uses the CID W-22 words in a closed message response set (Schultz and Schubert, 1969). Unlike the MRT, confusions in the MCDT can be made between either initial or final consonants within the same response set.

CALIFORNIA CONSONANT TEST (CCT): More recently Owens and Schubert (1977) published the *California Consonant Test* using a format similar to the MCDT. There are 100 test words with 3 foils in each response set, and like the MCDT, both initial and final positions are assessed. Although this test is time consuming, it is gaining in popularity for use in hearing aid evaluation and aural rehabilitation.

Sentence Materials

Sentence tests are not typically used to assess word recognition. However, it can be argued that clinicians should use larger linguistic units such as sentences, rather than single words, to assess intelligibility. The sentence is a much better representation of a sample of spoken communication and allows for linguistic features such as intonation patterns and co-articulatory effects not possible to achieve with a single word utterance. Although sentences are not frequently used by American audiologists for word recognition testing, they do deserve mention since they can be useful in certain clinical situations, especially aural rehabilitation.

CID EVERYDAY SENTENCES: The sentences most frequently used to assess speech intelligibility are commonly referred to in the USA as the 'CID everyday sentences' or the 'CHABA sentences' (Silverman and Hirsh, 1955). There are 10 sentences with a total of 50 key words. The subject must respond by repeating the entire sentence but is scored for only each key word correct. They are particularly useful for evaluation of the patient with severe recognition problems, such as the limited geriatric patient.

SYNTHETIC SENTENCE IDENTIFICATION TEST (SSI): This is a closed set sentence test comprised of third-order approximations of syntactically correct English sentences (Speaks and Jerger, 1965). The listener's task is to identify the test sentence from a group of 10 sentences on a response sheet. A message-to-competition ratio (MCR) of 0 (the competing message is a discourse on the life of Davey Crockett) results in performance-intensity (P-I) functions which are equivalent to P-I functions for PB words (Jerger, Speaks and Trammel, 1968). The SSI is currently used as part of the central auditory test battery and is sometimes used in hearing aid system assessment.

SPIN TEST: The speech perception in noise (SPIN) test utilizes the predictability of words in context as a factor in word recognition testing (Kalikow, Stevens and Elliot, 1977). There are eight sets of 50 sentences presented in a background of speech babble. Half the sentences contain *high* predictability test items and half contain *low* predictability test items. The subject's task is to identify the last word in each sentence. An overall score is derived from the difference between the scores on high and low predictability items. This test is beginning to gain clinical acceptance, especially for aural rehabilitation.

| | Surveys on Audiometric Practice | | | | | |
| | Martin and Pennington 1971 | | Martin and Forbis 1978 | | Martin and Sides 1985 | |
Number of Words	*Number*	%	*Number*	%	*Number*	%
50 for all patients	—	—	50	16.4	12	17.5
25 if patient answers first 25 correctly	—	—	125	40.8	70	31.7
25 for all patients	—	—	99	32.3	118	53.4
Other			30	9.8	21	9.5
More than one response	—	—	2	0.7	—	—
(Number of respondents)	—	—	(306)		(221)	

Table VII Number of words used to obtain a Word a Recognition Score (WRS)

METHODS: The most frequently used clinical method for assessing word recognition ability in the USA today includes the use of CID W-22 monosyllables in an open set paradigm (Table VI). Most clinicians use only half-lists (25 words) instead of full lists (50 words), see Table VII. The majority of audiologists use the speech recognition threshold (SRT) as the reference level for determining the level at which to administer the word recognition test (Table VIII). The words are usually administered monitored live voice (MLV), and each word is generally preceded by the carrier phrase 'say the word . . .' Contralateral masking of the non-test ear is typically employed with speech noise as the masker (Table IX).

| | Surveys on Audiometric Practice | | | | | |
| | Martin and Pennington 1971 | | Martin and Forbis 1978 | | Martin and Sides 1985 | |
Presentation Level	Number	%	Number	%	Number	%
— dB SL re. SRT	147	52.9	207	68.0	142	64.8
— dB HL	25	9.0	5	1.6	5	2.3
MCL	45	16.2	49	16.1	47	21.5
Obtain a P-I Function	9	3.2	15	4.9	8	3.7
Other	7	2.5	4	1.2	17	7.8
More than one response	45	16.2	25	8.2	—	—
(Number of respondents)	(278)		(305)		(219)	

Table VIII Level at which to obtain the Word Recognition Score (WRS)

| | Surveys on Audiometric Practice | | | | | |
| | Martin and Pennington 1971 | | Martin and Forbis 1978 | | Martin and Sides 1985 | |
Masking Criteria	Number	%	Number	%	Number	%
Mask all WR tests	—	—	14	4.5	16	7.1
Patient hears speech in nontest ear or in middle of the head	10	3.9	6	1.9	4	1.8
40 dB or greater difference between SRTS of each ear	66	25.7	188	61.0	53	23.7
40 dB or greater difference between presentation level of test and BC threshold of the nontest ear	132	51.4	51	16.6	117	52.2
Never	—	—	31	10.2	6	2.7
Other	23	8.9	6	1.9	28	12.5
More than one response	26	10.1	12	3.9	—	—
(Number of respondents)	(257)		(308)		(224)	

Table IX Masking criteria used to obtain a Word Recognition Score (WRS)

These clinical methods, and their limitations, are discussed below. In addition, methods used for the evaluation of the paediatric population are also discussed, although there are no reported data on frequency of usage for paediatric procedures.

HALF-LISTS VS WHOLE LISTS AND THE BINOMIAL DISTRIBUTION: Most audiologists use 25-word lists (see Table VII) with all patients regardless of the number of errors made in that half list (Martin and Sides, 1985). In 1978 Martin and Forbis reported that 40.8% of audiologists responding were qualifying their use of 25-word lists by presenting a full 50-word list if the patient missed a certain number of words in the first half of the list. That figure dropped to 31.7% in the more recent Martin and Sides (1985) report. We regret that there appears to be a move towards the use of half-lists without qualification. By applying the binomial distribution to the word recognition test score, Thornton and Raffin (1978) have demonstrated the need for frequent use of full lists. Studebaker (1982) suggests that lists even longer than 50 words may be necessary for reliable test scores. The formula for the standard deviation of a binomial distribution shows that when we increase the sample size (i.e. length of the word list), we decrease the standard deviation, or increase reliability. Specifically, a doubling of the number of words used, e.g. 50 instead of 25 words, results in a decrease in the standard deviation by the square root of two. In other words, variability is reduced by using full lists. What is also determined by the binomial distribution is that the largest standard deviations occur for word recognition scores in the mid-range, around 50%. It is true, therefore, that word recognition scores at either the upper limits (90 to 100%) or lower limits (0% to 10%) are the most reliable scores, so audiologists may have greater confidence in those scores after only 25 words are presented.

What we should have learned from considering speech recognition as a binomial distribution is that the audiologist should use careful judgement in order to determine what is an acceptable score with regard to a 'critical difference' as described by Thornton and Raffin. For example, a large sample size, or longer word lists, may be necessary in order to determine if hearing aids differ in their ability to provide optimum speech intelligibility. Indeed, Studebaker (1982) has shown that if a performance difference of 10% is obtained when comparing results of two word recognition tests, e.g. scores obtained with two different hearing aids, then 135 words must be presented in order to have an error rate no greater than 5%. In other words, in order to have 95% confidence that the two scores are different by 10%, 135 words must be presented. Furthermore, to achieve the accepted criterion difference of 6% with 95% confidence, 376 words must be presented (when comparing two word recognition scores for normal listeners). To make matters worse, if comparisons are made with more than two aids, the error rate increases further necessitating the use of still longer word lists.

The fact that audiologists in the USA have moved to the more frequent use of half-lists reflects a lack of understanding of the implications of Thornton and Raffin's application of the binomial distribution. Thus, the impact of their contribution is yet to be realized. Hopefully, clinical practice will soon benefit from the application of well-demonstrated theory.

PRESENTATION LEVEL: The majority of audiologists continue to use the speech recognition threshold (SRT) as a reference level for determining the level at which to present the word recognition test (see Table VIII). The next most frequently used level is MCL (most comfortable loudness). Infrequently used are a specific hearing level, or the attainment of a performance-intensity function for each patient. There are problems introduced by using any one of these particular methods to determine the presentation level. These problems can be reduced, however, if the factors which affect the WRS are understood by the clinician.

When examining the P-I functions in Figure 1, the practice of using the SRT as a reference level seems reasonable for normal hearing/conductive impaired listeners. For those patients, the average maximum score using CID W-22 monosyllables appears to be reached at 25–30 dB re. SRT; above that level the function then plateaus. However, the average optimum level changes for different stimuli, lists, recordings, etc. For example, the plateau (PB-max) for PB-50 monosyllables is reached at a higher level of approximately 33 dB. Knowledge of the psychometric function for the different materials available is thus essential in choosing a presentation level. It should be remembered, however, that average psychometric functions do not predict individual psychometric functions; individual P-I functions would be best. Still, audiologists typically use SRT plus 25-to-40 dB as presentation level since that level assumedly reaches plateau or maximum WRS (at least for persons with normal hearing or conductive hearing loss). Secondarily the choice of SRT plus 25-to-40 dB is made to reduce cross-hearing and thus reduce the need to mask the contralateral ear.

If we examine the P-I function for patients with sensorineural hearing loss, we can see that the use of any fixed reference level is not appropriate. The psychometric function for the sensorineural impaired listeners illustrates the decrement in performance which can occur at sound pressure levels greater than their level of maximum performance. The thoughtful audiologist will perform the word recognition test at more than one level if it is believed that the optimum score was not obtained. Still better, an individual P-I function should be obtained. This is rarely done in general clinical practice due to the limited time available. Perhaps a better use of clinic and patient time might be to omit the SRT, and obtain pure-tone thresholds and a complete P-I function.

Of course the audiologist must also keep in mind the relevance of the binomial distribution when comparing scores between tests presented at different levels. First, the WRS for the sensorineural patient is likely to be less than normal or less than 90%, therefore, the variability of that score will be great (Thornton and Raffin, 1978). For example, a patient who scores 50% on the first word recognition test must achieve a score on the second test which differs by more than 20% in order for that score to be considered statistically different within 95% confidence limits. Second, variability will increase as the number of comparison tests increases by the square root of the number of comparisons.

Another consideration when testing a patient with a sensorineural hearing loss is the configuration of the hearing loss. For persons with high frequency sensorineural hearing loss, we recommend accounting for the pure-tone threshold at either 2 or 3 kHz, since those frequencies are critical to consonant understanding. If possible, that is if not too uncomfortable for the patient and if hearing sensitivity permits, the word recognition test should be administered approximately 5 dB above the threshold of either of those frequencies. Optimally, obtaining a P-I function will assure that the maximum discrimination score under phones has been obtained, however, time constraints in a busy clinic may prevent the audiologist from obtaining the complete P-I function.

The use of MCL for speech as a strict determinant in choosing presentation level is not recommended since the level of maximum word recognition need not be equivalent to MCL in hearing-impaired patients (Posner and Ventry, 1977). For patients with recruiting ears whose severely limited dynamic range results in tolerance problems, the audiologist may have no choice but to deliver the speech stimuli at a comfortable level. It should be noted on the audiogram that MCL was chosen for that reason.

RECORDED VS. LIVE VOICE PRESENTATION: Most audiologists use monitored live voice presentation for word recognition testing (Martin and Pennington, 1971; Martin and Forbis, 1978), since, as discussed earlier, monitored live voice presentation does allow the audiologist greater flexibility during the evaluation. Because of the important use of the WRS as it relates to differential diagnosis, surgery, and amplification/aural rehabilitation, the audiologist is cautioned regarding the greater need for the standardization offered by recorded test materials in order to reduce variability. Inherent in the WRS is poor test-retest reliability. Variability can be as much as 48% in a sensorineural patient whose WRS is reduced to a mid-range score (Thornton and Raffin, 1978). When variability is a critical issue, it can be reduced by careful attention to test parameters, such as choosing recorded over monitored live voice presentation for the word recognition test.

CARRIER PHRASE: Most clinicians in the USA do use a carrier phrase for word recognition testing with monitored live voice presentation. 'Say the word . . .' is preferred by the majority of those who use a carrier phrase (Martin and Pennington, 1971; Martin and Forbis, 1978). There are arguments in the literature both for and against the use of a carrier phrase (Martin, Hawkins, and Bailey, 1962; Gladstone and Sieganthaler, 1971; Gelfand, 1975; Lynn and Brotman, 1981). In practice, the clinician chooses to use or not use a carrier phrase in accordance with the needs of the clinical situation and the patient. For example some children or geriatrics may be confused by the carrier phrase; on the other hand, some of these patients may require the carrier phrase as an alerting device. Indeed, some patients are annoyed by the carrier phrase.

MASKING: The majority of audiologists use contralateral masking when there is a specific ear difference. The criterion most often used (Table IX) is a 40 dB difference between the test presentation level and the best bone-conduction threshold of the non-test ear (Martin and Sides, 1985; Martin and Pennington, 1971). A greater number of audiologists continue to use speech noise as the contralateral masker. According to Martin and Sides (1985), 75% are currently using speech noise as a masker. There are no specific guidelines set forth by ASHA for determining the amount of noise necessary for suprathreshold masking. Clinicians in the USA typically use 40 to 50 dB as the amount of interaural attenuation for speech; they subtract the interaural attenuation value from the Hearing Level of the nontest ear and then add the largest air-bone gap of the non-test ear (Martin and Forbis, 1978; Martin and Sides, 1985). Simply stated, enough noise should be used to effectively mask out the amount of speech which may possibly crossover to the non-test ear, using the best bone-conduction threshold of the non-test ear as a reference. Effective masking levels are determined psychoacoustically by 33% of clinicians while 30% calibrate electroacoustically with the critical band formula (Martin and Sides, 1985).

Word Recognition Tests for Children

Choosing an appropriate word recognition test for a child is difficult because of the many factors which can affect the child's performance. Of primary importance are the child's receptive vocabulary, the response modality, and reinforcement techniques. We must be particularly careful in test selection for a child who has a significant hearing loss, since we cannot be certain to what extent the hearing loss has contributed to language delay; thus test scores may not reflect the child's auditory perceptual capabilities alone. There are, however, a few popular paediatric tests available which attempt to reduce the pragmatic and developmental problems inherent in this population. Although there are more paediatric tests available than are mentioned here, we have tried to present those which we believe are either commonly used or may be gaining in clinical popularity.

PBK-50 WORD LISTS: To overcome word familiarity problems imposed by adult PB monosyllables, PBK word lists were devised by Haskins (1949). They are composed of phonetically-balanced monosyllables selected from vocabulary word lists representative of kindergarten children's language. Use of this test is limited to children over $3\frac{1}{2}$ years old, since younger normal-hearing children do not achieve a maximum score (Sanderson-Leepa and Rintelmann, 1976).

229

WIPI: The *Word Intelligibility by Picture Identification* (WIPI) test was developed in a closed-set format to permit an alternate response mode for children (or any other difficult-to-test population) who have difficulty responding verbally (Lerman, Ross, and McLaughlin, 1965). The test has gained popularity in the USA because it provides the audiologist with four monosyllabic word lists which are easy to administer and score. The child must simply point to one of six pictures on a page. Pictures are colourful and for the most part easy to identify. Although vocabulary items were chosen for the paediatric population, this test (similar to the PBK word lists) is most appropriate for children whose receptive vocabulary is age 4 years or older. Clinically, we have observed that some of the test items are culturally biased, e.g. church, farm, barn. In spite of its limitations, the WIPI appears to have greater clinical popularity than other picture tests such as the DIP (Siegenthaler and Haspiel, 1966), NU-CHIPS (Katz and Elliott, 1978) and PSI (Jerger, *et al.*, 1980; Jerger, Jerger, and Lewis, 1981).

DIP: The *Discrimination by Identification of Pictures* (DIP) is a closed-set picture test. Limitations of this test are word familiarity problems and the small size of the closed set — a two picture matrix.

NU-CHIPS: The *Northwestern University Children's Perception of Speech* (NU-CHIPS) test was developed to assess the receptive vocabulary of 3-year old inner-city children. It is also a closed-set picture test of monosyllabic words which has the advantage of being appropriate for children as young as 3 years of age.

PSI: The newer *Paediatric Speech Intelligibility* (PSI) test is a picture test which uses both word and competing-message sentence materials. Sentences are broken into two groups: Format I sentences are for children with low receptive language ability and Format II sentences are for children with high receptive language ability. Thus there is the apparent advantage of controlling for the linguistic capabilities of the child.

SERT: The *Sound Effects Recognition Test* (SERT) is a nonlinguistic test (Finitzo-Hieber, Gerlin, Matkin, and Chernow-Skalka, 1980). This test, although not truly a word recognition test, was designed to assess the ability of the kindergarten child to recognize sounds within their own spontaneous language. It is a closed-set picture test in which the child must point to one of four pictures.

Methods

Presentation of test materials to children is usually performed using monitored live voice, if test materials permit. This format allows for the greater flexibility needed when working with a child. The audiologist can reinforce when indicated, use encouragement, change instructions, and otherwise do what is necessary to elicit responses. Obviously, certain tests, such as the SERT and PSI require recorded materials.

Informal assessment of word recognition by young children is also achieved by asking the youngster to point to various body parts. This can be done with a simple command or question or by playing the game 'Simple Simon says'.

Applications of Speech Audiometry to Aural Rehabilitation

Hearing Aid Evaluation and Selection

Traditionally the speech recognition threshold (SRT) and word recognition score (WRS) have been used in hearing aid evaluation and selection (Carhart, 1946a, b). The SRT is still used (although less frequently today) to choose the amount of gain of the hearing aid. This technique can lead to over-amplification, especially of the low frequencies. Pre- and post-evaluation comparisons of word recognition scores are still used to select the hearing aid system providing the maximum speech intelligibility score. Despite the fact that the WRS does not adequately discriminate one hearing aid from another (Shore, Bilger and Hirsch, 1960), the Carhart method has dominated clinical practice for over 40 years (Studebaker, 1980). This domination may exist because improvement in speech intelligibility is the primary goal of the hearing aid selection procedure. Fortunately, there has been a recent move away from using the word recognition test scores as the major determinant in hearing aid system selection. This move may be partially due to the greater understanding of the binomial distribution as it relates to reliability and paired-comparison variability issues (Studebaker, 1982). This move may be partially due also to research clarifying the contribution of the sound transmission characteristics of the external ear, its resonance, and eardrum impedance (Zwislocki, 1971; Djupesland and Zwislocki, 1972; Rabinowitz, 1981).

Methods other than comparison of word recognition test scores are gaining in clinical popularity for hearing aid system selection. Currently, some clinicians and clinical researchers have begun to use real-ear frequency specific methods hearing aid system selection (e.g. Pascoe, 1975; Byrne and Tonnisson, 1976; Berger, 1976; Lybarger, 1978). The hearing aid system selection procedures now emphasize comparison of unaided and aided pure-tone thresholds (functional gain), the application of prescriptive methods, and real-ear probe-microphone sound pressure measures of the patient. Alternative methods discussed by Studebaker (1982) include judgements of intelligibility, aided trials (Green and Ross, 1968; Gengel, Pascoe and Shore, 1971; Victoreen, 1973) and judgements of quality (Punch *et al.*, 1980). Although speech audiometry is still an important part of current research focussing on validation of different hearing aid system selection procedures, optimal hearing aid system selection methods are an enigma (Schwartz, 1982).

Rehabilitation

Until recently, the rehabilitation process had not received serious attention from either clinical or research audiologists. Traditional approaches focussed on speech reading emphasizing both phonetic and synthetic analysis of speech. Rehabilitation now covers a broader scope. It includes counselling, speech reading, and training to optimize the individual's ability to synthesize both auditory and visual cues. The development of new training techniques and new devices which enhance training have helped to improve the impaired listener's ability to make more and more complex phonemic distinctions.

PHONEME RECOGNITION: The use of monosyllabic word tests in aural rehabilitation is limited because they do not accurately reflect the individual's everyday communication ability. Other factors such as motivation, speech reading ability, intelligence, and language skill contribute to the individual's communicative success in real life situations. Most clinicians do use the CID W-22 or NU-6 monosyllabic word lists in order to assess word recognition ability, but these lists, used in their traditional open-set format do not allow for easy phoneme error analysis. As mentioned earlier, other types of tests such as the Modified Rhyme Test (MRT), and California Consonant Test (CCT) help in identifying those phoneme errors and confusions made by the hearing impaired listener. The Nonsense Syllable Test (NST) can be used when it is necessary to eliminate the problem of word familiarity and reduce memory effects. On the other hand when highly contextual material is needed, sentence materials such as the CHABA sentences are available. The SPIN test provides the clinician with a sentence test which varies in the amount of contextual cues offering both high- and low-predictability items.

Research on phonemic recognition (e.g. Miller and Nicely, 1955; Walden and Montgomery, 1975; Bilger and Wang, 1976) has revealed that certain distinctive features facilitate intelligibility: nasality, sonorance, voicing. Some consonants are more easily confused than others. Training programmes are being developed which focus on making same-different discriminations of consonant sounds in different word and sentence contexts, adjusting the level of complexity of the confusions to maximize learning (Kopra *et al.*, 1985).

More recently the major aim of an aural rehabilitation programme is towards synthetic analysis of connected discourse. Attention is still given to auditory and visual training using a more analytic approach but with the understanding that these two modalities are complimentary. Visual cues which are not distinguishable from each other, i.e. within group visemes (Woodward and Barber, 1960; Binnie, Montgomery, and Jackson, 1974) can be processed through the aid of auditory cues. On the other hand, auditory cues which are homophonous result in within-group confusions (Miller and Nicely, 1955) which can be resolved with visual input. For example, the homophones /p, t, k/ are visually recognizable due to differences in place of articulation, whereas the visemes /p, b, m/ are more easily differentiated auditorily. Thus, an aural rehabilitation programme must include phoneme recognition work to train across homophone and viseme boundaries. In addition, training must extend beyond phonemic recognition to include recognition of contextual, situational and pragmatic features of the communication process using both the auditory and visual modalities. The rehabilitation programme moves from easy or highly contextual materials, such as sentence materials, to more difficult or less contextual materials, such as monosyllables.

SPEECH TRACKING: A more recent approach which emphasizes the need for simultaneous analysis of visual and auditory cues is speech 'tracking' (De Filippo and Scott, 1978, Owens and Telleen, 1981). In this method the speaker and listener sit face-to-face so that the hearing-impaired patient is able to receive auditory, visual, and kinesthetic cues. The task of the patient is to repeat short segments of connected discourse spoken by the talker. Improvement is measured as an increase in speed of recognition in words per minute, or increased percent words correctly identifed. Passages are repeated at subsequent therapy sessions. The technique is gaining in popularity for the profoundly hearing impaired/deaf. The limitations to the procedure include no standardized materials or procedure, live-voice presentation, and tester/ therapist dependent modes of cueing the patient to repeat the connected discourse correctly.

MAC BATTERY: Another new series of tests has been developed for use with the severe-to-profound population. The *Minimal Auditory Capabilities* (MAC) battery (Owens *et al.*, 1981; revision: Owens *et al.*, 1985) is currently being used to evaluate potential candidates for a cochlear implant. The MAC consists of fourteen subtests (13 auditory and 1 lip reading) which include recognition of environmental sounds, phonemes, words, and sentences. These tests were designed to assess the auditory capabilities of those patients for whom routine speech recognition materials are too difficult and to provide a profile of those patients' speech recognition abilities which could be useful in the determination of an appropriate rehabilitation programme.

SELF-ASSESSMENT INVENTORIES: Interest in evaluating a patient's communication impairment in everyday life has led to the development of numerous hearing handicap inventories (Giolas *et al.*, 1979; Alpiner, 1978; Rupp, Higgins, and Maurer, 1977; Ventry and Weinstein, 1982; Weinstein and Ventry, 1982). A short description is presented of two useful scales, the Hearing Performance Inventory and the Hearing Handicap Inventory for the Elderly.

The Hearing Performance Inventory (HPI) is a questionnaire which permits the self-assessment of speech reception abilities (Giolas *et al.*, 1979). The individual is able to assess his/her own ability to understand speech in a variety of listening situations including speech in quiet, speech in noise, and speech with only auditory (no visual) cues available. Test items are divided

233

into six categories: understanding of speech, intensity, response, social, personal and occupational. The individual rates his/her behaviour in a particular everyday situation. Results from the HPI provide insight into the individual's own perception of communicative handicap but do not necessarily correlate well with speech recognition performance measures (Rowland, Dirks, Dubno and Bell, 1985).

The Hearing Handicap Inventory for the Elderly (HHIE) examines the patient's communication difficulties as well as the psychosocial effects of hearing loss on the patient's daily activities. A sample question on the HHIE is: 'Does a hearing problem cause you to visit friends, relatives, or neighbours less often than you would like?' (Ventry and Weinstein, 1982; Weinstein and Ventry, 1982). The HHIE provides a subjective evaluation of the patient's degree of handicap and can thus be helpful in predicting successful hearing aid use.

Research Directions

The directions for research in speech intelligibility are multifaceted. Some research will focus on the issues of validation and reliability of newly developed speech recognition tests with special relevance to hearing aid assessment and aural rehabilitation. Other current research includes a reinvestigation of the Articulation Index (AI). The AI is being evaluated for its predictive ability of the speech intelligibility of hearing impaired individuals (Pavlovic, Studebaker and Sherbecoe, 1985). The AI is also being compared with other prediction schemes such as the Speech Transmission Index (STI) as predictors of speech recognition performance in normal listeners (Humes, Boney and Ahlstrom, 1985) and hearing impaired listeners. Determination of hearing aid efficiency with an Articulation Index procedure is also being investigated (Marincovich and Studebaker, 1985).

Our society's current interest is in applications of high technology. There is ongoing research in the application of computers to clinical and educational programmes, particularly in the area of aural rehabilitation and real ear hearing aid fitting (Aitken and Bianco, 1985; Traynor *et al.*, 1985). For example, the winning scientific exhibit at the recent ASHA meeting was the application of the laser videodisc as an interactive system for computer-assisted instruction in speech reading (Kopra *et al.*, 1985). Computer use for the scoring of word recognition tests such as the SSW is also being evaluated (Condon, 1985).

A plethora of assistive listening devices has recently emerged on the market for hearing-impaired listeners. Some are directly coupled to the individual's hearing aid and others are independent. Research is beginning in areas of selection and fitting of these devices as well as in their use in therapy.

The use of speech materials in the development of hearing aid assessment procedures continues (Schum and Collins, 1985; Mintz, Johnson, Stach and Jerger, 1985; Neuman, Mills, and Schwander, 1985). Newer tests such as the PSI are also being evaluated for hearing aid use (Loiselle, 1985). Research in the area of aural rehabilitation is still focussed on developing and using new speech reading materials such as the Utah Vowel Imitation Test (U-VIT) as well as more traditional materials such as the CID W-22 mono-syllables (Koike, 1985; Spitzer *et al.*, 1985; Erb, 1985).

The development of new sensory aids for the severe and profoundly hearing impaired/deaf includes vibrotactile (Bernstein and Goldstein, 1985) and electrotactile devices (Saunders and Franklin, 1985). The work with cochlear implants has been the impetus for a significant amount of speech recognition research (Miller and Weisenberger, 1985; Carney, 1985; Weisen-berger *et al.*, 1985; Otto *et al.*, 1985; Brimacombe *et al.*, 1985; McCandless and Dankowski, 1985).

It is hoped that more research will be directed towards the development of clinical branching strategies which will improve the efficiency of speech audiometry procedures. Such strategies might include: more selective use of the SRT, appropriate use of pure-tone estimates of levels at which to present suprathreshold speech recognition materials, and increased use of perform-ance-intensity functions to assess speech intelligibility.

Chapter 12

The Scandinavian Approach to Speech Audiometry

S. Arlinger

The Scandinavian countries show many similarities with regard to how audiological service and practice are carried out. However, on closer inspection, when looking for a unified Scandinavian or Nordic approach to speech audiometry, one finds a considerable number of differences, the causes of which may be historical more often than being based on different scientific conclusions. The fact that Finnish belongs to the group of Finno-Ugric languages while Swedish, Norwegian and Danish are part of the Germanic languages also gives rise to some differences.

Naturally, it is impossible to be absolutely complete in trying to cover a subject of this nature. However, it is the intention to include the main aspects of speech audiometric testing for diagnostic and rehabilitative purposes as well as of technical equipment and principles of calibration. Also, some scientific projects concerning speech audiometry in Scandinavia will be discussed. Since the author's main experience stems from Sweden, that country will receive the most attention; I hope my fellow-Nordic colleagues will forgive me.

Routine Diagnostic Testing

Speech Reception Threshold

For the determination of Speech Reception Threshold, SRT, the most common test material is bisyllabic words, spondees. However, monosyllabic words and three-digit-combinations are also used.

In Sweden three lists of spondees are available, each containing 24 words. The words are presented alone without any carrier phrase. The interval between successive test words is about 5 seconds. The test lists used today were originally developed by Liden in his 1954 dissertation. The original version was recorded on gramophone records. In 1965 a revision was made by the Department of Technical Audiology, Karolinska Institute in Stockholm, when a number of test words were discarded as being too difficult semantically for hearing-impaired listeners. New recordings were made, this time on magnetic tape. The master tapes are stored at the Department of Technical Audiology, where all copies are produced for the clinics in Sweden. However, since copying a material recorded on magnetic tape is a simple procedure, a number of home-copied versions are obviously also in use in many clinics and hearing centres. Still, essentially all routine clinical speech audiometry in Sweden makes use of the same test material.

In Norway, bisyllabic test material is available in the form of twelve test lists of thirty words each, developed by Quist-Hanssen. However, SRT-values are usually not determined by means of those but instead a complete discrimination curve is usually determined using monosyllabic test words (see below).

In Denmark, up till now several sets of test lists have been in use at the different clinics and hearing centres. In the early 1950s, test lists were produced, which contained both one- and two-syllable words. Between 1970 and 1980 test lists were produced, based solely on monosyllabic test words and which gradually replaced the older material. No national standard material exists but at least three different sets of speech lists are being used at different clinics. However, at present, Elberling, Lyregaard and Ludvigsen are engaged in a project to produce a new test material to be recorded on Compact Disc and eventually to be used all over the country. For SRT-determinations, this material will make use of three-digit-combinations.

Finnish is a language which contains only a very few monosyllabic words. Thus, the test material that Jauhiainen developed for speech audiometry (1974) is based solely on bisyllablic words.

In Sweden, a standardized test procedure is used where the test words are first introduced at a level about 20 dB above the listener's pure tone average hearing threshold (0·5,1,2 kHz). The level is reduced in steps of 5 dB after a few test words have been presented until the patients start failing to identify the words correctly. Then ten test words are presented on that level. If five or more of the words were received correctly, the level is reduced by 5 dB and another set of ten test words are presented until a score of less than five out of ten is obtained. The SRT, defined as the level corresponding to a score of 50%, is determined by means of interpolation.

When contralateral masking is required to avoid the risk of cross-hearing, the commonly used clinical audiometers provide weighted noise with a slope of −12 dB/octave above 1 kHz. The necessary noise level, expressed in terms of effective masking level, is calculated as the speech level in the test ear minus 40 dB for the skull attenuation plus the average air-bone gap (0·5,1,2 kHz) for the masked ear. The masker level thus has to be changed when the speech level is changed during the testing.

Speech Discrimination

For the determination of Maximum Discrimination Score, monosyllabic test words are used in all Scandinavian countries except Finland since Finnish lacks such words in sufficient number.

In Sweden, twelve lists are available, originating from Liden (1954), each with 50 test words preceded by a carrier phrase: 'Now you'll hear . . .'. Each list is phonetically balanced and equalized. However, experience has shown that there are differences in degree of difficulty between the lists.

In Norway, fifteen lists of 35 monosyllabic test words each are available. They are presented without a carrier phrase, which has the consequence of a somewhat higher speech reception threshold. The usual clinical procedure is based on obtaining the complete discrimination curve by using these monosyllabic test words in groups of ten at each level tested. In addition, the discrimination curve obtained by means of digits as test words is recorded in a similar manner. Only if the levels corresponding to 50% correct for these two types of test words differ by more than 10 dB, is SRT determined by means of the spondee test lists. In other words, Norwegian speech audiometry clearly emphasizes the use of monosyllabic test words while spondees are used to a rather limited extent.

In Denmark speech discrimination scores are obtained by means of monosyllabic test-words. In the new test material being produced on compact discs, no phonetic balancing has been made in the recording, but each test-word is coded on the disc according to its phonetic content. Thus, this code can be used to organize test words in phonetically balanced lists at playback.

Finland, as already mentioned, lacks monosyllabic words which makes bisyllabic words the available alternative. The lists produced by Jauhiainen (1974) are six, each containing 25 test words preceded by a carrier phrase: 'You will hear the word . . .'.

The standardized Swedish clinical test procedure recommends a test level that the patient finds most comfortable. A starting level about 30 dB above the patient's SRT for the tested ear is usually suggested. If the patient wants a higher or lower test level, this is adjusted as required. A complete list of 50 monosyllabic test words is presented at the level chosen and the number of correctly identified and repeated test words is counted, each word corresponding to 2%. If the score is less than 70% other test levels are used to determine the shape of the curve, naturally with other test lists.

Since each complete list of 50 words is phonetically balanced, it is not recommended that only a part of a list is used. However, if after the first 25 words of a list the patient has missed at most one word, it is permissible to stop the test there in order to save time. The possible error is then considered negligible.

When contralateral masking is required, the same rules apply as for SRT-testing. When in some cases very high masking levels have to be used and the risk of over-masking appears, insert masking is recommended to reduce this risk. The insert ear-phone usually lacks reliable calibration. Therefore, in the calculation of necessary masking level the air-bone gap value of the ear to be masked is taken as the average difference at 0.5,1,2 kHz between air conduction thresholds, obtained with the particular insert ear-phone and ear-mould, and bone conduction thresholds.

Speech Audiometry in Rehabilitation Programmes

In addition to its use in measuring various characteristics of auditory physiology and patho-physiology, speech audiometry is an interesting tool to study the degree of handicap caused by a hearing impairment and the reduction in handicap offered by a hearing aid, other technical aids and various pedagogical rehabilitative measures.

This objective is usually based on a different test method as well as different speech material, as compared to diagnostic speech audiometry. The test is normally performed in a sound-field rather than by means of ear-phones. The purpose of the testing is to produce a measure of how the patient functions in a typical everyday listening situation. Thus, the sound-field often contains some degree of reverberation, i.e. a fairly normal room is preferred to an anechoic chamber. Normal speech is usually made up of relatively complete sentences. The ambient sound level is very rarely low but offers a relatively modest signal-to-noise ratio. Thus, the typical test material is based on sentences presented in a certain background noise. In a natural listening situation, the signal usually comes from a source with a specific location, towards which one tends to turn, while the ambient sound often originates from a number of different sources. Thus, the speech signal should be presented from a frontally located loudspeaker while the noise should be produced in other loudspeakers, located at different angles to the speech loudspeaker.

Speech audiometry is at present of rather limited use in rehabilitation programmes in Scandinavia. The probable reason for this is the relatively poor sensitivity of the method in differentiating between a better or a poorer hearing aid for a particular patient. This in turn may be due to the rather limited efforts put into developing special methods and test material specifically for this purpose. However, in some projects it has been shown to be capable of adding interesting information and has been sufficiently sensitive to show significant differences between group mean values. One example of this is the comparison in In-the-Ear and Behind-the-Ear hearing aids by Jerlvall *et al.* (1983).

Occasionally speech testing has been used to determine a listener's uncomfortable loudness level. Since the result of such a test is expressed in terms of hearing level for speech, it is rather difficult to apply to the choice or adjustment of hearing aids. This is due to the simple fact that hearing aid characteristics are usually expressed in terms based on pure tone or other narrow band signal measurements.

Recently, Hagerman (1982) has produced a new speech test material which might prove to be valuable with regard to hearing aid evaluation. It contains 12 lists, each list made up of ten five-word sentences. Each sentence contains one name, one verb, one digit, one adjective and one substantive, e.g. 'Gustav took eighteen black boxes'. Each list contains exactly the same words as the other lists but in different combinations and each list has a fairly good phonetic balance. Since the material is based on 50 words which all occur in all lists, only in different order, the lists are as equivalent as is possible.

The highest sensitivity in testing is obtained by presenting the word lists in a background of speech-shaped noise with the speech signal at a comfortable level. The background noise level is varied and the signal-to-noise ratio that gives 50% correct is determined (Hagerman, 1982, 1984). In normal hearing subjects he found a maximum slope of the discrimination function in speech-shaped noise of about 25% per dB change in signal-to-noise ratio.

In Denmark, considerable interest has been devoted to audio-visual speech perception with regard to hearing-aid performance and degree of hearing handicap. In the HELEN test (Ewertsen, 1973; Ludvigsen, 1974) the test material is based on sentences, and a correct score is based on whether the test subject understood the meaning of the sentence even if some words of minor importance are misunderstood. To avoid errors from tester bias, the sentences are formulated as questions, each to be answered by one single word. One example is the question: 'Which animal is biggest, a cat or a lion?' to be correctly answered by the single word 'Lion'.

Of course, in such speech material it is very difficult to obtain high equivalence between the various test lists. However, careful work has allowed the production of eight lists of 25 questions each with reasonable homogeneity and phonetic balance. Test material of this nature, intended to be used for auditory, visual and audio-visual presentation, is getting more attention lately in cochlear implant programmes.

Another application of speech audiometry to the measurement of degree of handicap, that should be included here, is the basic study by Aniansson (1974) concerning how even a rather small high frequency hearing loss contributes significantly to loss of speech discrimination in a noisy background. His results and those of additional studies have been of particular value in understanding the practical consequences of moderate degrees of noise induced hearing loss. His results have also been applied to define different degrees of handicap with regard to compensation for occupational hearing loss.

Distorted Speech Tests

In 1973, Margareta Korsan-Bengtsen published her dissertation on distorted speech audiometry. She applied a number of different distortions on her test material, consisting of sentences of 4–8 words each with four key words on which the scoring was based:

> interrupted speech with interruption rates of 4, 7 and 10 per sec and 50% duty cycle,
>
> frequency-distorted speech with a pass-band from 445 to 900 Hz time-compressed speech with speech rates at 220 and 290 words per minute.

In addition, she studied the effect of competing speech, in which test sentences were presented to the contralateral ear simultaneously with the presentation of a monosyllabic test word and its carrier phrase from the standard test lists for speech discrimination tests.

On subjects with normal hearing she found age to be a significant factor, which thus has to be taken into account in the clinical application of distorted speech tests. The main diagnostic aim of these tests is to detect central disorders that influence the information processing in the auditory pathways. Korsan-Bengtsen could show significantly reduced discrimination scores in patients with temporal lobe lesions involving the auditory cortex and with brainstem tumours involving the cochlear nuclei. She found interrupted speech and time-compressed speech to be the most sensitive test materials.

In a preliminary study on a group of patients with occupational exposure to industrial solvents of long duration, Ödkvist *et al.* (1982) found discrimination of distorted speech to be one of the few audio-vestibular tests that produced pathological results. This study is being continued and the results remain essentially stable: a significant effect is reduced discrimination of interrupted speech, interpreted as indicating a central neurological damage caused by the solvent exposure.

Speech Tests for Non-Organic Hearing Loss

Speech can also be used as a test signal in tests aimed at the detection of functional hearing loss, e.g., Stenger's test, Doerfler-Stewart's test and delayed-speech tests. However, particularly since the electrophysiological test methods became relatively common in the larger clinics, such speech tests are used very rarely.

Speech Audiometry for Children

Speech audiometry in children is naturally more difficult, since they are still developing their language skills and thus the construction of test material becomes rather more limited than with adult patients. Phonetic and linguistic requirements usually have to be reduced and more emphasis placed on the test words being simple and easy.

No standardized test material for children seems to exist in any Nordic country so far. In Sweden, taped test lists are commercially available, consisting of three-digit combinations and very simple mono- and bisyllabic test words. However, phonetic balance and equalization is not controlled. The Danish project of producing new standardized test material for speech audiometry also involves four test lists for children, each with 25 monosyllabic test words.

Technical Equipment

When speech audiometry started on a more regular scale in the 1950s, the gramophone record was the medium available. In Sweden, the records were used until around 1965, when tape recorders gradually took over as the revised test lists became available on regular $\frac{1}{4}$-inch magnetic tape. During the last few years, cassette recorders have gradually come into use in many clinics, replacing the older reel-to-reel recorders. The cassette offers a number of practical advantages: the cassettes by nature are very easy to put in and take out of the recorder. Each cassette can be given a tape length which exactly fits one test list whereby no winding needs to be done. One cassette for each test list means that all lists have essentially the same probability of being used and it is very easy to shift from one list to another with arbitrary combinations of lists. However, as can be expected the cassette recordings do have disadvantages also. The magnetic track on the tape is narrower, which makes the requirements on the recording or copying procedure quite severe. It is much easier to make a poor copy on cassette than on a $\frac{1}{4}$-inch tape with regard to signal-to-noise ratio, magnetic overload, and the general frequency characteristics of the recording. Thus, the new technique based on compact discs, where the signal stored is read by an optical detector based on a small laser, is of significant interest because it can offer both very high signal quality and easy handling. On the other hand, the recording is a more complex procedure with higher initial costs.

As already mentioned, a Danish project for nationally standardized speech test material will be recorded on compact disc. This approach is also being discussed in Sweden. In contrast to a tape recording, the compact disc is permanent and cannot be partially revised or edited. Thus, it is important that the test material to be recorded on compact disc should have a reasonable expected life.

Calibration

For the calibration of speech signal level, a test tone is usually recorded before or after the actual test list. On the Swedish lists, this is a 1 kHz tone with a level corresponding to the mean level of the test words as measured in dB C and time constant Fast. The strongest peaks of the test words may reach 10 to 15 dB above this level. When the speech audiometer is adjusted to correct level, an input level of this calibration tone that gives rise to a 0 dB reading on the VU-meter of the audiometer shall produce a sound level of 22 dB SPL when the TDH-39 ear-phone is placed on a 6 cc-coupler according to IEC 303 and the attenuator is set to 0 dB HL. So calibrated, a group of listeners with average pure tone hearing thresholds at 500 Hz, 1 kHz and 2 kHz (PTA) at 0 dB HL will have an average Speech Reception Threshold for spondees of 0 dB HL. The same reference level of 22 dB SPL for the calibration tone is then used for the monosyllabic test lists. This means that the average level necessary to reach 50% correct discrimination is around 5–6 dB HL (Liden, 1954).

On subjects with sensorineural hearing loss a slight difference between SRT and PTA may be expected. When the discrimination loss is of the order of 50%, an average SRT 5 to 6 dB above the PTA, both expressed in terms of dB hearing level, can be expected (Hagerman, 1979). On clinical patients this agreement between SRT and PTA is obtained with a standard deviation for the difference of the order of 5–7 dB (Hagerman, 1979).

In the Norwegian speech test material, a clear emphasis is placed on the monosyllabic test words. Thus the calibration of their speech audiometers refers to the 50% discrimination level for monosyllabic test words. The Norwegian calibration tone is recorded on a level 5 dB above the average level of the test words.

In the Finnish test lists, the 1 kHz calibration tone has been given a level equal to the average VU-meter reading of the first vowel of the test words. This is very close to the calibration tone level on the Swedish test lists. A reference level of 21 dB SPL for this tone, measured in a 6 cc-coupler, when the attenuator is set to 0 dB HL will give an average difference between SRT and PTA of zero on a group of normal-hearing listeners (Jauhiainen, 1974).

It is quite evident that although the differences in calibration rules are not large, the rules are still not identical. A standardization of the calibration tone level relative to the test word level, measured in a clearly defined way with regard to frequency weighting and time constant, is certainly desirable. The sound pressure level developed in the acoustic coupler with zero dB attenuator setting will of course have to differ, depending on language. A recommendation whether the calibration tone shall be adjusted with regard to the 50% discrimination level for that particular type of word or for bisyllabic words as the most common test material for SRT determination is of course also desirable.

Acknowledgement

Since very little has been published regarding the test material used in speech audiometry in Denmark and Norway, I turned to my two colleagues Carl Ludvigsen at the Children's Audiological Laboratory in Copenhagen and Arne Sundby at Ullevål Hospital in Oslo. For the very valuable information they provided, I am very grateful.

Chapter 13

Speech Audiometry in Australia

J. Bench

In writing for a book of speech audiometry which has a marked international flavour, it will be worth taking a little space to comment on some general characteristics of Australia and its population. Such characteristics will set a context for a discussion of Australian work in speech audiometry, and thereby assist the reader to appreciate the discussion which follows.

It is well known internationally that Australia occupies a very large land mass, which is approximately the same size as the United States of America. It is also well known that much of the country is desert or semi-desert (colloquial reference is made to the 'red centre') which is very sparsely populated. Most of the population lives close to the coast, especially the east and south-east coasts, which have hilly or mountainous regions close by (the Great Dividing Range), attract reasonable rainfall, and hence can support a population, which totals some fifteen million souls (Holmes, 1976). (The total population recently exceeded sixteen million).

What is much less well known is that the Australian population is heavily concentrated in the major eight city areas, which have grown up alongside the few great rivers. Hence the Australian population is heavily urbanized. About three quarters of the people lead an urban or suburban existence. They visit the deep country or desert areas relatively rarely, and then mainly for leisure purposes.

Immigration and Ethnicity

Population has always been an issue in Australia (Birrell and Birrell, 1981), usually on the grounds that there were not enough people, or that the rate of expansion of the population was too slow, or that the birthrate was falling. Australia has had a generous attitude to immigration, and this is reflected in its population growth. The population has now more than doubled from the 7.6 million of 1947 (Birrell and Birell, loc. cit.), mostly due to the encouragement of immigration. This emphasis on immigration has increasingly

247

emphasised immigration from Europe other than the United Kingdom and Eire, and from Asia. Thus about ten to fourteen per cent of the Australian population does not have English as a first language.

There is then a large minority of non Anglo-Australians comprised of ethnic groups. These ethnic people (and often their children) do not have English as their first language. This may not be appreciated by the non-Australian reader, who may have been led to expect that any lack of familiarity with English would be limited to the Aboriginal population. This latter population is, however, small (Cameron, 1985) albeit with a high incidence of middle ear disease, especially amongst its young children (Lewis, 1979). It amounts to just over 1% of the total population, and most of its members speak good or fair English. Aboriginal Health Workers are particularly aware of the value of early screening for hearing problems in children.

It might be thought that special efforts would have been made to develop materials and techniques in speech audiometry specifically for the ethnic population,and to train ethnic staff to administer and assess the results of such special speech audiometric tests. Such developments have frequently been discussed by audiologists and some teachers of the deaf. But these developments are only just beginning to be explored in a systematic way. The main reason is that the Anglo-Australians are by far the dominant social and cultural group, and acceptance of ethnic or cultural pluralism is a relatively recent phenomenon (Martin, 1978).

In this context, a current project (Osborn, 1985) is being conducted into speech audiometry for different ethnic groups at the Lincoln Institute in Melbourne. This project seeks to compare the responses of (1) monolingual (English-speaking), (2) monolingual (Greek or Vietnamese speaking) people who have attended language classes in English, and (3) bilingual (English and Greek or English and Vietnamese speaking) people, to Boothroyd word lists spoken by an Australian English speaker. The definitions of monolingual and bilingual used in this study are those suggested by Danhauer *et al.* (1984). The results of this study are awaited with interest.

The Provision of Audiological and Aural Rehabilitation Services

The Australian Bureau of Statistics has published surveys of 'Hearing and the Use of Hearing Aids' (1979), and 'Sight, Hearing and Dental Health' (1980) which provide a broad overview of the incidence of significant aspects of hearing impairment in Australia. These surveys cover hearing problems by age, sex, cause, age at first occurrence, surgical operations, possession of a hearing aid, prices of aids, types of aids, use and non-use of aids, recency of tests and types of tests (with or without an audiometer, but it is not possible to discover from the reports how many of the audiometric tests involved speech audiometry).

The main national agency for the provision of audiological services is the National Acoustic Laboratories (NAL), formerly the Commonwealth Acoustic Laboratories (CAL). NAL has its main base in Sydney, where its techniques are researched, and large centres in the major cities throughout the several States of the country. The very large cities, such as Melbourne, may have several NAL centres. NAL has been active for many years in audiological diagnostics, including speech audiometry, and in the design and supply of hearing aids (free for those under 21 years or over retiring age — adults of working age must pay for their hearing aids). More recently NAL has begun to consider services beyond the above, in aural rehabilitation and counselling.

Other main agencies providing audiological services are hospitals (especially the larger hospitals) and the Health Departments of the State Governments, but there are a large number of other agencies which provide some audiological services, the sum total of which is far from negligible (cf. Bench and Duerdoth, 1983).

These latter agencies make a considerable contribution to aural rehabilitation, covering counselling, education, training, and advice, as well as those aspects of aural rehabilitation immediately related to hearing impairment (e.g. how to get the best performance from a hearing aid). The provision of services through these agencies is a complex operation involving a large number of professional, semi-professional, ancillary and volunteer personnel (Bench and Duerdoth, 1983). Also, the types of agencies are quite different, involving public, private and charitable organisations. This results in the potential for communication problems between agencies and possible confusion for patients. To avoid these, most agencies are members of (or, in the case of some public agencies, have observer status in) the Australian Deafness Council, a charitable body which offers a coordinating umbrella function for all agencies offering services to hearing-impaired people in Australia.

Speech Audiometry and Australian English Usage

The assessment of hearing for speech is clearly dependent on the familiarity of the speech material to the listener. This means that the English content of material for speech audiometry in Australia should reflect Australian English usage. Australian English has a basic similarity to English as spoken in the United Kingdom, but increasingly reflects North American English usage, besides containing some expressions, phrases, and word usages which are essentially Australian (e.g., 'milk bar', very roughly equivalent to the American 'drug store' or the English 'corner shop'). Standard Australian English is very similar to standard English as regards grammar, but a minority of words (especially nouns or noun phrases and some verbs) as used in English may have a somewhat different meaning in Australia (Bench and Doyle, 1979). Thus whereas in Australia one 'barracks for' (i.e., expresses support), in the United Kingdom one 'barracks against' (i.e.; decries), a team or group. Interestingly, the verb 'to barrack' in the sense of 'decry' or 'jeer' as used in United Kingdom is Aboriginal Australian in origin, whereas, used in the sense of support, it is Irish in origin (Macquarie Dictionary). There has been something of a cross-over in usage between the two hemispheres.

For the reader who may wish to consider these matters further, the style and usages of Australian English have been reported by Blair (1977) and Mitchell and Delbridge (1965).

Word and Phoneme Tests and their Usage

The major audiological centres (NAL and audiology departments in the larger hospitals and in tertiary education institutions) make use of a variety of word and phoneme tests for clinical speech audiometry, most of which will be familiar to audiologists in English-speaking countries. Many of the more esoteric tests are used as screening tests (Wilde, 1985) for the more difficult-to-test patients, and as adjuncts to the clinical assessment of patients with central auditory problems.

Perhaps the most commonly used test (especially as an initial speech audiometry test) is the Boothroyd word lists (Boothroyd, 1968), usually scored by whole words reported correctly. The lists are available in Australia from recordings spoken with a middle Australian accent. Boothroyd's word lists are popular clinically because of their long history of usage, familiarity to all audiologists, convenient length, and convenience of scoring. Other tests used include the Kendall Toy Test (Kendall, 1956), the Word Intelligibility by Picture Identification (WIPI) Test (Ross and Lerman, 1970), the Modified Rhyme Test (House *et al.*, 1965), the CAL-PBM lists (Australian: Macrae *et al.*, 1963), the Clark PB word lists (Australian: Clark, 1981), the HRRC Rhyme Test (Eisenberg *et al.*, 1977) various nonsense syllable tests, the PLOTT Test (Australian: Plant, 1984b), and the Auditory Numbers (ANT) Test (Erber, 1980).

Of these the PLOTT Test, as developed by Plant and his colleagues in Sydney, is a recently devised comprehensive speech perception test, which requires a further period of time for thoroughgoing evaluation as a tool in speech audiometry. It consists of nine subtests for phoneme detection; number patterns; monosyllable, trochee, spondee and polysyllable distinctions; a picture vocabulary test; vowel length discrimination; vowel discrimination; initial voiced and voiceless stop consonant discrimination; consonant manner of articulation discrimination; and discrimination of place of articulation for consonants. The PLOTT test shows considerable promise in helping to decide whether a hearing-impaired person can perceive spectral information, or only time and intensity cues. Many children with hearing losses greater than 100 dB (ISO) were found by Plant (*loc. cit.*) to use spectral information in speech perception, and even those children who seemed to be limited to the use of time/intensity cues were able to distinguish between a number of vowel and consonant contrasts.

Upfold and Smither (1981) have outlined the use of the CUNY Nonsense Syllable Test (Levitt and Resnik, 1978), the Modified Rhyme Test, the Norton HRRC Rhyme Test, the Monosyllable, Trochee, Spondee Test (Erber and Alencewicz, 1976), and the SPIN Test (adapted for Australian speech characteristics) in a systematic Hearing-aid Fitting Protocol designed for use by NAL. This set of tests is designed for demonstration, counselling, training and potential verification of phonetic correlates of aided pure-tone information.

It is of interest that the CAL-PBMs and the Clark lists were especially designed for Australian usage, yet they are now infrequently used. Why should this be so?

The CAL-PBM lists consist of twelve lists each of 25 monosyllables, designed to be phonemically balanced across lists and to reflect common occurrence in Australian speech. However, Grant (1980) showed that, although 34% of the phonemes correlated well, 44% did not correlate well, with a sample of Australian speech. Further, across the lists, 29% of phonemes showed a wide range of occurrence, but 66% of phonemes did not occur in one or more lists. She concluded that the CAL-PBM lists could not be considered to be phonemically balanced.

Clark's word lists were derived from the Northwestern University Auditory Test No. 6, but were specially designed for Australian English. Clark's criteria for the design were: (i) monosyllabic CVC word structure; (ii) exact interlist phonological balance; (iii) minimal intralist phonotactic redundancy; (iv) high lexical familiarity; and (v) phonological distribution generally compatible with that for monosyllabic words in Australian English. Clark's lists do not appear to have been taken up by Australian audiologists to any great extent, despite their apparent virtues. The main reasons are clear: there are too few lists and each list is rather long (there are only four lists, each of 50 monosyllables).

It seems then that the CAL-PBM lists are phonemically suspect, and each list is relatively long (25 monosyllables compared with Boothroyd's twelve monosyllables), while the Clark lists are much too few, and each list is too long, for regular clinical use.

Byrne (1983) in Sydney has reviewed the area of word intelligibility in speech audiometry as it affects the assessment of speech-hearing in children. Byrne notes that a basic principle in designing word intelligibility tests is that the words should be familiar to the youngest age group for which the test is designed. He found that his youngest group of children tested ($4\frac{1}{2}$ to $6\frac{1}{2}$ years of age) performed at a poorer level than the next youngest group ($6\frac{1}{2}$ to 8 years), and both these groups performed more poorly than his oldest group (8 to 14 years), even though all the stimulus words, in a closed set. were known to the children. This finding confirms similar reports elsewhere (e.g., in the USA by Elliot *et al.*, 1983). It seems that knowledge of stimulus words is not enough; experience of the words is an important factor also, and such experience needs to be considered in divising speech audiometry materials (cf. Bench and Bamford, 1979). Byrne comments that speech perception thresholds calculated for young children, if interpreted according to expectations of adult performance, could be interpreted as a hearing loss for speech, when their performance fell inside the usual range for their age group. The implications for patient management of making such an error are clear, as is the need for a 'normal subjective calibration' of any speech test materials. In passing, we may note that a somewhat similar error may be incurred if the data of speech audiometric tests with words are interpreted as directly reflecting everyday hearing of spoken English (cf. Hood and Poole, 1971), because word lists do not contain grammatical and contextual cues.

Sentence Tests and Usage

Sentence lists and other suprasegmental tests are used relatively rarely in routine speech audiometry testing in Australia (as elsewhere). Some use is made of the SPIN Test (Kalikow *et al.*, 1977), where there is a need to control for context predictability, and the Minimal Auditory Capabilities (MAC) test battery (Owens *et al.*, 1980) is used in some centres (Blamey *et al.*, 1985). As Clark (*loc. cit.*) has pointed out, the choice between word lists and sentences as test material for speech audiometry depends upon the intended application and test stringency. Sentences offer high-level contextual linguistic cues in their semantic and syntactic structure, enabling a listener to predict a word relatively accurately with relatively little reliance on the acoustic information from the actual stimulus material. Words, however, require more stringent perceptual skills on the part of the listener in that the listener is forced to rely heavily on the acoustic information of the test words.

The only set of sentence lists designed for use in Australia and available for use are those developed by Tonisson (1977), although Bench and Doyle (*loc. cit.*), have prepared a set of BKB (Bench and Bamford, *loc. cit.*) sentence lists for use with hearing-impaired children which is currently being standardized in Australia and will be released shortly for use, and Dermody (1985) is currently preparing materials for assessing central auditory dysfunction. Tonisson's lists reflect the Central Institute of the Deaf (Davis and Silverman, 1970) Everyday Sentences. They consist of nine lists, each containing ten sentences or common phrases and 50 key words. The phraseology used and the length of the sentences makes these sentences appropriate for older children and adults, rather than the younger hearing-impaired child.

Clinical Practice and Reporting

It is disappointing that the results of most Australian standardization exercises for speech audiometry materials (both word and sentence lists) are difficult to find in easily accessible publications. Standardization data are readily available only for the word lists of Clark (*loc. cit.*). For most other test materials it resides in the vaults of various institutions or in the knowledge of the workers in those institutions. A similar comment could be made about the accessibility of reports of interesting clinical cases.

This reflects a considerable variation across the nation in the use of different kinds of speech audiometry tests even for similar purposes, and a relative paucity of systematic reporting of clinical findings which might be of use to colleagues. Exceptions to this situation as regards standardization would include the widespread use of the standardized Boothroyd word lists, and the standardized techniques of NAL which are developed in Sydney, and then put to use in the NAL centres throughout the country. In the latter context, reference has already been made to the work of Upfield and Smithers on the Hearing-aid Fitting Protocol.

This general situation is doubtless universal. A large number of speech audiometric tests in English have been developed over many years and are being used in many countries. Clinically, the audiologist practitioner cannot escape the 'tyranny of the particular' (Medawar, 1965). When faced with a variety of particular clinical cases and a shortage of time in which to assess and treat the patient, the audiologist will seek to use that test or approach, from amongst the large number available, which appears to offer the most useful information in the available time. This exigency encourages neither systematic reporting nor uniformity of procedure. The existence of NAL has had some unifying effect on a standardized approach to clinical work in speech audiometry in Australia, such that there may be a relatively more coherent approach to the area in Australia than in other countries. On the other hand, NAL publishes relatively little, apart from research papers and summary statistics.

Summary

Speech audiometry in Australia is conducted much like speech audiometry in other English speaking countries. The same kinds of tests are used, usually adapted for Australian needs, there is a wide range of such tests in use, the same techniques are employed, and the same problems are encountered. There is a lack of readily available public reports on the use of speech audiometry in Australia (as in other countries) which makes it difficult to tease out issues where Australian experiences may differ from experiences elsewhere.

One area where Australia has needs which would be rather different from some other English-speaking countries, is that of designing and using speech audiometry tests for its significant ethnic population, which comes mainly from Europe (excluding the UK and Eire) and from South East Asia. Work in this field is just beginning.

Australia differs too, in having a major national service, the National Acoustic Laboratories with centres distributed across the country. NAL allows of standardization of approach to speech audiometry and other services. It has the potential to provide clinical information for a large number of patients over a period of many years. It would be of great help and interest if this information could be collated and published. The following chapter by Dermody and Mackie goes some way to addressing this need.

Chapter 14

Speech Tests in Audiological Assessment at the National Acoustic Laboratories

P. Dermody and J. Mackie

The National Acoustic Laboratories consist of a research organization and a national network of Hearing Centres which provide audiological services to those under the age of 21 years as well as adults who receive government pension benefits including age pensions, sickness, supporting parents and veterans benefits. These categories collectively total about 7% of the Australian population who are entitled to audiological services from the National Acoustic Laboratories (NAL). In addition NAL sees several other classes of client including those seeking compensation from the government for noise induced hearing loss and aircraft pilots who require audiological assessment as part of their medical check.

As a consequence of this clinical caseload, NAL has requirements for speech tests for a range of audiological purposes including paediatric evaluations (NAL Paediatric Audiological Protocols Manual, 1984); hearing aid evaluations (Byrne, 1981); and evaluations for aural rehabilitation requirements (Upfold and Smither, 1981). However, the use of speech reception measures is restricted to assessment of communication adequacy, and does not include speech tests used for site-of-lesion evaluation in medical audiology. In Australia, medical audiology is typically carried out in hospital audiology clinics which are not connected to NAL.

Traditionally NAL has relied on research into speech tests available from audiological research overseas and has adapted these measures for its clinical requirements. This has usually involved development and standardization to meet the needs of dialect and local conditions. More recently and as part of the growing trend of disillusionment with traditional speech measures NAL has begun to investigate the use of new speech reception assessment techniques for clinical practice. In 1982 Mackie and Dermody published a report on the use of monosyllabic word tests in audiological assessment. This review discussed many of the problems in the traditional use of word tests and suggested the need for further research.

The present summary considers the traditional speech tests available for children and adults in NAL and their adaptation to local conditions. In addition, it discusses the recent developments that are at present under way to improve the speech reception assessment protocols available for clinical practice, and considers the future directions of this research.

Traditional Speech Reception Tests for Adults

Word Recognition Tests for General Adult Clinical Cases

Post-Second World War, developments produced several word lists for audiological application including the Psychoacoustic Laboratories (PAL) phonetically balanced (PB) lists (Egan, 1948) and the W-22 and W-2 lists (Hirsh, 1952). In the United Kingdom a set of lists based on 25 words (in contrast to the 50 words in the PAL PB lists) were also developed (Medical Research Council, 1947).

NAL (which was known as the Commonwealth Acoustic Laboratories — CAL — until the change of name in 1973) was influenced by these developments and during 1949–1951 recorded versions were made by an Australian speaker of the W-2 spondee word lists and 12 of the 20 PAL PB lists. These materials were recorded on 78 rpm records and in the case of the spondee words there was a 2 dB decrement in intensity every 4 words to aid in the determination of the 50% recognition threshold for the words.

The CAL Audiology Manual first published in 1953 indicated the need to perform recognition threshold tests with the spondee words to confirm pure-tone thresholds. In addition, PB words were presented at 110 dB SPL to indicate the word recognition performance plateau (the PB maximum score). It was also suggested that the results be used with the Social Adequacy Index (Davis, 1948).

By 1960 the CAL Audiology Manual adopted the use of 25 word lists as an alternative to the PAL PB lists to estimate PB max. These lists were based on the British lists (Medical Research Council, 1947) and were called the Phonetically Balanced Monosyllable (PBM) lists. To compensate for the reduced reliability of the 25 word lists, it was recommended that the lists be administered using 3 estimates of the performance-intensity (PI) curve. The initial presentation level was at 10 dB above the most comfortable listening level for speech. Another list was then presented at the most comfortable listening level while a third list was presented at 10 dB below the most comfortable level or at about the 50% recognition point if that could be estimated. Spondee lists were no longer recommended since it was felt that they provided little additional information to the puretone audiogram. Macrae, Woodroffe and Farrant (1963) recorded and standardized these lists, which have remained an integral part of speech discrimination evaluation of adult clients in NAL until recently.

In 1969 the CAL Audiology Manual changed the recommended adult speech test protocol, abandoning the PI function and recommending the use of average 3 frequency hearing loss for predicting presentation levels to obtain a PB max score. The recommendations included a presentation level of 90, 100, 110, 120 and 130 dB SPL for average hearing levels of 0–40, 41–60, 61–85, 86–100 and greater than 100 dB HL respectively. The use of the 50% spondee recognition score was not recommended. Because of the change from PI functions to single lists at only one level, it was suggested that less than 12% differences in the PBM list scores were non-significant and less than 20% were questionable. These estimates were based on the standardization data of Macrae *et al.* (1963). The change from PI function to single list produced a significant saving in clinical time but represented a much less reliable speech test methodology.

The practice of using a single list to determine PB max was maintained until about 1977 and used primarily for measuring perceptual differences in the ears that were not obvious from the pure tone audiogram and as a rough indication of the potential benefits of a hearing aid. The major reason for the shift away from the use of PB word lists was the adoption by NAL of a hearing aid selection procedure based on pure tone thresholds (Byrne and Tonnisson, 1976). This aid fitting procedure, developed at NAL, based aid selection on unaided tonal thresholds and confirmed the adequacy of the aid selection using aided tonal thresholds. Speech tests were not used as part of this procedure.

The reluctance to use speech tests was also reinforced by studies at NAL which highlighted the limitations of the NAL PBM word lists, consisting of only 25 items, to reliably measure anything but very gross differences in speech reception (Dermody and Byrne, 1975). Finally, a decision by NAL not to restandardize the PBM lists after the masters were found to be unusable led to a further decline in their clinical application. NAL, however, did rerecord the PBM lists, using the original speaker, and copies of the recordings were distributed as an unstandardized test.

The continuing need for speech tests in audiological assessment was however recognized and Upfold and Smither (1981) introduced a range of speech materials for clinical use. The philosophy used to generate these protocols reflected a significant change in the direction for the use of speech materials in NAL. The new protocols were developed as part of NAL's post hearing aid fitting programme for adult clients. The aim of the new protocols was to determine the success of the hearing aid fitting and/or to form the basis of decisions about requirements for aural rehabilitation, in addition to the hearing aid. Upfold and Smither did not recommend any speech tests as part of the audiological workup prior to fitting the aid except the PBM lists as required. However, a range of speech materials were advocated, post-fitting, to be used depending on the auditory receptive communication abilities of the client. The decision process and test options are presented in Figure 1. The

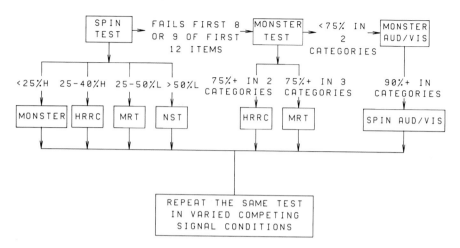

Figure 1.   Decision processes for speech tests post hearing aid fitting. The SPIN test used as the primary decision maker. Reproduced by kind permission of the authors.

protocol is based on the SPIN test (Kalikow, Stevens and Elliott, 1977) given live voice, at conversational level, with the client wearing hearing aids on the recommended settings.

The SPIN test requires the subject to repeat the final word of a sentence. In half the sentences the final word is highly predictable from the context and in the other sentences the final word has low predictability. Upfold and Smither suggest that clinicians use the SPIN test results as an indication of aided speech reception abilities, as well as the client's ability to use linguistic and contextual information. The SPIN results are also used to determine the difficulty of additional testing using speech reception assessment materials. The aim is to select materials on which the subject will perform at a level which reveals their difficulties with speech. The range of speech tests incorporated into the protocols includes the CUNY Nonsense Syllable Test (Levitt and Resnick, 1978); the modified Rhyme Test (House *et al.*, 1965); the Norton HRRC Rhyme Test (Eisenberg *et al.*, 1977); the Monosyllable, Trochee, Spondee Test — MONSTER (Erber and Alencewicz, 1976). These speech tests were chosen because they all use a closed set format to improve reliability and decrease the effects of linguistic factors. They also provide some data on phoneme reception abilities of the client as a basis for demonstration of speech cues, counselling on hearing aid use and hearing tactics, and auditory training.

These test protocols are currently used in NAL for general adult clinical cases. However, the procedures used in the protocols were adopted as an interim solution and the materials given live voice. No attempt has been made to record or standardize the materials.

Speech Tests with Other Adult Clinical Groups

The primary caseload at NAL is made up of elderly adults with hearing problems caused by aging, and to a lesser extent, those with noise induced hearing loss. Other adult clinical groups include those who are referred for either compensation or civil aviation testing. Speech tests are not used in the determination of work related hearing loss in Australia and consequently NAL has carried out no development of speech tests in that area.

The development of speech test measures for civil aviation has been carried out at NAL. Following general research on the use of speech tests to determine communicative efficiency in noise by Murray (1943), NAL became involved in civil aviation aircrew hearing tests in 1948. The International Civil Aviation Organization (ICAO) standards (1955) laid down that if a pilot failed to meet pure tone threshold requirements, a 'practical' test be completed to simulate 'radio telephony signals in a complex noise background'. In order to meet this requirement NAL recorded the PAL PB50 word lists and added electrical noise to the output. The noise used was developed to simulate the spectral composition of a DC3 engine and propellor noise. Carter and Farrant (1957) reported standardized data on this speech-in-noise for test for aircrew, but they also discussed dissatisfaction with the reliability and validity of the ICAO standards. They pointed out that if medical criteria were operating then the pure tone threshold results were adequate in themselves, but if the intention was to assess communication adequacy for either job selection or work performance then considerably more research would be required before speech tests were sufficiently reliable or valid. Despite these reservations the original recordings of the PAL PB50 word lists in noise were routinely used for aircrew failing puretone threshold criteria. In 1959 the PB word lists 2 and 3 were recorded with a mixture of white and line spectrum noise at +8 dB signal to noise ratio for presentation at 108 dB SPL (called the PBN lists). Macrae and Farrant (1961) restandardized the PBN lists combining PB lists 8 and 25 to give two 50 word lists. Current clinical practice for air personnel failing pure tone tests in NAL is to give both the speech in noise lists as well as a PBM list presented free field at 60 and 70 dB SPL to reflect across the table briefing.

Sentence Tests Used in NAL

Word tests have been used in audiology as a compromise between analytical assessment using speech elements and the assessment of everyday receptive communication ability. Analytical measures can be confounded by significant task effects (e.g. Walker, Bryne and Dillon, 1982) while measures of everyday communication like connected discourse are difficult to score or are subject to the effects of large individual differences in basic abilities such as listening comprehension. It also seems obvious that sentence tests when used with appropriate controls can provide measures of everyday speech reception abilities with greater face validity than word tests. However, in line with current audiological trends, NAL has investigated the use of word tests to a greater extent than sentence materials although sentence materials have been available for clinical application.

Dudley (1968) recorded lists of twenty-five sentences (100 target words) based on the sentence lists developed by Fry (1961). Dudley used a simple up–down adaptive test procedure with 5 dB steps (see next section for a description of adaptive test techniques). The study reported the results of 46 persons with a wide range of age and of hearing loss. While noise had been recorded on a second channel Dudley only reported the results for the adaptive level sentence test in quiet. He found that the performance-intensity function was very steep for most of the hearing impaired subjects ranging from 0% to 100% in 10–15 dB. Dudley recommended the procedure for clinical use but it has not been routinely employed.

Macrae and Brigden (1973) used the Central Institute for the Deaf (CID) everyday sentence test (Silverman and Hirsh, 1955; Davis and Silverman, 1970) in a study which investigated the relationship between the articulation index and receptive communication adequacy. Subsequently, Tonnisson (1976) carried out a standardization of an Australian recording of the CID sentences after making minor changes in the lists to make them consistent with Australian vocabulary usage. In this standardized recording Tonnisson also included a three minute passage of continuous speech which is the same average speech level as the sentences. Tonnisson recommended that for clinical applications the continuous passage be used to set the most comfortable loudness (MCL) level for the presentation of the lists. The CID recordings are used in NAL clinics for assessment of sentence reception under controlled listening conditions.

Recent Developments in Word Recognition Testing for Adults

Speech discrimination tests have many different applications in audiology and many of these applications involve comparison of the obtained test score in two or more different conditions. There has been an increasing awareness that PB word list scores are too variable to reliably reflect changes in listening conditions. One response to this, in NAL, was to reduce the rôle of speech tests in client assessments (Upfold and Smither, 1981), using speech tests qualitatively, as a tool in aural rehabilitation. However, NAL also investigated ways of quantifying the variability of speech tests to define more precisely the limitations of the clinical application of available test lists.

Several authors (Hagerman, 1976; Thornton and Raffin, 1978) have shown that the variability of speech discrimination test scores can be estimated by using a binomial model. Thornton and Raffin (1978) published confidence limits based on this model for word lists stating that variability depended only on the discrimination score obtained and the number of items in the test list. These data helped clinicians to quantify the variability in their test scores on individual clients. The research at NAL (Dillon 1982, 1983) further investigated the binomial model and its application to speech discrimination tests suggesting that if test scores were obtained in different test sessions then the binomial model may underestimate the variability for some individuals. The work of Thornton and Raffin (1978) and Dillon (1982, 1983) also emphasized the need to use more test items to improve test reliability. This work indicated that the 25 word lists were too variable to use to compare between conditions.

In addition to these attempts to quantify the variability of existing test lists, NAL has also investigated the use of other test methodologies, including the performance-intensity (PI) function and the use of adaptive speech test protocols. The aims of developing these methodologies was to improve the clinical reliability of speech tests.

Performance-Intensity Functions

A PI function is derived by testing speech discrimination at several presentation levels above the threshold of detection for speech. The information obtained from the PI function is useful for detecting differences in discrimination ability between the ears, not reflected in pure tone thresholds; for selecting which ear is selected for amplification; as a cross check on pure tone results; to assess the interaction of speech level and speech discrimination; and in determining the site of lesion in the central auditory nervous system. While the value of deriving a complete PI function has been generally acknowledged, it has not been regarded as clinically feasible at NAL because of time considerations. This objection has to a certain extent been met by the AB word lists (Boothroyd, 1968). Each list consists of 10 CVC words and there are 15 lists. The same 20 consonants and 10 vowels occur in each word list and the lists are scored phonemically, giving a maximum score of 30 items per list. The advantage of phoneme scoring is that it improves the reliability of the test by increasing the number of scorable items without increasing the test time. With these considerations in mind NAL have recorded and are currently standardizing the AB lists for Australian listeners after demonstrating that the lists have value in the evaluation of speech reception problems due to age (Dermody, Mackie and Anderson, 1984). This study showed that individual differences in PI function characteristics (slope, plateau and rollover) were related to age and may be of value in looking at difficulties in hearing aid use.

An important feature of the AB lists' standardization at NAL is the use of level equalization techniques as suggested by Lyregaard *et al.* (1976). In a study of different level equalization techniques (Dermody *et al.*, 1983a) found that Leq best reflected the listeners' judgements of loudness. The words in the Australian recording of the AB lists were digitally recorded and then equated for overall level using a Leq algorithm. This level equalization was done to decrease the variance in listener's responses caused by fluctuations in speaker voice level at the time of recording, thereby increasing the homogeneity of the items in the lists.

Adaptive Speech Test Protocols

Studies using adaptive speech tests have shown that they are reliable when used with normal hearing adults (Bode and Carhart, 1973; 1974; Levitt and Rabiner, 1967), hearing impaired adults (Dirks, Morgan and Dubno, 1982; Mackie and Dermody, 1982), and with young children (Mackie and Dermody, 1986). They can be used to evaluate performance with hearing aids (Tecca and Binnie, 1982); to estimate PB max (Kamm, Morgan and Dirks, 1983); and to estimate predetermined points on the PI function. Adaptive test methods involve changing the presentation level of the stimulus depending on the listener's response to the preceeding stimulus. A significant advantage of adaptive tests is that an estimate of the reliability of a subject's performance can be determined on a single test administration. Adaptive testing therefore offers a reliable technique for comparing a listener's performance in different conditions in a clinically feasible time.

NAL is currently investigating the use of the simple up–down adaptive procedure with both adults and children for evaluating hearing aid fitting. The simple up–down procedure determines the 50% recognition point and it is easy to administer manually. The tester must raise the presentation level after each incorrect response and lower the presentation level after each correct response. Figure 2 shows the results of a listener tested with a simple up–down adaptive procedure. In this example a step size of 2 dB is used. The first stimulus word is correctly identified and the presentation level is lowered by 2 dB. The testing is continued and the presentation level is decreased by 2 dB after each correct response until the first incorrect response after which the presentation level is increased by 2 dB. This is the first reversal. Testing continues until a predetermined number of reversals are completed or until the standard error falls within the tester's criterion. The 50% recognition threshold is the mean of the midpoints of each excursion. Standard error and confidence intervals are calculated at the end of each test based on the number of reversals and the standard deviation. In general, the greater the number of reversals, the smaller the standard error. Mackie and Dermody (1982) showed that the simple up–down technique was reliable when used

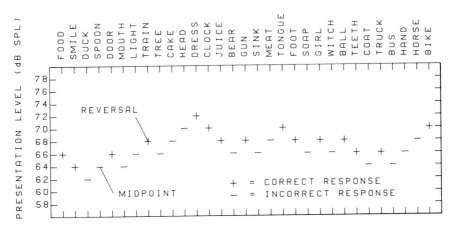

Figure 2.   Example of adaptive level speech testing using monosyllabic words.

with hearing impaired adults and the obtained threshold agreed closely with the 50% point obtained from a PI function. Because of the reliability of adaptive tests NAL is investigating their use in the evaluation of hearing aid fittings. A typical result obtained on a 70 year old male with a mild bilateral sensorineural hearing loss (average hearing loss of 28 dB HL) is presented in Table I. The testing was carried out in the free field using words from the NU-6 (Tillman and Carhart, 1966) lists. The test results indicate no aided advantage in the first aided condition. In this condition the subject was fitted with a low gain compression aid which had a low tone cut. The second aided condition uses the same aid fitted with an acoustic horn to increase the high frequency response of the aid. The adaptive test results indicate a significant shift in speech threshold with this aid. Adaptive speech tests can be used in this way to confirm aided advantage. This additional information is especially important in cases where the required aided tonal thresholds cannot be met at all frequencies by the available aids or in mild losses where valid aided tonal thresholds are sometimes not possible.

	50% recognition threshold (dB)	SE	CI (99%) (dB)
Unaided	39·5	0·35	38·4–40·5
Aided 1	38·4	0·35	37·3–39·5
Aided 2	30·2	0·56	28·5–31·9

Table I Results of adaptive speech testing comparing the speech thresholds, standard errors and confidence intervals of a listener unaided and with two hearing aids with different frequency responses.

Future Directions for Speech Tests in Adults with Mild to Moderate Hearing Loss

There are a number of requirements for assessment measures in adults with mild to moderate hearing loss. At NAL the primary group in this category are adults with hearing loss due to aging and the major reason for conducting speech assessment is to evaluate functional capabilities of the auditory system and for evaluation of the selected aid. With these goals in mind investigations are continuing at NAL to extend the available speech test options.

Recently, Dillon (1984) has suggested the use of subjective quality ratings for use in evaluating the overall performance of hearing aids. This procedure involves the use of speech material but it does not require the recognition of the words presented. The listener is only required to make a judgement of the relative quality of speech presented through different transmission systems. The use of quality judgements represents an important addition to clinical trials of hearing aids and might find use in general clinical assessment.

Other measures are also of interest. As Luce, Feustel and Pisoni (1983) point out there can be significant differences in cognitive processing of speech signals from different transmission sources even if the speech does not differ much in overall intelligibility. In the case of transmission loss due to hearing loss Stevenson and Martin (1977) showed that hearing impaired listeners produced slower reaction times to speech even when correct recognition occurred.

On the basis of these considerations NAL has begun a series of studies (e.g. Murray and Dermody, 1986) which are investigating the relationship between speech intelligibility scores or intelligibility judgements to cognitive processing factors of speech. The aim of the project is to develop speech transmission evaluation procedures (STEPs) for use in audiological settings. The present battery of measures for STEP include: the use of the PEST procedure (Taylor and Creelman, 1967) for obtaining the 70% recognition point on the PI function and a two alternative paired comparison technique for obtaining intelligibility ratings. The cognitive processing techniques include four classes of measures. The first set of measures extend the current speech recognition tests. These include presenting speech at a constant level (typically conversational level) and obtaining reaction times in a two alternative or multiple alternative response paradigm; and presenting words either in isolation or repeated three times on each trial. The one versus three repetition paradigm is based on the finding reported by Clark, Dermody and Palenthorpe (1985) that speech from degraded transmission sources does not show the same repetition effects as natural speech. The second set of measures look at speeded discrimination and classification tasks. These include a phoneme monitoring task and a speeded same-different classification task. The third set of measures are related to auditory memory and use a recognition memory task in which a string of speech sounds are presented followed by a probe for which the listener must decide whether it was an item in the string or not. Finally, linguistic processing abilities are measured. This is done with an auditory lexical decision task in which the listener must decide whether a sound string constituted an English word or not.

The preliminary results with these measures indicate that the cognitive processing tasks can be sensitive to differences in speech transmission sources or the effects of mild hearing loss even when no significant differences can be measured with the conventional intelligibility measures. We therefore expect some clinical application of these measures after further development.

Future Directions for Speech Tests in Adults with Severe to Profound Hearing Loss

NAL is at present developing protocols for complex adult case assessments. Procedures are to be developed for those persons with severe receptive communication problems caused by hearing loss who may require additional services to those provided by a conventional hearing aid.

Based on a number of investigations of measures used for assessment for rehabilitation (see the chapter by Plant in this volume for a discussion of the audio-visual tests investigated) Plant (1984a) developed a communication training programme for profoundly deafened adults (COMMTRAM). This programme also includes assessment procedures for use in decisions about which level is required for beginning rehabilitation. The present general criterion for inclusion in the programme is failure on the SPIN test as utilized in the procedure suggested by Upfold and Smither (1981). The COM-MTRAM assessment tests include a test of perception of the number of syllables in words; a vowel recognition test; and an initial consonant test. The NAL Lip reading Test (Plant and Macrae, 1981) is also used to provide information about audio-visual speech recognition performance.

These procedures represent the first stage in the development of speech recognition tests for severely and profoundly hearing impaired adults attending NAL Hearing Centres. However, given the present impetus provided by cochlear implant programmes there will be a continuing need to develop improved speech assessment measures for this group. It may also be possible to develop approaches combining verbal report data (e.g. continuous assessment diaries and questionnaires) with speech reception assessment (Dermody, 1982) to develop even more valid assessment procedures for adults with severe receptive communication difficults.

Traditional Speech Reception Tests for Children

NAL provides a full range of audiological services to children. These include hearing assessment for all ages including neonates, the provision of appropriate prosthetic devices (hearing aid, vibrotactile aid, FM aid), counselling of parents of hearing impaired children, and on-going monitoring of the child's auditory abilities, including a close liason with parents and teachers about the child's progress and advice about devices with which the child is fitted. NAL therefore has a need for paediatric speech tests appropriate to a wide range in age and degree of hearing loss.

Shortly after NAL was established, Murray (1952) developed a word intelligibility test for young children. This test, the Phonetically Balanced Objects (PBO) test was developed using the criteria that the stimuli were highly familiar monosyllabic words that could be represented by a simple object, that the objects have approximately similar visibility, and that the lists be phonemically balanced. Two lists of 25 words each were developed. These lists were used with hearing impaired children. Murray recommended that one of the lists be presented, live voice, at 75 dB SPL, and the other list visually alone, so that a ratio of auditory and visual scores could be determined. The primary limitation of the test was that, because of the requirements of phonemic balance, the child had to select a response from an array of 25 objects.

In addition to the PBO test, Murray (1955) also developed a test with a picture pointing response format. This test, the Phonetically Balanced Picture (PBP) Test consisted of four lists of 25 words each. Murray suggested that, as well as being a more convenient test form for children with sufficient vocabulary, the lists could be given as a group test for older children, who could mark each picture with an appropriate response number. Neither the PBO or PBP tests were standardized and monitored live voice presentation was recommended.

Byrne (1983) reported data on 94 normal-hearing children, aged four to 14 years using a recorded version of the PBP lists. His data indicate that the test results were significantly affected by age and presentation level for children up to eight years of age. This developmental effect was found despite the stimulus words all being within the receptive vocabulary of the children tested. Byrne attributes this developmental trend to the effects of receptive language abilities, although performance factors relating to the size of the response array may also play a significant role.

Recent Developments in Speech Intelligibility Tests for Children

A number of areas of investigation of speech tests for children are currently active at NAL. These will be considered in three separate sections related to tests for young children, assessment of mild to moderate hearing loss, and tests for children with profound hearing loss.

Speech Tests for Young Children

In clinical practice there are a number of reasons for assessing speech reception in young children, including confirmation of pure tone results; to assess areas of difficulty with speech discrimination and determine if speech reception abilities improve with increasing intensity; to confirm benefit in speech reception when aided; and as an indication of receptive efficiency in normal hearing children with receptive communication disorders. In addition, speech tests when given free field can also act as a rapport builder with a young child, prior to carrying out more formal assessment under earphones.

A concrete object speech test developed at NAL (Antognelli and Birtles, 1986) and modelled on the Kendall Toy Test (Kendall, 1953) is suitable for children aged 2 to 5 years. The test uses a closed response set of ten concrete objects which the child must be able to label appropriately. The test vocabulary of 15 words and the response objects were selected from an original 30 words and their objects which were presented to 74 children aged 2 to 5 years. The words and objects chosen for the test were spontaneously labelled by the children. The test has been developed using monitored live voice in the free field. In addition to the ten test items there are five supplementary items, which can be substituted for a test item, should the child have difficulty naming any item. The ten test words each contain one of five different vowels. The test is initially presented at 35 dBA and if the child makes three or more errors the presentation level is increased by 5 dB and another list presented. Successive lists are given at increasing levels until the child scores over 80% correct. This test has been used clinically with children as young as 2 years of age and the results obtained indicate a good correlation between the speech test score and hearing threshold levels for children with conductive hearing loss.

In order to provide additional measures for young children seen at NAL, NAL has recorded the Paediatric Speech Intelligibility (PSI) test (Jerger and Jerger, 1984; Jerger, Jerger and Abrams, 1983; Jerger, Jerger and Lewis, 1981) using an Australian speaker. The PSI materials were designed to provide a PI function for words and sentences in children as young as 2 years of age. The data collected on 30 children aged 2 to 4 years of age using the Australian recording gave results which were equivalent to those published on the American tape (Mackie, Jerger and Dermody, 1986).

The PSI test and the test developed by Antognelli and Birtles (1986) enable reliable speech tests to be carried out on very young children. This is possible because of their tight methodological controls, including a restricted message set, concrete word targets, and the use of the PI function. The PSI offers the additional advantage of allowing the clinician to compare performance on words versus sentences in quiet and at varying message to competition ratios.

NAL has also investigated the use of adaptive speech tests in young children (Mackie and Dermody, 1986). Words from the NU-CHIPS lists (Elliott and Katz, 1980) were recorded and presented to sixty children aged 3 to 7 years using a simple up–down adaptive procedure (see previous section on adaptive speech tests for adults for details of the adaptive test procedure). The results demonstrated that 3-year old children were able to complete the task with the same reliability as the 5- and 7-year olds. However, the actual 50% reception level was approximately 7 dB higher for the 3-year olds compared to the 7-year olds. Mackie and Dermody suggest that this relationship between age and speech threshold is not due to age related performance factors, but reflects the importance of receptive language abilities when speech recognition is tested in young children. That is, the raised threshold for the young children is due to their failure to use the partial cues that are available when listening to speech near threshold as a result of their relative inexperience with language (Elliott *et al.*, 1979). Mackie and Dermody also concluded that, providing appropriate age norms are obtained, the monosyllabic adaptive speech test (MAST) can be used with young children.

Speech Tests for Children with Mild to Moderate Hearing Loss

There is now ample evidence that children with mild to moderate hearing loss, including unilateral loss, high-tone bilateral sensorineural loss less than 25 dB HL, and in some cases long-standing conductive hearing impairment, are disadvantaged compared to their peers in language acquisition and school progress (see Dermody and Mackie, 1983a; 1983b, for reviews). The problems experienced by these children can be exacerbated by the fact that the hearing loss is usually identified late and even when it is identified there is often a reluctance on the part of the child to utilize a provided aid.

One of the difficulties facing the clinician in cases of very mild bilateral sensorineural hearing loss is to determine the extent of the communication handicap the child is experiencing and the intervention required. These children often reject hearing aids and it is valuable if an audiologist can demonstrate benefits from hearing aid evaluations to determine if it is worth persisting with the requirement for the child to wear hearing aids, at least at school. In order to determine if adaptive tests can be used as sensitive indicators of hearing aid performance in children with mild hearing loss, we have begun a study using the MAST procedure with NAL clinical cases. The test procedure uses the NU-CHIPS test presented in the free field (see Mackie and Dermody, 1986 for a full description of the test procedure) and a simple up–down test procedure. Table II reports the data of 2 children with mild bilateral sensorineural hearing losses, who have been fitted with binaural, behind the ear, compression hearing aids. Child 1 has a flat sensorineural loss, with a better ear three frequency average of 25 dB HL. The results of the MAST indicate an average 8.1 dB improvement in the speech threshold when the child is aided. Child 2 has a gently sloping bilateral sensorineural loss, with a three frequency average of 28 dB HL. This child also shows a marked improvement in speech threshold (9.6 dB speech gain) when aided. These results suggest that the hearing aids are providing significant benefit to these children even though their hearing loss is very mild.

	50% recognition threshold (dB)	*SE*	*CI (99%) (dB)*
Unaided	41·5	0·63	39·6–43·4
Child 1			
Aided	33·4	0·37	29·3–31·5
Unaided	41·0	0·74	38·9–43·1
Child 2			
Aided	31·4	0·59	29·7–33·1

Table II Results of adaptive speech testing for aid evaluation on two children with mild bilateral sensorineural hearing losses comparing their aided versus unaided speech thresholds, standard errors and confidence intervals.

Speech Assessment for Children with Severe to Profound Hearing Loss

NAL has a large caseload of children with severe and profound hearing losses. In response to the lack of available speech measures for these children Plant and Westcott (1982) and Plant (1984b) have developed a test (the PLOTT). The PLOTT test is based on the need identified by Erber (1974) to distinguish 'true' hearing from response to vibration in profound deafness. The PLOTT attempts to systematically explore the ability of each child to use either spectral or time/intensity cues available to them. The PLOTT consists of 9 subtests which cover a range of speech discrimination abilities. In subtest 1, the PLOTT measures a child's ability to detect the presence of the different vowels and consonants in a manner similar to Ling's 5 Sound Test (Ling and Ling, 1978). Subtests 2 and 3 are based on the Auditory Numbers Test (Erber, 1980) and the Children's Auditory Test (Erber and Alencewicz, 1976) and provide basic information about the child's ability to use spectral versus time/intensity cues. Subtest 4 is a twelve alternative monosyllabic discrimination test using highly familiar words which are non-confusable. Subtests 5 to 9 investigate vowel and consonant perception abilities using a picture pointing response. The contrasts tested include vowel length, vowel discrimination, consonant voicing and consonant manner and place of articulation. The results provide the audiologist with initial data about a child's use of speech cues and speech features when they are wearing their aid. This information can be used as the basis for planning auditory training.

The PLOTT has considerably improved our ability to assess speech recognition abilities in children with severe to profound hearing loss. Research is now being carried out to develop assessment measures of general receptive communication function. The investigations in this area began with clinical trials of the Test of Auditory Comprehension (TAC), (Trammel *et al.*, 1976). The TAC is made up of ten subtests assessing a range of auditory abilities, from gross discrimination to connected discourse comprehension in noise. The subtests are arranged in a hierarchical order and include: discrimination between speech and non-speech sounds; discrimination between speech, human non-speech and environmental sounds; discrimination of suprasegmental information; discrimination of monosyllabic and polysyllabic nouns; comprehension of spoken phrases; comprehension of sentences; comprehension of a three sentence story; comprehension of a five sentence story; comprehension of a three sentence story presented in noise; and comprehension of a five sentence story presented in noise.

Figures 3 to 6 show the results of two children tested with the TAC from a study reported by Mackie, Romanik and Dermody (1983). Figures 3 and 4 show the audiograms and Figures 5 and 6 the TAC results for two 12-year-old boys from the same school class. The TAC test was carried out free field in a sound treated room with the children wearing their hearing aids. The test uses a recorded male voice.

The audiograms indicate that child 1 (Figure 3) has slightly better pure-tone thresholds whereas the TAC results are significantly better for child 2 (Figure 6). This is especially evident in the latter subtests (subtests 4 to 9) which require auditory comprehension of phrases and stories. That is, for phrase and sentence understanding, the results for child 1 are significantly poorer than child 2 despite similar puretone thresholds. The speech understanding differences between the two children are not observed in the gross discrimination and word recognition subtests (subtests 1 to 4).

Mackie *et al.* (1983) concluded from their initial investigation using the TAC that measures which assess auditory comprehension in addition to speech discrimination and recognition are essential if we are to provide full assessments for children with severe to profound hearing loss on which to base habilitation programmes.

Future Directions for Speech Tests in Children with Mild to Moderate Hearing Loss

Procedures using adaptive test techniques like the MAST may provide more sensitive measures of speech reception for children with mild to moderate

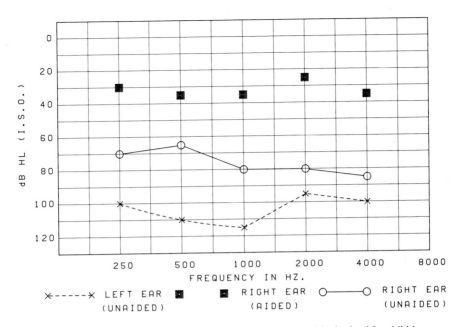

Figure 3. Puretone audiogram results and binaural aided thresholds obtained for child 1.

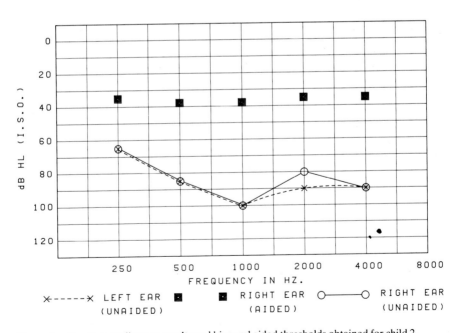

Figure 4. Puretone audiogram results and binaural aided thresholds obtained for child 2.

271

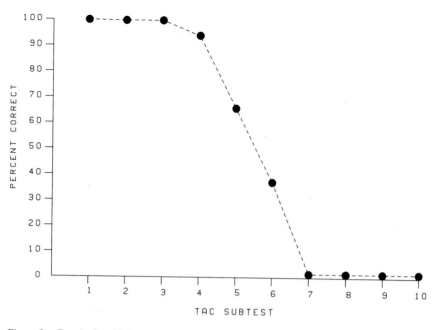

Figure 5.   Results for child 1 on the ten subtests of the TAC presented auditorally.

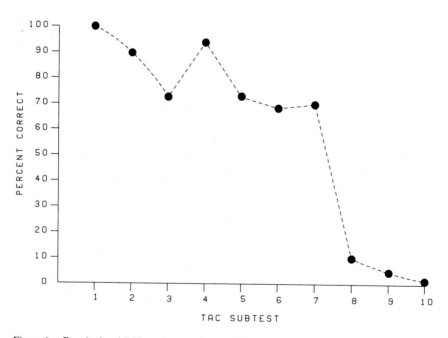

Figure 6.   Results for child 2 on the ten subtests of the TAC presented auditorally.

hearing loss. However, there is increasing concern that losses due to conductive impairment (Jerger *et al.*, 1983) or unilateral hearing loss (Bess, 1982) may also have effects on the receptive language process. In order to investigate these effects and provide early intervention where required it is necessary to extend the range of current speech reception assessment measures to include assessment of auditory receptive language learning and acquisition in young children.

In 1980, NAL commenced studies on the use of measures which could identify children with auditory receptive communication disorders at school entry (age 4·6 to 6·6 years) and thereby provide early intervention for this group before the auditory language learning disorder produced later related problems in verbal skills such as reading. The studies were based on the findings that children with language related disorders such as reading problems demonstrate auditory processing disorders (e.g., Dermody and Mackie, 1980; Dermody, Mackie and Katsch 1983; Dermody, Katsch and Mackie 1983).

The early identification studies produced procedures which have come to be known as the National Acoustic Laboratories Tests of Auditory Language Learning for Kindergarten (NALTALLK) and include measures of: phonological processing in which the child must demonstrate his/her knowledge of sounds in words; auditory vocabulary acquisition which tests the child's knowledge of words presented auditorally; and listening comprehension which assesses the child's ability to retain and understand speech. The measures for NALTALLK were generated from an auditory language acquisition model and based on observations about the types of problems demonstrated by language disordered children in the classroom.

These measures provide information relevant to planning intervention/habilitation programmes for normal-hearing children with language/learning disorders in addition to children with mild to moderate hearing loss who have not acquired normal receptive language proficiency (Dermody, Cowley and Mackie, 1982; Dermody and Mackie, 1982).

The NALTALLK measures are being used in two longitudinal studies in which we are looking at the relationship between these auditory language abilities at school entry and later verbal abilities, including reading. The data for the first three years of the study indicate there is a high correlation between listening abilities in kindergarten and later verbal abilities and reading skills. These results indicate that the NALTALLK measures can be used for early identification of children with receptive language disorders. Further studies are at present under way to investigate the use of these procedures in the assessment of the specific problems in receptive language acquisition experienced by children with mild to moderate hearing loss.

Future Directions for Speech Tests in Children with Severe to Profound Hearing Loss

At NAL we have identified the need for developing speech measures for monitoring a child's progress in auditory skills and for assessment on which to base auditory training programmes. The PLOTT and the TAC both represent useful clinical measures to meet these needs. Work is currently in progress to extend these measures to provide a more in-depth measure of speech reception and develop parallel auditory and auditory-visual forms for testing sentence understanding capacities. The project known as the Hearing Impaired Tests of Receptive Communication (HITORC) is only in its initial stages but two developments will be discussed here.

In order to investigate a potential task for monitoring the speech reception abilities of the hearing impaired, Mackie *et al.* (1983) included in their study an additional measure of auditory comprehension (the Token Test) to compare with the TAC results of children with severe to profound hearing loss. The Token Test was originally developed by DeRenzi and Vignolo in 1962 to assess mild receptive language disorders in adult aphasics. The Token Test has gained wide acceptance in aphasia clinics but has not previously been used with hearing impaired children. The test consists of five sections which all use a restricted vocabulary based on tokens which have different shapes (squares or circles), different colours (red, blue, green, white, and yellow) and different sizes (large and small). The token are placed in front of the listener and instructions are given about operations to be performed with the tokens (e.g. point to the big green circle). The instructions increase in complexity during the test and the later sections are sensitive to mild auditory reception difficulties. Mackie and Dermody (1981) published developmental data on the Token Test for normal-hearing children and found that the Token Test was sensitive to differences in verbal abilities in these children.

Figures 7 and 8 show Token Test results for the same children whose audiograms and TAC results are presented in Figures 3 to 6. The results for the Token Test reflect the differences in auditory reception performance between child 1 and 2 which were found on the TAC. Child 2 is significantly better in overall listening performance than child 1.

The Token Test easily lends itself to multiple forms which can be presented to compare auditory alone, audio-visual and total communication presentation. Figures 7 and 8 also show the audio-visual presentation results from the Token Test for the two children. Again we see a significant difference in the performance of the two children which suggests that it is not the auditory reception differences alone that differentiate the speech reception of the two boys. Child 1 also has significantly poorer abilities than child 2 for audio-visual presentation which indicates that child 1 may have generally poorer receptive communication abilities despite unilateral hearing thresholds better than child 2. This type of information can be extremely

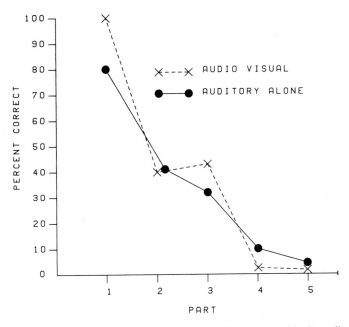

Figure 7. Results for child 1 on the 5 sections of the Token Test presented in the auditory alone and audio-visual conditions.

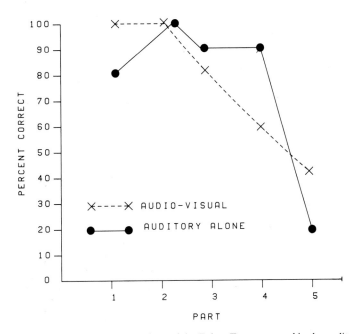

Figure 8. Results for child 2 on the 5 sections of the Token Test presented in the auditory alone and audio-visual conditions.

useful to teachers involved in planning and justifying habilitation programmes. We have generally found a good correspondence between performance on the Token Test and overall TAC scores which means that the Token Test may come to play a rôle in monitoring the auditory reception performance of children with severe to profound hearing loss.

Another HITORC project at present under way is the development of an audio-visual version of the TAC battery. Initial studies have retained the present TAC subtests but divided the items between auditory-alone and audio-visual presentation. The results for three children (child 3, 4 and 5 respectively) on this measure are presented in Figures 9, 10 and 11. Only the results for subtests 4 to 8 are presented since only the later sections of TAC permit audio-visual presentation. The speech in noise sections were not included in the testing of child 3 because of the child's problems with discrimination in quiet. The results in Figure 9 are those of a 10-year-old girl (child 3) with an average hearing loss of 93 dB HL. Figure 10 shows the results of a girl, 9 years and 10 months of age (child 4), with an average hearing loss of 95 dB HL. It can be seen from a comparison of these results that there is a striking difference in both the auditory-alone and audio-visual performance of the two children. This difference is not evident in subtests 4 and 5 presented audio-visually but is significant for all other subtests presented audio-visually and for all the subtests presented in the auditory alone

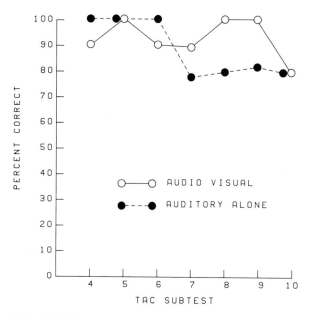

Figure 9. Results for child 3 (9 years 10 months), on the TAC subtests 4 to 10 presented in the auditory alone and audio-visual conditions.

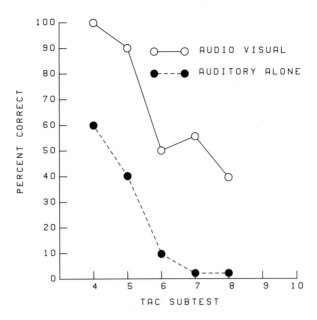

Figure 10. Results for child 4 (aged 10 years) on the TAC subtests 4 to 8 presented in the auditory alone and audio-visual conditions.

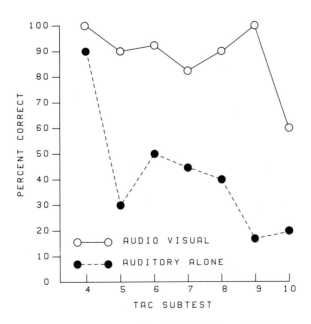

Figure 11. Results for child 5 (aged 12 years) on the TAC subtests 4 to 10 presented in the auditory alone and audio-visual conditions.

condition. We are at present investigating the rôle that this sort of result might play in habilitation programmes for the children.

The results in Figures 9 and 10 reflect the large individual differences in auditory reception capacity that can be obtained in children who are the same age and have the same degree of hearing loss. Figure 11 shows the very large intra-subject differences that can occur in a child with auditory-alone and audio-visual presentations. These results are from a 12-year-old boy with an average hearing loss of 108 dB HL (child 5). There are large performance differences between the two presentation conditions indicating that the child has very poor auditory-alone abilities using his hearing aid except for simple sound discrimination. However his audio-visual abilities are quite good even for connected sentence comprehension. This information is clearly of use in planning the required emphasis for individual instruction programmes.

A great deal more needs to be accomplished in the HITORC project before a full set of procedures are available. However, the potential clinical value of this work has been demonstrated and suggests that considerably improved measures can be developed in the future for use with severe to profoundly hearing-impaired children.

Conclusions

The present status of speech tests for elderly and paediatric cases at NAL reflects the recent uncertainty in audiology about the purpose, choice and use of speech reception assessment techniques. While it is recognized and accepted that speech tests are an essential and integral part of audiological testing, it is also clear that in the past we have adopted simplistic notions about how speech tests might best be incorporated into clinical practice. Appropriate speech tests can perform a number of critical functions in audiological assessment ranging from processing assessment of the peripheral auditory system to measures of auditory receptive communication efficiency for occupational placement. However, before these functions can be fully incorporated into clinical protocols it is necessary to clearly define our objectives for the tests and to improve the reliability and validity of the measures. The research and development of speech tests at NAL is likely to remain an active area for some time.

Chapter 15

Some Aspects of Speech Tests in Non-European Languages

J. J. Knight

The testing of telephone links with English speech was introduced over 75 years ago by engineers in the USA (Campbell, 1910; Fletcher, 1929). Often the speech was in the form of nonsense syllables. The same procedures were later applied for assessing the degree of disability of hearing-impaired people especially in the rehabilitation of American servicemen who had suffered noise-induced hearing losses in the course of their participation in the Second Word War (Egan 1948). This involved the evaluation of the benefit of hearing aids or the value of auditory training. While the telephone tests had used nonsense syllables with trained crews of both listeners and speakers using live voice, for audiological applications the accuracy and repeatability of the tests was improved by using sound recordings of simple words or sentences to prevent chance variations occurring in the presentation of the speech material. It was necessary to take great care with the preparation of the recordings to ensure uniformity and good fidelity of reproduction of the speech.

Selection of Speech Material for Tests

The first important use of recorded speech test material in Britain was for research with potential hearing aid users to determine the requirements of hearing aids for the National Health Service (Medical Research Council, 1947). It was decided at the outset to prepare test lists of monosyllabic words having the approximate distribution of speech sounds from everyday normal English speech. There was available much experience from the wartime work of the Psycho-Acoustic Laboratory at Harvard University later described by Egan. A vocabulary of 1200 monosyllabic words had been grouped into 24 lists of 50 words and then re-ordered and adjusted so that the final 20 lists satisfied the criteria of equal average difficulty, equal phonetic composition (or balance), composition representative of English speech, and only containing words in common use. Exceptionally easy words had been discarded from

279

the original 1200. It was found by the Harvard experimenters that attempts to satisfy the above requirements with lists of only 25 words failed, and that 50 words were necessary. In the British Medical Research Council work first 20 disc records were prepared of 50 familiar monosyllabic words, 25 spoken by a male voice and 25 by a female; the words were selected for phonetic balance (PB) by Fry, who earlier had produced sentence material for speech tests for live voice (Fry and Kerridge, 1939). These sentence lists were also used to assess the prototype hearing aids. At a later stage in the original hearing aid researches, Fry further amended the Harvard vocabulary and re-selected the words for approximate phonetic balance in groups of 25 (rather than 50) words for a third series of 20 MRC disc records in 1945. At this time a series of modified Fry–Kerridge sentence lists was recorded at the same sound level by a male speaker who had recorded the word lists. Further investigations led to the conclusion that a 40 per cent word articulation score corresponds to 90 per cent sentence intelligibility and that therefore the 40 per cent word score is a critical one. Later, the 50 per cent word score was adopted as it is more representative of giving practically complete sentence intelligibility. This has led to the concept of 'Hearing Loss for Speech' (Hirsh, 1952) often being taken at the 50 per cent word score for the decibel difference between the speech levels required by the average normal ear and the defective ear to attain that score.

By the early 1950s the use of speech audiometry with disc records had become an established clinical procedure in Britain and the USA and it had reached the standard text books (Hirsh, 1952; Watson and Tolan, 1949). A detailed evaluation of the third series of MRC word lists with male speakers together with a design for a simple speech audiometer for clinical use, was reported by Knight and Littler in 1953. Speech audiometry was then starting in several European countries using the same basic techniques for preparing recorded speech material. In 1961 Fry revised the British monosyllabic PB word and sentence lists and issued them on reel-to-reel magnetic tape. So much preparation and care went into the production of the Series 3 MRC and Fry word lists that, after more than 25 years they have not been bettered and are used extensively in Britain for routine clinical speech audiometry.

As with English-speaking and European countries, the above principles need to be applied in the setting up of routine speech audiometry in other languages. In the absence of detailed analyses of languages for which speech audiometric material is to be prepared, the frequency of occurrence of the phonemes must be estimated using a selection of simple written texts and articles. An alternative is by analysis of recordings of radio transmissions of news bulletins. For completeness, brief mention is also made of another development with English word lists to which reference is made later in this chapter, in respect of its application to Cantonese speech audiometry. For many years speech tests have been available for measurement of phonemic differentiation by choosing the right word from as many as six rhyming alternatives. Foster and Haggard in 1979 devised a Four Alternative Auditory Feature (FAAF) test that is based on similar principles. Its object is to measure the word identification score with precision in the region of the maximum score as a function of the spectral variables. The test uses 25 sets of 4 minimally-paired words giving 100 different words. Recordings were made of the key words with male and female voices and response sheets are used containing 25 items to a page.

Recording Requirements and Standardization

Before proceeding to an account of some of the less well-known speech test materials that have been produced in non-European languages, it may be helpful to refer to some necessary requirements in recording the test sounds. The first need is for the availability of a suitable broadcasting talks studio or at least a quiet non-reverberant room equipped with high quality sound recorders for magnetic tape. In order to ensure that the master tape produced is not the weakest link in the chain of the speech audiometric system, the overall frequency response of the recorder and microphone should be substantially flat in at least the range 100 to 8000 Hz and should not rise at any frequency outside this band by more than 3 decibels relative to the response at 1 kHz. The recording system should have minimum harmonic distortion and a high signal-to-noise ratio.

The test words are usually spoken with intervals of 4 seconds but first the speaker should practice reading the words clearly to give an approximately constant peak level as indicated by a sound level meter set to the 'C' or 'Linear' scale and 'Fast' response, and placed alongside the recording microphone.

When a test list has been recorded satisfactorily it is necessary to measure the peak level of each recorded word with a view to re-recording or adjusting any that are markedly different. Next, listening tests are conducted with normally-hearing subjects to identify any differences in shape of curve of word or phoneme score versus sound level for individual lists; also to equalize the average difficulty of the lists as required for Egan's criteria already cited.

Finally it is necessary to record a calibration tone on each recording for use in setting up the speech audiometer to a standard condition. Usually a 15 seconds or more duration of a pure tone of 1 kHz, or a narrow band of noise centred on this frequency, is recorded at the average peak level of the words as measured above. However, Fuller and Whittle in 1982 investigated the acoustic measure which corresponded best with the speech detection threshold over a wide range of sound level meter weighting networks and response times. The meter response times were found to affect the correlations much less than the weighting networks; the highest correlations were obtained with the 'A' network and 'Impulse Hold'. Results are awaited of a similar investigation concerning the hearing loss of speech at 50 per cent score.

Recent proposals by a Working Group on Speech Audiometers of the International Electrotechnical Commission have suggested that the zero of the hearing level control should in future correspond to the average normal threshold level (50 per cent score) for monaural listening for all speech test recordings. Also that, for uniformity, at this zero setting the calibration signal should produce a sound pressure level of 20 decibels at the listening test position in a free field; with earphone presentation the coupler measurements should be referred to the free field.

Non-European Languages

The speech material in the English language described above is basically suitable for hearing tests on an estimated 300 million people speaking English within the world population of 4,000 million. However, there are more than 3,000 known living languages, the great majority of which can be ascribed to about 12 main language families. More than half the world's population can be reached by as few as 13 languages. Chinese is spoken by the greatest number of people followed by English, Hindi, Russian, Spanish, Japanese, German, French, Italian, Malay, Bengali and Portuguese.

Considerable technical and other resources are needed to prepare suitable material for speech audiometry for countries outside Europe and the USA in which some 90% of the world population do not speak English. In some of these countries, the necessary resources have not been readily available and, in recent years, some students from abroad studying audiology at British Universities have applied themselves to producing speech test material in their own languages. This has proved to be a useful subject for research projects, often leading to a postgraduate degree. The accounts of speech audiometry for the non-European languages that follow are necessarily incomplete but those included mostly originate from projects with which the present author was connected, either as a collaborator at the University of London, or as an external examiner to the Universities of Manchester or Southampton.

Languages of India and Pakistan

India is the second most populous country with 684 million inhabitants in 1981 (China has 1,010 million). While Hindi is the vernacular language of India, English remains an official language and 14 regional languages are also recognized for adoption as official state languages covering 90% of the Indian population. Roughly one third speak Hindi, other popular languages being Telugu, Bengali, Marathi, Tamil, Urdu, Gujarati, Kannada, Malayalam,

Orriya, Punjabi, Assamese, Kashmiri and Sanskrit. Pakistan, with a population of 84 million, has Urdu and Bengali as state languages.

Speech audiometry in India was started in 1966. By 1971 the Rehabilitation Unit in Audiology and Speech Pathology at the All-India Institute of Medical Sciences, New Delhi, had prepared PB monosyllabic and Spondee word lists in the Hindi local dialect. De Sa followed in 1973 by publishing further PB word lists for speech audiometry in Hindi. Kapur (1971) referred to lists in Malayalam, Tamil and Telugu.

Arabic Test Lists

Arabic, the major Semitic language, is spoken by some 75 million inhabitants living South and East of the Mediterranean. Countries in which it occupies official status include Algeria, Egypt, Iraq, Israel, Jordan, Kuwait, Lebanon, Libya, Morocco, Saudi Arabia, Syria and North and South Yemen. It can be taken that African speech audiometry began when Messouak (1956) produced word lists in Moroccan colloquial Arabic. Alusi *et al.* followed at London University in 1974 with a compilation and evaluation of recorded monosyllabic and disyllabic word lists in the literary or 'classical' Arabic language. Six lists each of 25 monosyllabic words were recorded in a Baghdad accent by a male speaker. The words were phonetically balanced for vowels but the balance was not perfect for consonants due to their unevenness of distribution in Arabic. These authors introduced the concept of plotting the speech audiogram on arithmetical probability paper to give a straight line plot rather than the usual sigmoid-shaped curve which results from use of the traditional linear co-ordinates. As yet this potential innovation has received no support in the clinical field. Recently there have been other productions of Arabic word lists by Ashoor and Prochazka (1982, 1985) for testing hearing of adults and children with speech in Saudi Arabia, again with Modern Standard (classical) Arabic. For adults, this material comprises 6 lists of 20 PB nouns and, for children, 8 lists of 10 PB mono- and disyllabic nouns. Onsa, in 1984 at Manchester University, developed the first speech test material in standard Sudanese Arabic, the dialect of central Sudan, for use in local audiology clinics. Several 20 PB word lists and ten 10 word lists were produced using monosyllabic words. The latter were tested on normally-hearing Sudanese subjects and found to be satisfactory as regards inter-list consistency and sensitivity.

Other African Languages

Although Arabic is used extensively in the countries of North Africa, the 'lingua franca' of Southern Africa is Swahili. However, Muyunga in 1974 working at London University on the development of speech audiometric material for Zaire, (population 30 million) reported that the great majority of the Zairian languages are Bantu languages; of the four official vernacular languages Lingala is spoken by 8.4 million, Swahili by 6.3 million, Ciluba by 4.3 million and Kikongo by 2.8 million. He applied himself to developing speech audiometry in Lingala as a priority, for it is the language of Kinshasa, the capital, and of the National Army. It is also used in Congo-Brazzaville and in the Central African Republic. Ciluba was included in the study as it was the mother tongue of the investigator. Twelve PB lists of 25 Lingala disyllabic words and 14 similar lists of Ciluba words were produced. Three lists for each language were tape recorded using male speakers. The usual recording and equalization procedures were applied and a 1 kHz tone was added for standardization purposes during replay. The speech recordings were evaluated with several normally-hearing groups of subjects with comparable results to those obtained with English speech audiometry. Hinchcliffe (1968) found, with two Indian languages (Hindi and Tamil), that knowledge of the language is not an important factor in speech audiometry, providing sufficient co-operation and understanding of the test situation is obtained from the subject. This was confirmed by Muyunga through tests on subjects to whom Lingala and Ciluba were unknown languages, with results that were reliable, particularly in respect of the maximum word score and the threshold of detectability. He concluded that this finding would help to overcome the problem of speech audiometry with the many languages used in Zaire.

Cantonese

Finally for the purposes of this chapter, reference is made to speech audiometry in Cantonese. Mandarin as spoken in Beijing is now the national language of China's 1,010 million inhabitants and so is spoken by three times the number of people who speak English. Unlike in India and Africa, it is only in the South-Eastern maritime provinces of China that several mutually intelligible dialects are spoken and one of them is Cantonese (population of Canton is 5 million). Kam, a postgraduate student from nearby Hong Kong (population 5 million), in 1982 at the University of Southampton, developed and evaluated a forced-choice Cantonese speech test. It used monosyllabic words and was produced specifically for audiological diagnostic purposes. The design was based on that of the FAAF test except that a three alternative closed response set was necessary with the phonological constraints imposed by Cantonese. 120 test items were chosen to be presented in 4 lists of 30 words.

Present and Future Studies

Similar studies to those referred to above have commenced in Britain for the languages of Uganda and Zambia. The task for future workers is now lightened by the many papers already mentioned and the availability of more comprehensive accounts in unpublished theses accepted by Universities. From these accounts it will be understood that pre-requisites for the extension of speech audiometry to further languages are:

1. A thorough knowledge of the language and access to the advice of a professional expert in the language. In several of the studies listed, invaluable advice has been obtained from the willing co-operation of experts at the School of Oriental and African Studies, University of London.
2. Access to a quiet recording studio with high-quality recording facilities.
3. Small teams of volunteers who will co-operate as listeners for the trial recordings, to assess them in order to test and if necessary adjust the equality of difficulty of the test lists.

Equipment for Speech Audiometry:

A Draft Standard

This Appendix gives a draft version of a proposed Part 2 of IEC Standard 645 Audiometers. Part 1 deals with pure tone audiometers while Part 2 will cover the requirement for speech audiometers. This draft is based entirely on the work of IEC TC29 Working Group 19 but should not be taken to represent the views of any member of that working group or the IEC. In due course a final version will appear, first for comment and then for voting on by National Committees and only after a majority vote in favour will it become an International Standard. However, this version does indicate the direction of thinking and may serve to guide those who are considering the purchase or the manufacture of speech audiometers.

1. Introduction

This standard describes an audiometer which is specifically designed for speech audiometric purposes. Part 1 of IEC 645 details the requirements for pure tone audiometers in terms of the performance of each component module. Many of these modules are common to speech audiometers, e.g., the output level control, but Part 1 does not specify the requirements with speech as a signal source. This second part of the standard specifies the requirements for an audiometer where speech is used as a signal source; however, to avoid duplication, it does not specify those elements that are common to both pure tone and speech audiometers.

Performance requirements are given for both live voice and recorded speech inputs. Although live speech audiometry may not be capable of meeting the object of this standard, it is widely practised, particularly with children, and therefore a specification is included in order to ensure as high a level of repeatability as possible.

The standard does not specify the speech material that is used for test purposes or the required acoustic properties of the test room.

287

2. Scope

This standard specifies requirements for audiometers designed to provide means for quantitatively measuring the response of a test subject to speech sounds, or for those parts of other types of audiometer, i.e., pure tone audiometers, that are also used for speech testing purposes.

3. Object

The purpose of this standard is to ensure that tests of hearing using speech as the test stimulus, on a given human ear performed with different audiometers which comply with this standard, shall give substantially similar results.

Audiometers are classified into two types; Type A instruments provide the fullest range of facilities while Type B provides only basic facilities.

4. Related Standards

IEC 318: An IEC artificial ear, of the wideband type, for the calibration of earphones used in audiometry.

IEC 268–7: Headphones and Headsets.

IEC 645–1: Audiometers. Part 1 Pure tone Audiometers.

IEC 651: Sound level meters.

5. Explanation of Terms

5.1 Speech Audiometer

An instrument for the measurement of hearing for speech test material.

5.2 Hearing Threshold Level for Speech

The sound pressure level measured in a specified manner corresponding to the level at which 50 per cent of a specified speech test material can be recognised correctly by monaural listening using a specified scoring method.

5.3 Average Hearing Threshold Level for Speech

The average value of the hearing threshold level for speech derived from testing an adequately large number of otologically normal subjects of a specified age group.

6. General Requirements

All requirements not stated in this standard are given in IEC 645 Part 1.

7. Minimum Requirements For Specific Types of Audiometer

Two types of audiometer are specified and the requirements for minimum mandatory facilities are given in Table 1. Other facilities are not precluded.

Table 1 Minimum Facilities for Speech Audiometers

	Type A	Type B
SIGNAL OUTPUT		
Earphones	X	X
Bone Vibrator	X	
Loudspeaker	X	X
Electrical Signal Output	X	X
Monitor Loudspeaker/Earphone for Test Material	X	X
SIGNAL INPUT		
Speech Replay Device[1] or Electrical Signal	X	X
Input for Recorded Material	X	X
Microphone Input for Live Voice Test Material	X	
MASKING NOISE		
Broad Band	X	X[2]
Speech Weighted	X	X[2]
Input for external masking signal	X	
ROUTING OF MASKING NOISE		
Contralateral Earphone/2nd Loudspeaker	X	X
Ipsilateral Earphone/Loudspeaker	X	
HEARING LEVEL CONTROL	X	X
INTERRUPTER SWITCH	X	
SIGNAL LEVEL INDICATOR	X	X
INPUT FOR COMMUNICATION WITH TEST SUBJECT	X	
TALK BACK SYSTEM	X	

Notes
1. The replay device is not normally supplied by the manufacturer of the audiometer.
2. Either a broad band or a speech weighted masking noise may be used.

8. Specification of Acoustic Output

8.1 Earphone Output

The acoustic output and overall frequency response characteristic are specified in terms of sound pressure level measured in an IEC 318 ear simulator.

8.2 Loudspeaker Output

The acoustic output and overall frequency response of the loudspeaker shall be measured at an angle of incidence of zero degrees in a free field at a distance of 1 metre.

Note. The performance may be substantially different in a sound field other than a free field.

8.3 Bone Vibrator Output

No specification is given for the bone vibrator output. The manufacturer shall state the method of measurement used when a bone vibrator is provided.

8.4 Equivalent Free Field Output

In order to provide values for equivalent free field listening conditions the methods described in IEC 268–7 shall be used.

9. Signal to Noise Ratio

9.1 Overall Signal to Noise Ratio

The overall signal to noise ratio shall be measured with the replay system operating. The signal to noise ratio shall be better than 45 dB.

9.2 Amplifier Signal to Noise Ratio

With the output of the audiometer and the input socket loaded with an appropriate impedance, the signal to noise ratio of the audiometer amplifier shall be better than 70 dB.

10. Overall Characteristics

10.1 With Microphone (Live Voice) Input

10.1.1 The overall frequency response characteristic of the live voice channel shall be measured with the signal level indicator set to its reference point. The free field sound pressure level developed by the loudspeaker at a stated distance, or the sound pressure level developed by the earphone in the ear simulator, at least at the frequencies 125, 250, 500, 1000, 2000, 4000 and 6000 Hz shall not differ from that at 1000 Hz by more than ±5 dB, and shall not rise at any frequency outside this band by more than 5 dB, relative to the level at 1000 Hz. The manufacturer shall state how the microphone is to be used, e.g., angle of incidence, to achieve the indicated performance.

The manufacturer shall provide details of the electrical characteristics of the microphone input socket and the input electrical signal required to meet the above requirements for both earphone and loudspeaker output.

Note. True free-field measurements cannot be made in rooms that are not anechoic.

10.2 With Recorded Speech Input

10.2.1 Integral Replay System

If the audiometer has the means of replaying recorded speech material as an integral part of it, the following shall apply. The requirements below relate to both the replay device and the audiometer.

The frequency response characteristic shall be such that with an appropriate test material, the sound pressure level developed by the loudspeaker at a stated distance, or the sound pressure level developed by the earphone in the ear simulator, at least at the frequencies 125, 250, 500, 1000, 2000, 4000 and 6000 Hz, shall not differ from that at 1000 Hz by more than ±5 dB, and shall not rise at any frequency outside this band by more than 5 dB relative to the level at 1000 Hz.

10.2.2 External Replay System

If the replaying equipment is not an integral part of the audiometer the requirements of clause 10.2.1 shall be met but the manufacturer shall specify how conformity is to be established.

10.3 Harmonic Distortion

10.3.1 Earphone Output

The total harmonic distortion for the earphone output shall not exceed the corresponding pure tone values given in IEC 645 Part 1, Table IV. This shall be measured with a pure tone input set to give an indication 9 dB above the reference zero position of the signal level indicator, clause 13.

10.3.2 Loudspeaker Output

With the same input conditions as in 10.3.1, up to a setting that will give 80 dB SPL at 1 metre in a free field, the total harmonic distortion shall not exceed 3 per cent. This shall be measured for input signals of 250, 500 and 1000 Hz. The total harmonic distortion shall be less than 10 per cent at 100 dB sound pressure level for the same frequencies.

11. Reference Equivalent Threshold Calibration Level for Speech Audiometers

As it is not possible for the manufacturer of a speech audiometer to specify the sound pressure level for the average normal threshold for different recorded speech test materials, the reference equivalent threshold calibration level is given as a single value of 20 dB SPL.

At the reference indication of the hearing level control, the calibration signal shall produce a sound pressure level of 20 dB ± 2 dB in the ear simulator or in a free field at 1 metre from the loudspeaker, when the calibration signal causes the level indicator to be at its reference point.

Note. The producer of the recorded speech test material recording should specify the relationship between the calibration tone on the recording, the speech material and the method of measurement in order that the output level of the test material may be related to the reference equivalent threshold calibration level.

12. Tests for Conformity

12.1 Frequency Response

12.1.1 Frequency Response of Earphone Output

The sound pressure level shall be measured in a specified acoustic coupler or ear simulator at least at the following frequencies: 125, 250, 500, 1000, 2000, 4000 and 8000 Hz with a constant signal input level.

12.1.2 Frequency Response of Loudspeaker Output

The sound pressure level produced by the loudspeaker, for a constant signal input level, shall be measured at least at the frequencies 125, 250, 500, 1000, 2000, 4000 and 8000 Hz by a Type 1 Sound Level Meter, IEC 651 Sound Level Meters, using the C or Linear frequency weighting network. The measurement shall be made in a free field at a zero degree incidence at a distance of 1 metre.

13. Hearing Level Control

13.1 The hearing level control shall have only one scale and one reference point. It shall be calibrated in intervals of 5 dB or less.

13.2 The hearing level control shall be capable of controlling the output over at least the range from −10 to 80 dB for loudspeakers and −10 to 100 dB for earphones with reference to the reference equivalent threshold calibration level for speech audiometers.

14. Signal Level Indicator

14.1 A signal level indicator shall be provided to monitor both speech and calibration input signals.

The level indicator shall have a reference point towards the maximum of the scale and have the characteristics of a meter known as a VU meter. This meter has an integration time of 165ms and a time to reach 99 per cent of the final reading of 300ms. The time to return to zero is 165ms.

14.2 The signal level indicator shall be connected at a point in the circuit before the hearing level control. Provision shall be made in the amplifier for easy adjustment of its gain to cover a range of at least 20 dB in the level of input signals. It shall be possible to readjust the level of the calibration signal with an accuracy of ±1 dB.

15. Masking Sound

15.1 The masking sound from the audiometer shall consist of a weighted random noise and/or, where appropriate, white noise, as specified in clause 7.3.2 of IEC 645 Part 1.

The weighted random noise shall have a spectrum level that is constant from 250 to 1000 Hz and fall at 12 dB/octave from 1000 to 6000 Hz. This characteristic shall be met within ±5 dB. Below 250 Hz the level shall not rise above that at 250 Hz.

15.2 The masking level control shall be calibrated to the reference equivalent threshold calibration level for speech audiometers.

15.3 The masking sound shall be controlled over at least the range 0–80 dB for loudspeaker outputs and 0–100 dB for earphone outputs.

16. Monitor Earphone or Loudspeaker

The sound pressure level produced by the monitor earphone or loudspeaker shall be adjustable to meet the needs of individual testers, i.e., 50 to 90 dB SPL. The sound output of the earphone shall be independent of the setting of the hearing level control and shall not have any influence on the test signals.

17. Talkback System

In order to hear the subject's verbal responses to the test material, a microphone shall be placed near to the subject, feeding an amplifier with either an earphone or loudspeaker output for the tester to use. This shall not be required when the tester and subject are in the same room. No specification is given for this facility, but it should have sufficiently good reproducing qualities to enable a wide range of speech level to be clearly heard.

18. Interrupter Switch

An interrupter switch for the test material shall have the same characteristics as the tone interrupter switch specified in IEC 645 Part 1, clause 8.6.

19. Instruction Manual

The audiometer shall be supplied with an instruction manual which shall contain, in addition to the appropriate requirements of Part 1 of this standard, the following information:

(a) The specified distance and angle of incidence for loudspeaker testing.
(b) The coupler or ear simulator type used for the calibration of the earphones.
(c) The transfer characteristics from the ear simulator to other acoustic couplers.
(d) The coupler or ear simulator sound pressure levels corresponding to equivalent free field conditions.

References

Aitken, S. and Bianco, C. (1985) *Computerized instruction for hearing-impaired pre-schoolers*. Presented at the American Speech-Language-Hearing Association's Annual Convention in Washington, D.C.

Alpiner, J. G. (1978) *Handbook of adult rehabilitative audiology*. Williams and Wilkins, Baltimore.

Alusi, H. A., Hinchcliffe, R., Ingham, B., Knight, J. J. and North, C. (1974) Arabic speech audiometry. *Audiology* 13, 212–220.

American National Standards Institute. (1969) American national standard specification for audiometers. *ANSI* S3.6–1969. New York.

American Speech-Language Hearing Association. (1979) Guidelines for determining the threshold level for speech. *ASHA* 21, 353–355.

Anderson, C. M. B. and Whittle, L. S. (1971) Physiological noise and the missing 6 dB. *Acoustica*, 24(5), 261–272.

Andrianjatovo, J. (1972) *Audiométrie Vocale en Langue Malgasy*. Paris: Compagnie Française d'Audiologie.

Aniansson, G. (1974) Methods for assessing high frequency hearing loss in every-day listening situations. *Acta Otolaryngologica*, Suppl. 320.

Antognelli, P. and Birtles, G. (1986) *The Kendall toy test revisited: the development of an Australian version*. Paper presented at Australian Audiological Society 7th National Conference, Ballarat, Victoria.

Aplin, D. Y. and Kane, J. M. (1985) Variables affecting pure tone and speech audiometry in experimentally simulated hearing loss. *British Journal of Audiology*. 19, 219–228.

Asher, J. W. (1958) Intelligibility tests: A review of their standardization, some experiments, and a new test. *Speech Monographs*, 25, 14–28.

Ashoor, A. A. and Prochazka, T. (1982) Saudi Arabic speech audiometry, *Audiology*, 21, 493–508.

Ashoor, A. A. and Prochazka, T. (1985) Saudi Arabic speech audiometry in children. *British Journal of Audiology*, 19, 229–238.

Australian Bureau of Statistics (1979) *Hearing and the Use of Hearing Aids (Persons Aged 15 Years or More) September 1978*, Canberra: Australian Bureau of Statistics.

Australian Bureau of Statistics (1980) *Sight, Hearing and Dental Health (Persons Aged 2 to 14 Years), February–May 1979*, Canberra: Australian Bureau of Statistics.

Barfod, J. (1973) Intelligibility scores and confidence intervals. *Proceedings, Speech Intelligibility Symposium, Liege*: 25–33.

Beattie, R. C. and Edgerton, B. J. (1976) Reliability of monosyllabic discrimination test in white noise for differentiating among hearing aids. *Journal of Speech and Hearing Disorders*, 41, 464–476.

Beattie, R. C., Edgerton, B. J. and Svihovee, D. V. (1975) An investigation of Auditec of St Louis recordings of Central Institute for the Deaf spondees. *Journal of the American Audiology Society*, 1, 97–101.

Beattle, R. C., Svihovee, D. V. and Edgerton, B. J. (1975) Relative intelligibility of the CID spondees as presented via monitored live voice. *Journal of Speech and Hearing Disorders*, 40, 84–91.

Bench, J. and Bamford, J. (1979) *Speech Hearing Tests and the Spoken Language of Hearing Impaired Children*, New York and London: Academic Press.

Bench, J. and Doyle, J. (1979) *The BKB/A (Bamford Kowal Bench) Sentence Lists for Speech Audiometry — Australian Version*, Lincoln Institute, Victoria, Australia.

Bench, J., Kowal, A. and Bamford J. M. (1979) The BKB (Bamford-Kowal-Bench) sentence lists for partially hearing children. *British Journal of Audiology*, 13, 108–112.

Bench, R. J. and Duerdoth, J. C. P. (1983) *Victorian Demographic Study of Hearing Impairment, Vol. 1. Services and Facilities for Hearing Impaired People in Victoria*, Deafness Foundation (Victoria), Australia.

Berger, K. W. (1971) Speech Audiometry. In D. E. Rose (Ed.), *Audiological Assessment*. New Jersey, Prentice-Hall, Inc.

Berger, K. W. (1976) Prescription of hearing aids: a rationale. *Journal of the American Audiology Society*, 2, 71–78.

Berger, K., Hagberg, N. S. and Rane, R. L. (1977) *Prescription of hearing aids*. Kent OH: Herald Publishing Co.

Berkowitz, A. and Hochberg, I. (1971) *Self assessment of hearing handicap in the aged*. *Archives of Otolaryngology*, 93, 25–28.

Bernstein, C. (1981) *Use of speech discrimination in predicting hearing handicap in the elderly*. Paper presented at the New York State Speech-Language Hearing Association Convention.

Bernard, J. R. L. (1970) A cine x-ray study of some sounds of Australian English, *Phonetica*, 21, 138–50.

Bernstein, L. E., Schecter, M. B. and Goldstein, M. H. (1985) Vibrotactile sensitivity thresholds of hearing children and of profoundly deaf children. *Journal of the Acoustical Society of America*, 78, Suppl. 1.

Berry, B. F., John, A. J. and Shipton, M. S. (1979) A computer controlled audiometry system. *Proceedings of Institute of Acoustics Spring Conference, Southampton*.

Bess, F. H. (1982) Basic Hearing Measurement. In N. J. Lass, L. V. McReynolds, J. L. Northern, D. E. Yoder (Eds), *Speech, Language and Hearing*. Philadephia: W. B. Saunders Co.

Bess, F. H. (1982) Children with unilateral hearing loss. *Journal of the Academy of Rehabilitation Audiology*, 15, 131–144.

Bess, F. H. (1983) Clinical assessment of speech recognition. In D. F. Konkle and W. F. Rintlemann (Eds) *Principles of Speech Audiometry*. Baltimore: University Park Press.

Biesalski, P., Leitner, H., Leitner, E. and Gaugel, D. (1974) Der Mainzer Kindersprachtest. Sprachaudiometrie im Vorschulalter (The Mainz speech test for preschool-age children). *HNO* (Berlin) 22, 160–161.

Bilger, R. C. and Wang, M. D. (1976) Consonant confusions in patients with sensorineural hearing loss. *Journal of Speech and Hearing Research*, 19, 718–748.

Binnie, C. A., Montgomery, A. A. and Jackson, P. L. (1974) Auditory and visual contributions to the perception of consonants. *Journal of Speech and Hearing Research*, 17, 619–630.

Birrell, R. and Birrell, T. (1981) *An Issue of People: Population and Australian Society*, Melbourne: Longman Cheshire.

Black, J. W. (1952) Accompaniments of word intelligibility. *Journal of Speech and Hearing Disorders*. 17, 409–418.

Blair, D. (1977) *Judging the Varieties of Australian English*, Working Papers, Speech and Language Research Centre, Sydney: Macquarie University, 109–111.

Blamey, P. J., Dowell, R. C., Brown, A. M. and Clarke, G. M. (1985) Clinical results with a hearing aid and a single-channel vibrotactile device for profoundly deaf adults, *British Journal of Audiology*, 19, 203–210.

Bocca, E., Calearo, C. and Cassinari, V. (1954) A new method for testing hearing in temporal lobe tumours. *Acta Otolaryngologica*, 44, 219–221.

Bode, D. and Carhart, R. (1973) Measurement of articulation functions using adaptive test procedures. *IEEE Transactions on Audio and Electroacoustics* AU21, 196–201.

Bode, D. and Carhart, R. (1974) Stability and accuracy of adaptive tests of speech discrimination. *Journal of Acoustical Society of America*, 56, 963–970.

Bonding, P. (1979) Frequency selectivity and speech discrimination in sensorineural hearing loss. *Scandinavian Audiology*, 8, 205–215.

Boothroyd, A. (1968) Developments in speech audiometry. *Sound*, 2, 3–10.

Borg, E. (1982) Correlation between auditory brainstem response (ABR) and speech discrimination scores in patients with acoustic neurinoma and in patients with cochlear hearing loss. *Scandinavian Audiology*, 11, 245–248.

Bosatra, A. and Russolo, M. (1982) Comparison between central tonal tests and central speech tests in elderly subjects. *Audiology*, 21, 334–341.

Brady, P. T. (1971) The need for standardization in the measurment of speech level. *Journal of the Acoustical Society of America*, 50, 712–714.

Brandy, W. T. (1966) Reliability of voice tests of speech discrimination. *Journal of Speech and Hearing Research*, 9, 461–465.

Brimacombe, J. A., Danhauer, J. L., Mecklenburg, D. J. and Prietto, A. L. (1985) *Cochlear implant patient performance on the MAC Battery*. Presented at the American Speech-Language-Hearing Association Annual Convention in Washington, D.C.

Brinkmann, K. (1974a) The new recording of 'Words for Testing Hearing with Speech', *Journal of Audiological Technique*, 13, 12–40.

Brinkmann, K. (1974b) The new recording of the Marburg sentence intelligibility test. *Journal of Audiological Technique*, 13, 190–206.

Brinkmann, K., Diestel, H.-G., Mrass, H. (1969a) Tests with the Speech Audiometer. Part I: Properties of the word lists. *Journal of Audiological Technique*, 8, 38–51.

Brinkmann, K., Diestel, H.-G., Mrass, H. (1969b) Tests with the Speech Audiometer. Part II: Electro-acoustical transmission properties. *Journal of Audiological Technique*, 8, 126–142.

Brinkmann, K., Diestel, H.-G. (1970) Tests with the Speech Audiometer. Part III: The result of hearing tests. *Journal of Audiological Technique*, 9, 114–126.

Brinkmann, K., Richter, U. (1983) Determination of the normal threshold of hearing by bone conduction using different types of bone vibrators. *Audiological Acoustics*, 22, 62–85 and 114–122.

British Standards Institution BS 4668 (1971) *Specification for an acoustic coupler (IEC reference type) for calibration of earpones used in audiometry*.
BS 4669 (1971) *Specification for an artificial ear of the wide-band type for the calibration of earphones used in audiometry*.
BS 2497 (1972) *Specification for a reference zero for the calibration of pure-tone audiometers, parts 1–4*.

BS 4009 (1975) *An artificial mastoid for the calibration of bone vibrators used in hearing aids and audiometers.*

BS 5966 (1980) *Specification for audiometers.*

Broadbent, D. E. (1967) Word frequency effect and response bias. *Psychological Review*, 74, 1–15.

Brunt, M. (1978) Chapter 23 in *Handbook of Clinical Audiology* (2nd edition, Katz, J. (Ed.) Baltimore: Williams and Wilkins.

Bryant, W. S. (1904) A phonographic acoumeter, *Archives of Otolaryngology*, 33, 438–443.

Byrne, D. (1981) Selective amplification: some psychoacoustic considerations. In F. Bess, B. Freeman and J. Sinclair (Eds) *Amplification in Education.* Chapter 17. Washington: A. G. Bell Association for Deaf.

Byrne, D. (1983) Theoretical prescriptive approaches to selecting the gain and frequency response of a hearing aid. *Monographs in Contemporary Audiology*, 4, No. 1.

Byrne, D. (1983) Word familiarity in speech perception testing of children, *British Journal of Audiology*, 5, 77–80.

Byrne, D., Tonisson, W. (1976) Selecting the gain of hearing aids for persons with sensorineural hearing impairments. *Scandinavian Audiology*, 5, 51–59.

Cameron, R. J. (1985) *Year Book of Australia 1985*, Canberra: Australian Bureau of Statistics.

Campbell, G. A. (1910) Telephonic intelligibility. *Philosophical Magazine*, 19, 152–159.

Campbell, R. A. (1974) Computer Audiometry. *Journal of Speech and Hearing Research*, 17, 134–140.

Carhart, R. (1946a) Selection of hearing aids. *Archives Otolaryngology*, 44, 1–18.

Carhart, R. (1946b) Tests for selection of hearing aids. *Laryngoscope*, 56, 780–794.

Carhart, R. (1946) Speech reception in relation to pattern of pure tone loss. *Journal of Speech Disorders*, 11, 97–108.

Carhart, R. (1951) Basic principles of speech audiometry. *Acta Otolaryngologica*, 40, 62–71.

Carhart, R. (1965) Problems in the measurement of speech discrimination. *Archives of Otolaryngology*, 82, 253–260.

Carhart, R. (1971) Observations on relations between thresholds for pure tones and for speech. *Journal of Speech and Hearing Disorders*, 36, 476–483.

Carhart, R. and Porter, L. S. (1971) Audiometric configuration and prediction of threshold for spondees. *Journal of Speech and Hearing Research*, 14, 86–495.

Carney, A. E. (1985) Tactile aids: A comparison of single and multichannel devices. *Journal of the Acoustical Society of America*, 78, Suppl. 1, S16.

Carroll, J. B., Davies, P. and Richman, B. (1971) *Word Frequency Book.* New York: American Heritage Publishing Co. Inc.

Carter, N. and Farrant, R. (1957) *Australian Application of ICAO Aircrew Hearing Standards.* Commonwealth Acoustic Laboratories Report No. 12. Sydney: NAL.

Chaiklin, J. B. (1959) The relation among three selected auditory speech thresholds. *Journal of Speech and Hearing Research*, 2, 237–243.

Chaiklin, J. and Ventry, I. (1964) Spondee threshold measurement. A comparison of 2 and 5 dB methods. *Journal of Speech and Hearing Disorders*, 10, 141–145.

Chaiklin, J., Font, J. and Dixon, R. (1967) Spondee thresholds measured in ascending 5 dB steps. *Journal of Speech and Hearing Disorders*, 10, 141–145.

Chilla, R., Gabriel, P., Kozielski, P., Bäusch, D. and Kabas, M. (1976) Der Göttinger Kindersprachverständnistest (The Göttingen speech test for children). *HNO* (Berlin) 24, 342–346.

Clark, J. E. (1981) Four PB word lists for Australian English, *Australian Journal of Audiology*, 3, 21–31.

Clark, J., Dermody, P. and Palethorpe, S. (1985) Cue enhancement by stimulus repetition: natural and syntehtic speech comparisons. *Journal of the Acoustical Society of America*, 78, 458–462.

Coles, R. R. A. (1972) Can present day audiology really help in diagnosis? — An otologist's question. *Journal of Laryngology and Otology*, 86, 191–224.

Coles, R. R. A. (1982) Chapter 10 in *Otolaryngology 1: Otology* Gibb, A. G. and Smith, M. F. W. (Eds) London: Butterworth Scientific.

Coles, R. R. A., Markides, A. and Priede, V. M. (1973). In *Disorders of Auditory Function*, Taylor, W. (Ed.) London: Academic Press.

Coles, R. R. A. and Priede, V. M. (1974) *Derivations of formulae for masking of the non-test ear in speech audiometry*. ISVR Memorandum No 448, Institute of Sound and Vibration Research, University of Southampton.

Coles, R. R. A. and Priede, V. M. (1975) Masking of the non-test ear in speech audiometry. *Journal of Laryngology and Otology*, 89, 217–226.

Commonwealth Acoustic Laboratory Audiology Training Manual (1953) Sydney: NAL.

Commonwealth Acoustic Laboratory Audiology Training Manual (1961) Sydney: NAL.

Commonwealth Acoustic Laboratory Audiology Training Manual (1969) Sydney: NAL.

Condon, M. (1985) *Efficacy of microcomputer scoring of the Staggered Spondaic Word Test*. Presented at the American Speech-Language Hearing Association's Annual Convention in Washington, D.C.

Conklin, E. S. (1917) A method for determination of relative skill in lip-reading. *Volta Review*, 19, 216–220.

Craig, W. N. (1964) Effects of preschool training on the development of reading and lipreading skills of deaf children. *American Annals of Deaf*, 109, 280–296.

Creelman, C. D. (1957) Case of the unknown talker. *Journal of the Acoustical Society of America*, 29, 655.

Cutting, J. A. and Pisoni, D. B. (1978) In *Speech and language in the laboratory, school and clinic*. Kavanagh, J. F. and Strange, W. (Eds) Cambridge: MIT Press.

Danhauer, J. L., Crawford, S. and Edgerton, B. J. (1984) English, Spanish and bilingual speakers' performance on a nonsense Syllable Test (NST) of speech sound discrimination, *Journal of Speech and Hearing Disorders*, 49, 164–169.

Darbyshire, J. O. (1970) A technique for the application of speech audiometry to severely hearing impaired subjects. *The Teacher of the Deaf*, 68, 99–103.

Davis, A. C. (1983) Hearing disorders in the population. First phase findings of the MRC National Study of Hearing. In *Hearing Science and Hearing Disorders* Lutman, M. E. and Haggard, M. P. (Eds) London: Academic Press.

Davis, H. (1948) The articulation area and the Social Adequacy Index for hearing. *Laryngoscope*, 68, 761–778.

Davis, H. and Silverman, R. S. (1970) *Hearing and Deafness*. New York: Holt, Rinehart and Winston.

Davis, H. and Silverman, R. S. (1978) *Hearing and Deafness*, 4th Ed. New York: Holt Rinehart and Winston.

Davis, R. J., Kastelanski, W. and Stephens, S. D. G. (1976) Some factors influencing the results of speech tests of central auditory function. *Scandinavian Audiology*, 5, 179–186.

Day, H. E., Fusfeld, I. S. and Pintner, R. (1928) *A Survey of American Schools for the Deaf*. Washington: National Research Council.

De Filippo, C. L. and Scott, B. L. (1978) A method for training and evaluating the reception of ongoing speech. *Journal of the Acoustical Society of America* 63, 1186–1192.

Denes, P. B. (1963) On the statistics of spoken English. *Journal of the Acoustical Society of America*, 35, 892–904.

Denes, P. B. and Pinson, E. M. (1963) *The Speech Chain*. New Jersey: Bell Telephone Laboratories, Murray Hill.

Department of Immigration (1978) *Consolidated Statistics*, 10, Canberra: Australian Government Publishing Service.

DeRenzi, E. and Vignolo, L. (1962) The Token Test — a sensitive test to detect receptive disturbances in aphasics. *Brain* 85, 665–678.

Dermody, P. (1982) *Assessing and evaluating audiological assessment and evaluation.* Paper presented at Audiological Society of Australia 5th National Conference, Leura, N.S.W.

Dermody, P. (1985) Personal Communication.

Dermody, P. and Byrne, D. (1975) *Variability in speech test performance for binaural hearing aid evaluations.* National Acoustic Laboratories Report No. 62. Sydney: NAL.

Dermody, P., Cowley, J. and Mackie, K. (1982) *Language disorders and academic failure in kindergarten children: possible identification procedures.* Paper presented at Australian Psychological Society Conference, Melbourne.

Dermody, P. and Mackie, K. (1980) *Auditory memory deficits in language disordered children.* NAL Report 81. Sydney: NAL.

Dermody, P. and Mackie, K. (1982) An initial assessment battery for measuring auditory receptive language in children. *Australian Journal of Audiology, Supplement 1*, p. 6.

Dermody, P. and Mackie, K. 1983a) Problems in establishing tympanometric screening criteria: Experience with a language/learning disordered population. *Australian Journal of Human Communication Disorders*, 11, 41–50.

Dermody, P., Katsch, R. and Mackie, K. (1983a) Amplitude equalisation techniques for speech intelligibility testing. *Proceedings of the 11th International Congress of Acoustics* 4, 45–48.

Dermody, P., Katsch, R. and Mackie, K. (1983b) Auditory processing limitations in low verbal children: Evidence from a two response dichotic listening task. *Ear and Hearing*, 4, 272–277.

Dermody, P. and Mackie, K. (1983b) Effects of mild to moderate hearing loss on educational achievement. In H. Milne, C. Campbell and S. Payne (Eds). *Proceedings of the 8th National Conference of the Australian Association of Special Education.* Volume 2. Brisbane: AASE.

Dermody, P. Mackie, K. and Anderson, M. (1984) *Investigation of an Australian recording of the AB speech lists with elderly hearing impaired persons.* Paper presented at the 6th National Conference Australian Audiological Society, Greenmount. Qld.

Dermody, P., Mackie, K. and Katsch, R. (1983) Dichotic listening in good and poor readers. *Journal Speech and Hearing Research*, 26, 341–348.

De Sa, N. (1973) Hindi PB lists for speech audiometry and discrimination test. *Indian Journal of Otolaryngology*, 25, 67–75.

Dewey, G. (1923) *Relative frequency of English speech sounds*. Cambridge, Mass: Harvard University Press.

DiCarlo, L. and Kataja, R. (1951) An analysis of the Utley lipreading test. *Journal of Speech and Hearing Disorders*, 16, 226–240.

Dillon, H. (1982) A quantitative examination of the sources of speech discrimination test score variability. *Ear and Hearing*, 3, 51–58.

Dillon, H. (1983) The effect of test difficulty on the sensitivity of speech discrimination tests. *Journal of Acoustical Society of America*, 73, 336–344.

Dillon, H. (1984) *A procedure for subjective quality rating of hearing aids.* NAL Report No. 100. Sydney: NAL.

Deutsche Industrie-Norm DIN 45621 (1961, 2nd edition 1973): *Wörter für Gehörprüfung mit Sprache* (Word lists for intelligibility test).

DIN 45621-2 (1980): *Sprache für Gehörprüfung; Sätze* (Sentence lists for intelligibility test).

DIN 45621-3 (1985): *Sprache für Gehörprüfung; Wörter für die Gehörprüfung bei Kindern* (Speech material used in audiology; word lists for intelligibility testing in paediatric audiology).

DIN 45624 (1976): *Sprachaudiometer; Begriffe, Anforderungen, Prüfung* (Speech audiometers; terminology, requirements, testing).

DIN 45626 (1976): *Tonträger zum Prüfen des Hörvermögens; besprochen mit Wörtern nach DIN 45621 (Aufnahme 1969)* (Sound carrier for the hearing test using speech in accordance with DIN 45621 (recording 1969)).

DIN 45626-2 (1980): *Tonträger mit Sprache für Gehörprüfung; Tonträger mit Sätzen nach DIN 45621-2 (Aufnahme 1973); Anforderungen* (Sound recording medium for the hearing test using speech in accordance with DIN 45621-2 (recording 1973); requirements).

DIN 45633-2 (1969): *Präzisionsschallpegelmesser; Sonderanforderungen für die Anwendung auf kurzdauernde und impulshaltige Vorgänge (Impulsschallpegelmesser)* (Precision sound level meter; special requirements for the application to impulsive sounds and sounds of short duration (Impulse sound level meter)).

DIN 45619-1 (1975): *Kopfhörer; Bestimmung des Freifeld-Übertragungsmaßes durch Lautstärkevergleich mit einer fortschreitenden Schallwelle* (Earphones; determination of the free field sensitivity level by loudness comparison with a progressive sound wave).

DIN 45619-2 (1975): *Kopfhörer; Bestimmung des Freifeld-Übertragungsmaßes durch Lautstärkevergleich mit einem Bezugs-Kopfhörer* (Earphones; determination of the free field sensitivity level by loudness comparison with a reference earphone).

Dirks, D. D., Kamm, C., Bower, D. and Betsworth, A. (1977) Use of performance-intensity functions for diagnosis. *Journal of Speech and Hearing Disorders*, 42, 408–415.

Dirks, D., Morgan, D. and Dubno, J. (1982) A procedure for quantifying the effects of noise on speech recognition. *Journal of Speech and Hearing Disorders*, 47, 114–123.

Dirks, D. D., Stream, R. W. and Wilson, R. H. (1972) Speech audiometry: Earphone and sound field. *Speech and Hearing Disorders*, 7, 162–176.

Dirks, D. D. and Wilson, R. H. (1980) Binaural hearing in sound field. In E. Libby (Ed.) *Binaural Hearing and Amplification. V. I.* Zenetron Hearing Instruments, Inc., Chicago.

Dix, M. R., Hallpike, C. S. and Hood, J. D. (1949) 'Nerve' deafness: Its clinical criteria, old and new. *Proceedings of the Royal Society of Medicine*, 42, 527–536.

Djupesland, G. and Zwislocki, J. J. (1972) Sound pressure distribution in the outer ear. *Scandinavian Audiology*, 1, 197–203.

Dodds, J. (1972) An object puzzle as an indicator of hearing acuity in children from a mental age of three. *Sound* 6, 49–55.

Dreschler, W. A. and Plomp, R. (1980) Relation between psychophysical data and speech perception for hearing-impaired subjects. *Journal of the Acoustical Society of America*, 68, 1608–1615.

Dubno, J. R. and Dirks, D. D. (1982) Evaluation of hearing-impaired listeners using a nonsense-syllable test. I. Test reliability. *Journal of Speech and Hearing Research*, 25, 135–141.

Dubno, J. R., Dirks, D. D. and Langhofer, L. R. (1982) Evaluation of hearing-impaired listeners using a nonsense-syllable test. II. Syllable recognition and consonant confusion patterns. *Journal of Speech and Hearing Research*, 25, 141–148.

Dudley, P. (1968) *The development of a speech hearing test using recorded sentences.* CAL Report No. 5. Sydney: NAL.

Duquesnoy, A. J. and Plomp, R. (1983) The effect of a hearing aid on the speech-reception threshold of hearing-impaired listeners in quiet and in noise. *Journal of the Acoustical Society of America*, 73, 2166–2173.

Edgerton, B. J. and Danhauer, J. L. (1979) *Clinical implications of speech discrimination testing using nonsense stimuli.* Baltimore: University Park Press.

Egan, J. P. (1948) Articulation testing methods. *Laryngoscope*, 58, 955–991.

Eisenberg, L. S., Luckley, R. S., Norton, N. B. and Berlinger, K. I. (1977) *A speech discrimination task for profoundly deafened adults: HHRC Rhyme Test.* Paper presented at ASHA Convention, Chicago.

Elliott, L., Conners, S., Kille, E., Levin, S., Ball, K. and Katz, D. (1979) Children's understanding of monosyllabic nouns in quiet and in noise. *Journal of the Acoustical Society of America*, 66, 12–21.

Elliott, L. and Katz, D. (1980) *Development of a New Children's Test of Speech Discrimination.* Auditec, St Louis.

Elliot, L. L., Clifton, L. B. and Servi, D. G. (1983) Word Frequency Effects for a Closed-Set Word Identification Test, *Audiology* 22, 229–240.

Elphick, R. (1984) Comparison of live and video presentation of a speech reading test with children. *British Journal of Audiology*, 18, 109–116.

Erb, L. L. V. (1985) *Homophonous monosyllabic words used as a lipreading test.* Presented at the American Speech-Language-Hearing Association's Annual Convention in Washington, D. C.

Erber, N. P. (1972) Auditory, visual and auditory-visual recognition of consonants by children with normal and impaired hearing. *Journal of Speech and Hearing Research*, 15, 143–422.

Erber, N. P. (1974) Pure tone thresholds and word recognition abilities of hearing impaired children. *Journal of Speech and Hearing Research*, 17, 194–202.

Erber, N. P. (1977) Evaluating speech perception ability in hearing impaired children. In F. H. Bess (Ed.) *Childhood Deafness: Causation, Assessment and Management.* New York: Grune and Stratton.

Erber, N. P. (1980) Use of the auditory numbers test to evaluate speech perception abilities of hearing impaired children. *Journal of Speech and Hearing Disorders*, 45, 527–532.

Erber, N. (1980) Use of the auditory numbers test to evaluate speech perception abilities of hearing impaired children. *Journal of Speech and Hearing Disorders*, 41, 256–267.

Erber, N. and Alencewicz, C. (1976) Audiologic evaluation of deaf children. *Journal of Speech and Hearing Disorders*, 41, 256–267.

Ewertsen, H. W. (1973) *Auditive, visual and audio-visual perception of speech.* The Helen Group, State Hearing Centre, Bispebjerg Hospital, Copenhagen.

Ewertsen, H. W. (1974) Auditory and audio-visual speech perception related to hearing disorders. *Scandinavian Audiology* Supplement 4, 76–82.

Ewertsen, H. W. and Birk-Nelson, H. (1973) Social hearing handicap index: social handicap in relation to hearing impairment. *Audiology* 12, 180–187.

Fairbanks, G. (1958) Test of phonemic differentiation: The Rhyme Test. *Journal of the Acoustical Society of America*, 30, 596–600.

Fant, G. (1960) *Acoustic Theory of Speech Production*. The Hague: Mouton.

Fant, G. (1967) Auditory patterns of speech. In W. Wathen-Dunn (Ed.) *Models for the Perception of Speech and the Visual Form*, Cambridge.

Farrimond, T. (1959) Age differences in the ability to use visual aids in auditory communications. *Language and Speech*, 2, 179–192.

Feldman, H. (1960) A history of audiology: A comprehensive report and bibliography from the earliest beginnings to the present. (Translated by J. Tonndorf from: Die geschichtliche Entwicklung der Horprufungsmethoden, kuze Darstellung und Bibliographie von der Anfongen bis zue Gegenwart, in Zwanglose Abhandungen aus dem Gebeit der Hals-Nasen-Ohren-Heilk-unde. H. Leicher, R. Mittermaiser, and G. Theissing (Eds). Georg Theime Verlag, Stuttgart, 1960) *Translation: Beltone Institute of Hearing Research*, 22, 1–111.

Festen, J. M. and Plomp, R. (1983) Relations between auditory functions in impaired hearing. *Journal of the Acoustical Society of America*, 73, 652–662.

Finitzo-Heiber, T., Gerli, I. J., Matkin, N. D. and Cherow-Skalka, E. (1980) A Sound effects recognition test for paediatric evaluation. *Ear Hear*, 1, 271–276.

Fisher, J., King, A., Parker, A. and Wright, R. (1983) Assessment of speech production and speech perception as a basis for therapy. In Hochberg, I. *et al.* (Eds). *Speech of the Hearing Impaired*. Baltimore MD: University Park Press.

Fletcher, H. (1929) *Speech and Hearing*. New York: D. Van Nostrand Co.

Fletcher, H., Steinberg, J. C. (1929) Articulation Methods. *Bell Systems Technical Journal*, 8, 806–854.

Fletcher, H. (1950) A method of calculating hearing loss for speech from an audiogram. *Journal of the Acoustical Society of America*, 22, 1–10.

Foster, J. R. and Haggard, M. P. (1979) (FAAF) An efficient analytical test of speech perception. *Proceedings of the Institute of Acoustics*, IA3, 9–12.

Foster, J. R. and Haggard, M. P. (1984) *Introduction and Test Manual for FAAF II*. Nottingham: MRC Institute of Hearing Research.

Foster, J. R., Haggard, M. P. and Iredale, F. E. (1981) Prescription of gain-setting and prognosis for use and benefit of post-aural hearing aids. *Audiology* 20, 157–176.

Fourcin, A. J. (1976) Speech pattern tests for deaf children. In Stephens, S. D. G. (Ed.) *Disorders of Auditory Function, II*. London: Academic Press.

Fourcin, A. J. (1979) Chapter 9. In Beagley H. A. (Ed.), *Auditory investigation: the scientific and technological basis*. Oxford: Clarendon Press.

French, N. R. and Steinberg, J. C. (1947) Factors governing the intelligibility of speeh sounds. *Journal of the Acoustical Society of America*, 19, 90–119.

French, N. R., Carter, C. W. Jr. and Koenig, W. Jr. (1930) The words and sounds of telephone conversations. *Bell System Technical Journal*, 9, 290–324.

Fry, D. B. (1947) The frequency of occurrence of speech sounds in Southern English. *Archives Néerlandaises de Phonétique Expérimentale* 20, 103–106.

Fry, D. B. (1961) Word and sentence tests for use in speech audiometry. *Lancet*, 2, 197–199.

Fry, D. B. (1964) Modifications to speech audiometry. *International Audiology*, 3, 227–236.

Fry, D. B. (1979) *The Physics of Speech*. Cambridge: Cambridge University Press.

Fry, D. B. and Kerridge, P. M. T. (1939) Tests for hearing of speech by deaf people. *Lancet*, 1, 106–111.

Fuller, H. C. (1983) Speech level standardization in audiometry. *Proceedings of the 11th International Congress of Acoustics, Paris*, 3, 205–208.

Fuller, H. C. and Moss, I. K. (1985) A survey of speech audiometry in the National Health Service. *National Physical Laboratory, Acoustics Report Ac 105.*

Fuller, H. C. and Whittle, L. S. (1982) The measurement of speech levels for audiometry. *Proceedings of Institute of Acoustics Spring Conference, Guildford.*

Gatehouse, S. and Haggard, M. P. (1987) The effects of air-bone gap and presentation level on auditory disability. In press, *Ear and Hearing.*

Gelfand, S. A. (1975) Use of the carrier phrase in live voice speech discrimination testing. *Journal of Auditory Research*, 15, 107–110.

Gengel, R. W., Pascoe, D. and Shore, I. (1971) A frequency-response procedure for evaluating and selecting hearing aids for severely hearing impaired children. *Journal Speech and Hearing Research*, 36, 341–353.

Gerber, S. E. and Fisher, L. B. (1979) Prediction of hearing aid users' satisfaction. *Journal of the American Audiological Society*, 5–1, 35–40.

Gimson, A. C. (1980) *An Introduction to the Pronunciation of English* 3rd edition. London: Edward Arnold.

Giolas, T. G., Owens, E., Lamb, S. H. and Schubert, E. D. (1979) Hearing performance inventory. *Journal of Speech and Hearing Disorders*, 29, 215–230.

Gladstone, V. A. and Siegenthaler, B. M. (1971) Carrier phrase and speech intelligibility test score. *Journal of Audiology Research*, 11, 101–103.

Grant, J. M. (1980) The CAL-PBM's a Misnomer?, *Australian Journal of Audiology*, 2, 19–21.

Green, D. S. and Ross, M. (1968) The effect of a conventional versus a non-occluding (CROS-type) earmold upon the frequency response of a hearing aid. *Journal of Speech and Hearing Research* 11, 638–647.

Green, R. J. and Bamford, J. (1986) A comparative investigation into clinical hearing aid selection procedures. (In preparation).

Gruber, J. (1891) *A textbook of the diseases of the ear.* New York: D. Appleton and Co.

Hagerman, B. (1976) Reliability in the determination of speech discrimination. *Scandinavian Audiology*, 5, 219–228.

Hagerman, B. (1979) Reliability in the determination of speech reception threshold (SRT). *Scandinavian Audiology*, 8, 195–202.

Hagerman, B. (1982) Sentences for testing speech intelligibility in noise. *Scandinavian Audiology*, 11, 79–87.

Hagerman, B. (1984) Clinical measurements of speech reception threshold in noise. *Scandinavian Audiology*, 13, 57–63.

Haggard, M. P., Foster, J. R. and Iredale, F. E. (1981) Use and benefit of postaural aids in sensory hearing loss. *Scandinavian Audiology*, 10, 45–52.

Haggard, M. P., Lindblad, A. C. and Foster, J. R. (1986) Psychoacoustical and audiometric prediction of auditory disability at listener-adjusted presentation levels. *Audiology*, 25, 277–298.

Haggard, M. P., Wood, E. S. and Carroll, S. (1984) Speech, admittance and tone tests in school screening. Reconciling economics with pathology and disability perspectives. *British Journal of Audiology*, 18, 133–153.

Hahlbrock, K.-H. (1970) 2nd edition. Sprachaudiometrie (Speech audiometry). Stuttgart: Georg Thieme Verlag.

Haskins, H. A. (1949) *A phonetically balanced test of speech discrimination for children.* Masters Thesis. Northwestern University, Evanston, Illinois.

Hawley, M. (Ed.) (1977) *Speech Intelligibility and Speaker Recognition.* Stroudsburg PA: Dowden Hutchinson and Ross.

Hayes, D. and Jerger, J. (1979) Aging and hearing aid use. *Scandinavian Audiology*, 8, 33–40.

Hazan, V. (1986) *Speech pattern audiometric assessment of hearing-impaired children.* Ph.D Thesis. University of London.

Hazan, V. and Fourcin, A. J. (1985) Microprocessor controlled speech pattern audiometry. *Audiology,* 24, 5, 325–35.

Heider, F. and Heider, G. (1940) An experimental investigation of lipreading. *Psych. Monograph,* 124–153.

High, W. S., Fairbanks, C. and Glorig, A. (1964) Scale of self assessment of hearing handicap. *Journal of Speech and Hearing Disorders,* 29, 215–230.

Hinchcliffe, R. (1968) Report on audiology in India. *Sound,* 2, 59–68.

Hinkle, R. R. and Binnie, C. A. (1979) *List equivalency CID sentences presented in three sensory conditions.* ASHA Convention Atlanta.

Hirsh, I. J. (1952) *The measurement of hearing.* New York: McGraw-Hill.

Hirsh, I. J., Davis, H., Silverman, S. R., Reynolds, E. G., Eldert, E. and Benson, R. W. (1952) Development of materials for speech audiometry. *Journal of Speech and Hearing Disorders,* 17, 321–337.

Hirsh, I. J., Reynolds, E. G. and Joseph, M. (1954) Intelligibility of different speech materials. *Journal of the Acoustical Society of America,* 26, 530–538.

Hirsh, I. J. (1964) Clinical audiometry and the perception of speech and language. *Review Laryngology,* 85, 453–460.

Holmes, J. W. (1976) *Water Resources of Australia and the Pattern of Population Concentrations,* Research Report No. 4, Canberra: Australian Government Publishing Service.

Holsgrove, G. and Halden, J. (1984) Speech tests of hearing. Some new test material. *Journal of the British Association of Teachers of the Deaf,* 8, 16–18.

Hood, J. D. (1957) The principles and practice of bone conduction audiometry: A review of the present position. *Proceedings of the Royal Society of Medicine,* 50, 689.

Hood, J. D. (1981) Chapter 16 in *Audiology and Audiological Medicine,* Vol. 1 Beagley, H. A. (Ed.) Oxford: Oxford University Press.

Hood, J. D. (1984) Speech discrimination in bilateral and unilateral hearing loss due to Meniere's disease. *British Journal of Audiology,* 18, 173–177.

Hood, J. D. and Poole, J. P. (1971) Speech audiometry in conductive and sensorineural hearing loss. *Sound,* 5, 30–38.

Hood, J. D. and Poole, J. P. (1977) Improving the reliability of speech audiometry. *British Journal of Audiology,* 11, 93–102.

House, A. S., Williams, C. E., Hecker, M. H. L. and Kryter, K. D. (1963) Psychoacoustic speech tests: a Modified Rhyme Test. U.S. Air Force Systems Command. Hanscom Field, Electronics Systems Division, *Technical Document Report* ESD-TDR-63-403.

House, A. S., Williams, C. E., Hecker, M. H. L. and Kryter, K. D. (1965) Articulation testing methods: consonantal differentiation with a closed-response set, *Journal of the Acoustical Society of America,* 37, 158–166.

Howes, D. (1957) On the relation between the intelligibility and frequency of occurrence of English words. *Journal of the Acoustical Society of America,* 29, 296–305.

Howes, D. (1966) A word count of spoken English. *Journal of Verbal Hearing and Verbal Behaviour,* 5, 572–607.

Hudgins, C. V. (1949) A method of appraising the speech of the deaf. *Volta Review,* 51, 597–601.

Hudgins, C. V., Hawkins, J. E. Jr., Karlin, J. E. and Stevens, S. S. (1947) The development of recorded auditory tests for measuring hearing loss for speech. *Laryngoscope,* 57, 57–89.

Huff, S. J. and Nerbonne, A. (1982) Comparison of the American Speech-Language-Hearing Association and revised Tillman-Olsen methods for speech threshold measurement. *Ear Hear.* 3, 335–339.

Hughson, W. and Thompson, E. A. (1942) Correlation of hearing acuity for speech with discrete frequency audiograms. *Archives Otolaryngologica*, 36, 526–540.

Humes, L. E., Boney, S. and Ahlstrom, C. (1985) *Comparisons of two schemes for predicting speech recognition in normals.* Presented at the American Speech-Language-Hearing Association's Convention in Washington, D.C.

Hurley, R. M. (1980) Chapter 8 in *Speech Protocols in Audiology.* Rupp, R. R. and Stockdell, K. G. (Eds). New York: Grune and Stratton.

International Civil Aviation Organisation Report (1955) *Special meeting on hearing and visual requirements for personnel licensing.* London: ICAO.

International Electrotechnical Commission (IEC)94 (1968) *Magnetic recording and reproducing systems.*

IEC 268–7 (1984) *Sound system equipment.* Part 7: *Headphones and headsets.*

IEC 303 (1970) *IEC provisional reference coupler for the calibration of earphones used in audiometry.*

IEC 318 (1970) *An IEC artificial ear, of the wide-band band type for the calibration of earphones used in audiometry.*

IEC 373 (1971) *An IEC mechanical coupler for the calibration of bone vibrators having a specified contact area and being applied with a specific static force.*

IEC 645 (1979) *Audiometers.*

IEC 651 (1979) *Sound level meters.*

IEC 711 (1981) *Occluded-ear simulator for the measurement of earphones coupled to the ear by ear inserts.*

International Organization for Standardization (ISO) 389 (1985) with addendum 1: *Acoustics — Standard reference zero for the calibration of pure-tone audiometers.*

ISO 6189 (1983) *Acoustics — Pure-tone air conduction threshold audiometry for hearing conservation purposes.*

ISO 7566 (1987) *Acoustics — Standard reference zero for the calibration of pure-tone bone-conduction audiometers.*

Jauhiainen, T. (1974) *An experimental study of the auditory perception of isolated bi-syllable Finnish words.* Academic dissertation, The Institute of Physiology, University of Helsinki.

Jeffers, J. (1977) *A re-evaluation of the Utley lipreading sentence test.* Paper presented at 1967, ASHA convention, Chicago.

Jeffers, J. and Barley, M. (1971) *Speechreading (Lipreading).* Springfield: Charles C. Thomas.

Jerger, J. (1973) Audiological findings in aging. *Advances in Oto-Rhino-Laryngology*, 20, 115–124.

Jerger, J. and Hayes, D. (1976) Hearing aid evaluation: clinical experience with a new philosophy. *Archives of Otolaryngology*, 102, 214–225.

Jerger, J. and Jerger, S. (1971) Diagnostic significance of PB word functions. *Archives of Otolaryngology*, 93, 593–580.

Jerger, J., Speaks, C., Malquist, C. (1966) Hearing-aid performance and hearing-aid selection. *Journal of Speech and Hearing Research*, 9, 136–149.

Jerger, J., Speaks, C. and Trammell, J. L. (1968) A new approach to speech audiometry. *Journal of Speech and Hearing Disorders*, 33, 318–328.

Jerger, J., Weikers, N. J., Sharbrough, F. W. III. *et al.* (1969) Bilateral lesions of the temporal lobe: A case study. *Acta Otolaryngologica* Supplement 258, 1–51.

Jerger, S. and Jerger, J. (1976) Estimating speech threshold from the PI-PB function. *Archives of Otolaryngology*, 102, 487–496.

Jerger, S. and Jerger, J. (1979) Quantifying auditory handicap. A new approach. *Audiology*, 18, 225–237.

Jerger, S. and Jerger, J. (1982) Paediatric Speech Intelligibility Test: Performance-Intensity Characteristics. *Ear and Hearing*, 3–6, 325–334.

Jerger, S. and Jerger, J. (1984) *Paediatric Speech Intelligibility Test.* Auditec of St Louis.

Jerger, S. and Jerger, J. (1985) Paediatric hearing aid evaluation: Case reports. *Ear and Hearing*, 6–5, 240–244.

Jerger, S., Jerger, J. and Abrams, S. (1983) Speech audiometry in the young child. *Ear and Hearing*, 4, 56–66.

Jerger, S., Jerger, J., Alford, B. and Abrams, S. (1983) Development of speech intelligibility in children with current otitis media. *Ear and Hearing*, 4, 138–145.

Jerger, S., Jerger, J. and Lewis, S. (1981) Paediatric speech intelligibility test. II. Effect of receptive language age and chronological age. *International Journal of Paediatric Otorhinolarnygology*, 3, 101–118.

Jerger, S., Lewis, S. Hawkins, J. and Jerger, J. (1980) Paediatric Speech Intelligibility test. I. Generation of test materials. *International Journal of Paediatric Otorhinolaryngology*, 2, 217–230.

Jerlvall, L., Almqvist, B., Ovegård, A. and Arlinger, S. (1983) Clinical trial of In-the-Ear hearing aids. *Scandinavian Audiology*, 12, 63–70.

Johnson, D. R. (1976) Communications characteristics of a young deaf adult population: Techniques for evaluating their communication skills. *American Annals of the Deaf*, 409–424.

Jupiter, T. (1982) *Audiometric and speechreading correlates of hearing handicap in the elderly.* Unpublished doctoral dissertation, Teachers College, Columbia University.

Kalikow, D. N., Stevens, K. N. and Elliot, L. L. (1977) Development of a test of speech intelligibility in noise using sentence materials with controlled word predictability. *Journal of the Acoustical Society of America*, 61, 1337–1351.

Kam T. P. K. (1982) *Speech audiometric test material in Cantonese.* Unpublished M.Sc. dissertation, University of Southampton.

Kamm, C., Morgan, D. and Dirks, D. (1983) Accuracy of adaptive procedure estimates of PB Max level. *Journal of Speech and Hearing Disorders*, 48, 202–209.

Kapur, Y. P. (1971) *Needs of the speech and hearing handicapped in India.* Christian Medical College and Hospital, Vellore, India.

Katz, J. (1962) The use of staggered spondaic words for assessing the integrity of the central auditory nervous system. *Journal of Auditory Research*, 2, 327–337.

Katz, J. (1977) Chapter 4 in *Central Auditory Dysfunction* Keith, R. W. (Ed.) New York: Grune and Stratton.

Katz, D. R., Elliot, L. L. (1978) *Development of new children's speech discrimination tests.* American Speech-Language-Hearing Association. Chicago.

Keith, R. W. (1977) Chapter 3 in *Central Auditory Dysfunction* Keith, R. W. (Ed.) New York: Grune and Stratton.

Kendall, D. C. (1953) Audiometry for young children: Part 1. *Teacher of the Deaf*, 51, 171–178.

Kendall, D. C. (1954) Audiometry for young children *Teacher of the Deaf*, 52, 18–23.

Kendall, D. C. (1956) On the management of deafness in the young child. *Proceedings of the Royal Society of Medicine*, 49, 463–467.

Kendall, M. G. and Stuart, A. (1958) The Advanced Theory of Statistics. Vol. 1, London: Griffin.

Klein, W., Plomp, R. and Pols, L. C. W. (1970) Vowel spectra, vowel spaces, and vowel identification. *Journal of the Acoustical Society of America*, 48, 999–1009.

Knight, J. J. and Littler, T. S. (1953) The technique of speech audiometry and a simple speech audiometer with masking generator for clinical use. *Journal of Laryngology.* 67, 248–265.

Koike, J. J. M. (1985) *The development of the Utah Vowel Imitation Test. (U-VIT).* Presented at the American Speech-Language-Hearing Association's Annual Convention in Washington, D.C.

Kopra, L. L., Dunlop, R. J., Kopra, M. A. and Abrahamson, J. E. (1985) *Laser videodisc interactive system for computer-assisted instruction in speechreading.* Scientific Exhibit at ASHA Convention, Washington, D.C.

Korsan-Bengtsen, M. (1973) Distorted speech audiometry. *Acta Otolaryngologica* Suppl. 310.

Kruel, E. J., Bell, D. W. and Nixon, J. C. (1969) Factors affecting speech discrimination test difficulty. *Journal of Speech and Hearing Research,* 12, 281–287.

Kruel, E. J., Nixon, J. C., Kryter, K. D., Bell, D. W. and Lang, J. S. (1968) A proposed clinical test of speech discrimination. *Journal of Speech and Hearing Research,* 11, 536–552.

Kryter, K. D. (1962a) Methods for the calculation and use of the articulation index. *Journal of the Acoustical Society of America,* 34, 1689–1697.

Kryter, K. D. (1962b) Validation of the articulation index. *Journal of the Acoustical Society of America,* 34 1698—1702.

Kryter, K. D., Williams, C. and Green, D. M. (1962) Auditory acuity and the perception of speech. *Journal of the Acoustical Society of America,* 34, 1217–1223.

Ladefoged, P. (1962) *Elements of Acoustic Phonetics.* Chicago: University of Chicago Press.

Ladefoged, P. (1982) *A Course in Phonetics* (2nd Ed.) New York: Harcourt Brace Jovanovich.

Lehiste, I. and Peterson, G. E. (1959) Linguistic considerations in the study of speech intelligibility. *Journal of the Acoustical Society of America,* 31, 280–286.

Lehmann, R. (1962) *Étude psychophysique de l'intelligibilité du langage.* Theses de l'Université de Paris, Éditions de la Revue d'Optique Théorique et Instrumentale.

Lerman, J. W., Ross, M. and McLauchlin, R. M. (1965) A picture-identification test for hearing-impaired children. *Journal of Audiological Research,* 5, 273–278.

Leshowitz, B. (1977) Speech intelligibility in noise for listeners with sensorineural hearing damage. *IPO Annual Progress Report,* 12, 11–23.

Levitt, H., Collins, M. J., Dubno, J. R., Resnick, S. B. and White, R. E. C. (1978) *Development of a protocol for the prescriptive fitting of a wearable hearing aid.* (Communication Sciences Laboratory Report No. 11). New York: City University of New York.

Levitt, H. and Rabiner, L. (1967) Use of a sequential strategy in speech intelligibility testing. *Journal of Acoustical Society of America,* 42, 609–612.

Levitt, H. and Resnick, S. (1978) Speech perception by the hearing impaired: methods of testing and the development of new tests. In C. Ludwigen and J. Barfod (Eds) Sensorineural Hearing Impaired and Hearing Aids. *Scandinavian Audiology* Suppl. 6, 107–128.

Lewis, A. N. (1979) Educational consequences of otitis media ear disease in aboriginal children. *Proceedings of the Australian Deafness Council Seminar, October, Melbourne, 17–18.*

Lidén, G. (1954) Speech audiometry. *Acta Otolaryngologica* Suppl. 14, 1–45.

Lidén, G. (1971) The use and limitations of the masking noise in pure-tone and speech audiometry. *Audiology,* 10, 115–128.

Ling, D. (1978) Auditory coding and reading — an analysis of training procedures for hearing impaired children. In Ross, M. and Giolas, T. G. (Eds) *Auditory Management of Hearing Impaired Children*. Baltimore: University Park Press.

Ling, D. and Ling, A. (1978) *Aural Habilitation: The Foundation of Verbal Learning in Hearing Impaired Children*. Washington: Alexander Graham Bell Association for the Deaf.

Loiselle, L. H. (1985) *Use of the PSI for paediatric hearing aid evaluations*. (A miniseminar). Presented at the American Speech-Language-Hearing Association's Annual Convention in Washington, D.C.

Lowell, E. L. (1957) *A film test of lipreading*. John Tracy Research Papers II. John Tracy Clinic, Los Angeles.

Lowell, E. L. (1974) Auditory and visual perception of different units of speech. *Scandinavian Audiology* Suppl. 4, 31–37.

Luce, P., Feustel, T. and Pisoni, D. (1983) Capacity demands in short term memory for synthetic and natural word lists. *Human Factors* 25, 17–32.

Ludvigsen, C. (1974) Construction and evaluation of an audio-visual test (the Helen test). *Scandinavian Audiology* Suppl 4, 67–75.

Lutman, M. E. (1987) *Psychoacoustical characterisation of sensorineural hearing loss*. (In preparation).

Lutman, M. E., Brown, E. J. and Coles, R. R. A. (1986) Self-reported disability and handicap in the population in relation to pure-tone threshold, age, sex and type of hearing loss. *British Journal of Audiology*, 21, 45–58.

Lutman, M. E. and Clark, J. (1986) Speech identification under simulated hearing aid frequency response characteristics in relation to sensitivity frequency resolution and temporal resolution. *Journal of the Acoustical Society of America*, 80, 1030–1040.

Lybarger, S. F. (1978) Selective amplification — A review and evaluation. *Journal of the American Audiological Society* 3, 258–266.

Lynn, G. E. and Gilroy, J. (1977) Chapter 6 in *Central Auditory Dysfunction* Keith, R. W. (Ed.) New York: Grune and Stratton.

Lynn, J. M. and Brotman, S. R. (1981) Perceptual significance of the CID W22 carrier phrase. *Ear and Hearing*, 2, 95–99.

Lyregaard, P. E. (1973) On the statistics of speech audiometry data. Teddington: NPL Acoustics Report AC 63.

Lyregaard, P. E. (1976) On the relation between recognition and familiarity of words. Teddington: NPL Acoustics Report AC 78.

Lyregaard, P. E., Robinson, D. W. and Hinchcliffe, R. (1976) A feasibility study of diagnostic speech audiometry. Teddington: NPL Acoustics Report Ac 73.

McCandless, G. A. and Dankowski, N. K. (1985) *Factors which determine speech discrimination in a multichannel cochlear implant*. Presented at the American Speech-Language-Hearing Association's Annual Convention in Washington, D. C.

McCormick, B. (1977) The toy discrimination test: an aid for the screening of hearing of children above the mental age of 2 years. *Public Health, London*, 67–69.

McCormick, B. (1979a) The skill of lipreading — a review. *Hearing* 34, 126–130.

McCormick, B. (1979b) A comparison between a two-dimensional and a three-dimensional lipreading test. *IRCS Medical Sciences Journal (Biomedical Technology)* 7, 324.

McGurk, H. and Macdonald, J. (1976) Hearing lips and seeing voices. *Nature* 264, 746–8.

Mackie, K. and Dermody, P. (1981) A normative study of the Token Test. *Australian Journal of Human Communication Disorders*, 9, 14–23.

Mackie, K. and Dermody, P. (1982) *Adaptive speech testing with hearing impaired adults*. Paper presented at Audiological Society of Australia 5th National Conference, Leura. N.S.W.

Mackie, K. and Dermody, P. (1982) *Word intelligibility tests in audiology for the assessment of communication adequacy*. NAL Report No. 89. Sydney: NAL.

Mackie, K. and Dermody, P. (1986) Use of a monosyllabic adaptive speech test (MAST) with young children. *Journal Speech and Hearing Research*, 29, 275–281.

Mackie, K., Jerger, S. and Dermody, P. (1986) *Results of an Australian recording of the Paediatric Speech Intelligibility Test*. Paper presented at Audiological Society of Australia 7th National Conference, Ballarat, Victoria.

Mackie, K., Romanik, S. and Dermody, P. (1983) Audiological assessment of auditory receptive language in severely and profoundly hearing impaired children. In H. Milne, C. Campbell and S. Payner. *Proceedings of the 8th National Conference of the Australian Association of Special Education. Volume 2*. Brisbane: AASE.

Macrae, J. and Brigden, D. (1973) Auditory threshold impairment and everyday speech reception. *Audiology*, 12, 272–290.

Macrae, J. and Farrant, R. (1961) *Standardisation of the CAL revised (33rpm) recordings of the PBN word lists nos. 2, 3, 4, 5, 8 and 9 used in testing civil aviation aircrew*. CAL Report No. 21 Sydney: CAL.

Macrae, J., Woodroffe, P. and Farrant, R. (1963) Standardisation of the Commonwealth Acoustic Laboratories' recordings of phonetically balanced monosyllabic word lists. *Journal of the Oto-Laryngological Society of Australia*, 1, 197–203.

Marincovich, P. J. and Studebaker, G. A. (1985) *Calculation of hearing aid efficiency with an Articulation Index procedure*. Presented at the American Speech-Language-Hearing Association's Annual Convention in Washington, D.C.

Markides, A. (1978) Speech discrimination functions for normal hearing subjects with AB isophonemic word lists. *Scandinavian Audiology*, 7, 239–245.

Markides, A. (1980) Best listening levels of hearing impaired children. *Journal of the British Association of Teachers of the Deaf*, 6, 117–124.

Markides, A. (1980) The relationship between hearing loss for pure tones and hearing loss for speech among hearing-impaired children. *British Journal of Audiology*, 14, 115–121.

Markides, A. (1980) The Manchester Speech reading (Lipreading) Test. In Taylor, I. G. and Markides, A. (Eds) *Disorders of Auditory Function III*. London: Academic Press.

Martin, F. N. and Forbis, N. K. (1978) The present status of audiometric practice: a follow-up study. *ASHA*, 20, 531–541.

Martin, F. N., Hawkins, R. R. and Bailey, H. A. T. (1962) The nonessentiality of the carrier phrase in phonetically balanced (PB) word testing. *Journal of Auditory Research*, 2, 319–322.

Martin, F. N. and Pennington, C. D. (1971) Current trends in audiometric practices. *ASHA* 13, 671–677.

Martin, F. N. and Sides, D. G. (1985) Survey of current audiometric practices. *ASHA* February, 1985, 29–36.

Martin, J. I. (1978) *The Migrant Presence*. Sydney: George Allen and Unwin.

Martony, J. (1974) On speechreading of Swedish consonants and vowels. *STL-QPSR (Royal Institute of Technology, Stockholm)* 2–3, 11–33.

Mason, M. K. (1943) A cinematographic technique for testing visual speech comprehension. *Journal of Speech Disorders*, 8, 271–278.

Matzker, J. (1959) Two new methods for the assessment of central auditory functions in cases of brain disease. *Annals of Otology, Rhinology and Laryngology* 68, 1185–1197.

Medawar, P. B. (1965) *The great problems: a program for the natural sciences.* Address given at Cornell University.

Medical Research Council (1947) Special Report Series No. 261 *Hearing aids and audiometers.* London: HM Stationery Office.

Messouak, H. (1956) *Audiométrie Vocale en Arabic Maghrebin.* Les cahiers de la CFA No. 4. Paris: Compagnie Française d'Audiologie.

Miller, G. A., Heise, C. A. and Lichten, D. (1951) The intelligibility of speech as a function of the context of the test material. *Journal of Experimental Psychology,* 41, 329–335.

Miller, G. A. and Nicely, P. (1955) An analysis of perceptual confusions among some English consonants. *Journal of the Acoustical Society of America,* 27, 338–352.

Miller, J. D. and Weisenberger, J. M. (1985) The case of tactile aids. *Journal of the Acoustical Society of America* Suppl. 1. S16.

Milner, P. and Flevaris-Phillips, C. (1985) Speech reception in deaf adults using vibrotactile aids for cochlear implants. *Journal of the Acoustical Society of America* 78, Suppl 1, S17.

Mines, M. A., Hanson, B. F. and Shoup, J. E. (1978) Frequency of occurrence of phonemes in conversational English. *Language and Speech* 21, 221–241.

Mintz, S. L., Johnson, K. C., Stach, B. A. and Jerger, J. F. (1985) *Adaptive Speech audiometry for hearing evaluations.* Presented at the American Speech-Language-Hearing Association's Annual Convention in Washington, D.C.

Mitchell, A. G. and Delbridge, A. (1965) *The Speech of Australian Adolescents,* Sydney: Angus and Robertson.

Mitchell, A. G. and Delbridge, A. (1965) *The Pronounciation of English in Australia.* Australia: Angus and Robertson.

Moncur, J. P. and Dirks, P. (1967) Speech intelligibility in reverberation. *Journal of Speech and Hearing Research,* 10, 186–195.

Montgomery. A. A., Walden, B. E., Schwartz, D. M. and Prosek, R. A. (1984) Training auditory-visual speech reception in adults with moderate sensori neural hearing loss. *Ear Hear* 5, 30–36.

Moore, B. C. J. (1982) *An Introduction to the Psychology of Hearing.* London: MacMillan.

Morkovin, B. (1947) Rehabilitation of the aurally handicapped through the study of speech reading in life situations. *Journal of Speech Disorders,* 12, 363–368.

Murray, N. M. and Dermody, P. (1986) *Development of lists for auditory lexical decision tasks.* Paper presented at Audiological Society of Australia 7th National Conference, Ballarat.

Murray, N. (1943) *Articulation tests in flight.* ATL Informal Report No. IR-9. Sydney: CAL.

Murray, N. (1952) *The CAL PBO speech perception tests for deaf children.* Commonwealth Acoustic Laboratory Report No. 4. Sydney: CAL.

Murray, N. (1955) *The CAL PBP speech perception tests for deaf children.* Commonwealth Acoustic Laboratory Report No. 9. Sydney: CAL.

Muyunga, Y. K. (1974) *Development and application of speech audiometry using Lingala and Ciluba word lists.* Unpublished Ph.D. Thesis. University of London.

Myatt, B. and Landes, B. (1963) Assessing discrimination loss in children. *Archives of Otolaryngology,* 77, 359–362.

National Acoustic Laboratories Paediatric Audiological Protocols Manual. (1984) Field Services Section. Sydney: NAL.

Newby, H. A. (1958) *Audiology: Principles and Practice.* New York: Appleton-Century Crofts.

311

Neuman, A. C., Mills, R. C. and Schwander, T. J. (1985) *Noise reduction: Effects on consonant perception by normal hearing listeners.* Presented at the American Speech-Language-Hearing Association's Annual Convention in Washington, D.C.

Niemeyer, W. (1967) Sprachaudiometrie mit Sätzen (Speech audiometry using sentences). *HNO* (Berlin) 15, 335–343.

Noble, W. G. (1978) *Assessment of impaired hearing.* New York: Academic Press.

Noble, W. G. and Atherley, G. R. C. (1970) The hearing measurement scale: A questionnaire for the assessment of auditory disability. *Journal of Auditory Research*, 10, 229–250.

Ödkvist, L. M., Bergholtz, L. M., Åhlfeldt, H., Andersson, B., Edling, C. and Strand, E. (1982) Otoneurological and audiological findings in workers exposed to industrial solvents. *Acta Otolaryngologica* Suppl. 386, 249–251.

Olsen, W. O. and Matkin, N. D. (1979) Speech audiometry. In Rintleman, W. F. (Ed.) *Hearing Assessment.* Baltimore: University Park Press.

Olsen, W. O., Noffsinger, D. and Carhart, R. (1976) Masking level differences encountered in clinical populations. *Audiology*, 15, 287–301.

O'Neill, J. J. and Oyer, H. J. (1981) *Visual Communication for the Hard of Hearing* (2nd edition). Englewood Cliffs: Prentice-Hall.

Onsa, S. A. (1984) *The development of material for speech audiometry in Sudanese Arabic.* Unpublished M.Sc. Thesis. University of Manchester.

Osborn, R. (1985) Personal Communication.

Otto, S. R., Tyler, R. S., Preece, J. P. and Lansing, C. R. (1985) *Consonant recognition with single and multichannel cochlear implant systems.* Presented at the American Speech-Language-Hearing Association's Annual Convention in Washington, D.C.

Owens, E. (1961) Intelligibility of words varying in familiarity. *Journal of Speech and Hearing Research*, 4, 113–129.

Owens, E., Kessler, D. K., Raggio, M. W. and Schubert, E. D. (1985) Analysis and revision of the Minimal Auditory Capabilities (MAC) battery. *Ear and Hearing*, 6(6), 280–290.

Owens, E., Kessler, D. K., Telleen, C. C. and Schubert, E. (1980) *The Minimal Auditory Capabilities Battery.* Auditec of St Louis.

Owens, E., Kessler, D. K., Telleen, C. C. and Schubert, E. (1981) The minimal auditory capabilities (MAC) battery. *Hearing Aid Journal*, 34, 9–34.

Owens, E. and Telleen, C. C. (1981) Tracking as an aural rehabilitative process. *Journal of the Academy of Rehabilitation Audiology*, 14, 259–273.

Owens, E., Benedict, M. and Schubert, E. D. (1972) Consonant phoemic errors associated with pure tone configurations and certain kinds of hearing impairment. *Journal of Speech and Hearing Research*, 15, 308–322.

Owens, E. and Schubert, E. D. (1968) The development of the California Consonant Test. *Journal of Speech and Hearing Research*, 20, 463–474.

Pascoe, D. P. (1975) Frequency responses of hearing aids and their effects on the speech perception of hearing-impaired subjects. *Annals of Otorhinolaryngology* Suppl. 23, 84, 1–40.

Patterson, R. D., Nimmo-Smith, I., Weber, D. L. and Milroy, R. (1982) The deterioration of hearing with age: Frequency selectivity, the critical ratio, the audiogram and speech threshold. *Journal of the Acoustical Society of America*, 72, 1788–1803.

Pavlovic, C. V., Studebaker, G. A. and Sherbecoe, R. L. (1985) *Method for predicting speech discrimination of the hearing impaired.* Presented at the American Speech-Language-Hearing Association's Annual Convention in Washington, D.C.

Perry, F. R. (1979) *Monash diagnostic test of lipreading ability*. Australian Council for Education Research, Melbourne.

Pestalozza, G. and Shore, I. (1955) Clinical evaluation on the basis of different tests of auditory function. *Laryngoscope* 65, 1136–1163.

Peterson, G. E. and Lehiste, I. (1962) Revised CNC lists for auditory tests. *Journal of Speech and Hearing Disorders*, 27, 62–70.

Pickett, J. M. (1980) *The Sounds of Speech Communication*. Baltimore: University Park Press.

Pickett, J. M., Revoile, S. G. and Danaher, E. M. (1983) Speech-Cue Measures of Impaired Hearing. In *Hearing Research and Theory, Volume 2*. Tobias, J. V. and Schubert, E. D. (Eds), New York: Academic Press.

Plant, G. (1984a) *COMMTRAM — A Communication Training Program for Profoundly Deafened Adults*. Sydney: NAL.

Plant, G. (1984b) A diagnostic speech test for severely and profoundly hearing impaired children. *Australian Journal of Audiology*, 6, 1–9.

Plant, G. (1986) *A single-transducer vibrotactile aid to lipreading*. STL-QPRS (Royal Institute of Technology, Stockholm) In press.

Plant, G. and Macrae, J. (1977) Visual identification of Australian consonants vowels and diphthongs. *Australian Teacher of the Deaf*, 18, 46–50.

Plant, G. and Macrae, J. (1981) The NAL lipreading test: development standardization and validation. *Australian Journal of Audiology*, 3, 49–57.

Plant, G. and Macrae, J. (1985) *The PLOTT test*. Paper presented at the NAL Hearing Aid Conference, Sydney.

Plant, G., Macrae, J. and Pearce, J. (1980) Performance on Lipreading test by native and non-native speakers of English. *Australian Journal of Audiology*, 2, 25–29.

Plant, G., Macrae, J., Dillon, H. and Pentecost, F. (1984) Lipreading with minimal auditory cues. *Australian Journal of Audiology*, 6, 65–72.

Plant, G., Phillips, D. and Tsembis, J. (1982) An auditory-visual speech test for the elderly hearing-impaired. *Australian Journal of Audiology*, 4, 62–68.

Plant, G. and Westcott, S. (1982) A diagnostic speech perception test for severely and profoundly hearing impaired children. *Australian Journal of Audiology* Suppl 1, 9.

Plomp, R. and Duquesnoy, A. J. (1982) A model for the speech-reception threshold in noise with and without a hearing aid. *Scandinavian Audiology* Supplement 15, 95–111.

Plomp, R. and Mimpen, A. M. (1979) Improving the reliability of testing the speech-reception threshold for sentences. *Audiology*, 18, 43–53.

Pollack, I. (1959) Message uncertainty and message reception. *Journal of the Acoustical Society of America*, 31, 1500–1508.

Pollack, I., Rubenstein, H. and Decker, L. (1959) Intelligibility of known and unknown message sets. *Journal of the Acoustical Society of America*, 31, 273–279.

Posner, J. and Ventry, I. M. (1977) Relationships between comfortable loudness levels for speech and speech discrimination in sensorineural hearing loss. *Journal of Speech and Hearing Disorders*, 42, 370–375.

Priede, V. M. and Coles, R. R. A. (1976) Speech discrimination tests in investigation of sensorineural hearing loss. *Journal of Laryngology and Otology*, 90, 1081–1092.

Pronovost, W. and Dumbleton, C. (1954) A picture type speech sound discrimination test for children. *Journal of Speech and Hearing Research*, 19, 360–366.

Prosek, R. A. (1981) Some effects of training on speech recognition by hearing-impaired adults. *Journal of Speech and Hearing Research*, 24, 207–216.

Punch, J. L. (1980) Multidimensional scaling of quality judgments of speech signals processed by hearing aids. *Journal of the Acoustical Society of America*, 68–2, 458–466.

Punch, J. L. and Beck, E. L. (1980) Low-frequency response of hearing aids and judgments of aided speech quality. *Journal of Speech and Hearing Disorders*, 45, 325–335.

Rabinowitz, W. M. (1981) Measurement of the acoustic input immittance of the human ear. *Journal of the Acoustical Society of America*, 70, 1025–1035.

Reed, M. (1959) A verbal screening test of hearing. *Proceedings of the III World Congress of the Deaf, Wiesbaden (Germany)*. Herausgegeben vom Deutschen Gehorlosen-Bund e.v, Frankfurt am Main.

Resnick, D. M. and Becker, M. (1963) Hearing aid evaluation — a new approach. *ASHA* 5, 659–699.

Resnick, S. B., Dubno, J. R., Hoffnung, S. and Levitt, H. (1975) Phoneme errors on a nonsense syllable test. *Journal of the Acoustical Society of America*, 58 (Suppl. 1) 114.

Resnick, S. B., Dubno, J. R., Howie, D. G., Hoffnung, S., Freeman, L. and Slosberg, M. (1976) *Phoneme identification on a closed response nonsense syllable test*. Houston: American Speech Hearing Language Association.

Richards, D. L. (1973) Telecommunication by Speech. London: Butterworth.

Richter, U. (1976) Klirrfaktoren verschiedenartiger Schallsender (Harmonic distortion of sound sources of different kind). 5. DAGA — Tagung, Heidelberg, *VDI-Verlag*, Düsseldorf 1976, 479–482.

Richter, U. and Brinkmann, K. (1976) The sensitivity level of bone-conduction receivers. *Journal of Audiological Technique*, 15, 2–15.

Richter, U. and Brinkmann, K. (1977) Speech audiometry via bone-conduction. *Proceedings of the Ninth International Congress on Acoustics*, Madrid, Vol. 1, 403.

Rosen, J. K. (1978) The evaluation of handicap secondary to acquired hearing impairment. *Journal of the Academy of Rehabilitative Audiology*, 11(2), 2–9.

Rosen, S. and Corcoran, T. (1982) A video-recorded test of lipreading for British English. *British Journal of Audiology*, 16–4, 245–254.

Rosen, S. and Fourcin, A. J. (1983) When less is more: further work. University College, London. *Speech, Hearing, and Language: Work in progress*. 1, 1–27.

Rosen, S., Fourcin, A. and Moore, B. (1981) Voice pitch as an aid to lipreading. *Nature*, 291, 150–152.

Rosen, S., Moore, B. C. J. and Fourcin, A. J. (1979) Lipreading with fundamental frequency information. *Proceedings of the Institute of Acoustics. Autumn Conference*, paper 1A2, 5–8.

Rosenzweig, M. R. and Postman, L. (1958) Frequency of usage and the perception of words. *Science*. 127, 263–266.

Ross, M. (1978) Hearing aid evaluation. In *Handbook of Clinical Audiology*. Jack Katz (Ed.) Baltimore: Williams and Wilkins Co.

Ross, M. and Lerman, J. W. (1970) A picture identification test for hearing impaired children. *Journal of Speech and Hearing Research*, 13, 44–53.

Rowland, J. P., Dirks, D. D., Dubno, J. R. and Bell, T. S. (1985) Comparison of speech recognition-in-noise and subjective communication assessment. *Ear and Hearing*. 6(6), 291–296.

Rudmose, W. (1964) Concerning the problem of calibrating TDH-39 earphones at 6 kHz with a 9A coupler. *Journal of the Acoustical Society of America*, 36, 1049(A).

Rupp, R. R. (1980) Chapter 4 in *Speech Protocols in Audiology*. Rupp, R. R. and Stockdell, K. G. (Eds) New York: Grune and Stratton.

Rupp, R. R., Higgins, J. and Maurer, J. F. (1977) A feasibility scale for predicting hearing aid use (FSPHAU) with older individuals. *Journal of the Academy of Rehabilitation Audiology*, 10, 81.

Rupp, R. R. and Stockdell, K. G. (1980) Chapter 2 in *Speech Protocols in Audiology*. Rupp, R. R. and Stockdell, K. G. (Eds) New York: Grune and Stratton.

Sanderson-Leepa, M. E. and Rintelmann, W. F. (1976) Articulation function and test-retest performance of normal-learning children on three speech discrimination tests: WIPI, PBK50, and NU Auditory Test No. 6. *Journal of Speech Disorders*, 41, 503–519.

Saunders, F. A. and Franklin, B. (1985) Field tests of a wearable 16-channel electro-tactile sensory aid in a classroom for the deaf. *Journal of the Acoustical Society of America*, 78, Suppl. 1, S17.

Savin, H. B. (1963) Word frequency effects and errors in the perception of speech. *Journal of the Acoustical Society of America*, 35, 200–206.

Schmitz, H. D. (1980) Hearing aid selection for adults. In *Amplification for the Hearing-Impaired*. Michael C. Pollack (Ed.) New York: Grune and Stratton.

Schultz, M. C. and Schubert, E. D. (1969) A multiple choice discrimination test (MCDT). *Laryngoscope* 79, 382–399.

Schum, D. J. and Collins, M. J. (1985) *Test-Retest reliability of two paired-comparison hearing aid evaluations*. Presented at the American Speech-Language-Hearing Association's Annual Convention in Washington, D.C.

Schwartz, D. (1982) Hearing Aid Selection Methods: An Enigma. In *The Vanderbilt Hearing Report* Studebaker, G. A. and Bess, F. H. (Eds). Upper Darby, Pa: Monographs in Contemporary Audiology.

Shannon, C. E. (1948) A mathematical theory of communication. *Bell System Technical Journal*, 27, 379–423 and 623–656.

Shapiro, I. (1976) Hearing aid fitting by prescription. *Audiology* 15, 163–173.

Shoop, C. (1978) *Training effects of CV syllables instruction on the geriatric population*. ASHA Convention. San Francisco.

Shoop, C. and Binnie, C. A. (1979) The effect of age on the visual perception of speech. *Scandinavian Audiology*, 8, 3–8.

Shore, I., Bilger, R. C. and Hirsh, I. J. (1960). Hearing aid evaluations: reliability of repeated measures. *Journal of Speech and Hearing Disorders*, 25, 152–170.

Siegenthaler, B. and Haspiel, G. (1966) *Development of two standardized measures of hearing for speech by children*. U.S. Department of Health, Education, and Welfare. Project No. 2372. Contract No. OE-5-10-003.

Silverman, S. R. and Hirsh, I. (1955) Problems related to the use of speech in clinical audiometry. *Annals of Otology, Rhinology and Laryngology*, 64, 1234–1244.

Skamris, N. (1977) Personal communication.

Skamris, N. (1974) Assessment of lipreading ability of deafened persons. *Scandinavian Audiology*. Supplement 4, 128–135.

Sortini, A. and Flake, C. (1953) Speech audiometry testing for pre-school children. *Laryngoscope*, 63, 991–997.

Speaks, C. and Jerger, J. (1965) Method for measurement of speech identification. *Journal of Speech and Hearing Research*, 8, 185–194.

Spitzer, J. B., Leder, S. B., Flevaris-Phillips, C. and Milner, P. (1985) *Standardization of videotaped tests of speechreading ranging in task difficulty*. Presented at the American Speech-Language-Hearing Association's Annual Convention in Washington, D.C.

Stein, L. and Zerlin, S. (1963) Effect of circumaural earphones and earphone cushions on auditory threshold. *Journal of the Acoustical Society of America*, 35, 1744–1745.

Stevenson, P. W. (1973) *An automated system for speech audiometry*. Ph.D Thesis, University of Essex, UK.

Stevenson, P. and Martin, M. (1977) *Phonemic discrimination difficulties and sensori-neural hearing loss*. London: Royal National Institute of the Deaf.

Stream, R. W. and Dirks, D. D. (1974) Effects of loudspeaker position on differences between earphones and free-field thresholds (MAP) and (MAF) *Journal of Speech and Hearing Research*, 17, 549–568.

Studebaker, G. A. (1980) Fifty years of hearing aid research: an evaluation of progress. *Ear and Hearing*, 1, 57–62.

Studebaker, G. A. (1982) Hearing aid selection: an overview. In *The Vanderbilt Hearing Aid Report*. Studebaker, G. A. and Bess, F. H. (Eds). Upper Darby, Pa: Monographs in Contemporary Audiology.

Studebaker, G. A., Bissett, J. D. and Van Ort, D. (1982) Paired comparison judgments of relative intelligibility in noise. *Journal of the Acoustical Society of America*, 72–1, 80–92.

Summerfield, A. Q. (1983) Audio-visual speech perception, lipreading and artificial stimulation. In *Hearing Science and Hearing Disorders*. Lutman, M. E. and Haggard, M. P. (Eds).

Summerfield, A. Q. and Foster, J. (1983) Assessing audiovisual speech-reception disability. In: *High Technology Aids for the Disabled*. Perkins, W. J. (Ed.) London: Butterworth.

Taylor, M. and Creelman, C. (1967) PEST: efficient estimates on probability functions. *Journal of the Acoustical Society of America*, 41, 782–787.

Tecca, J. and Binnie, C. (1982) The application of an adaptive procedure to the California Consonant Test for hearing aid evaluation. *Ear and Hearing*, 3, 72–76.

Thompson, G. and Lassman, F. (1969) Relationship of auditory distortion test results to speech discrimination through flat versus selective amplification systems. *Journal of Speech and Hearing Research*, 12, 594–686.

Thorndike, E. L. and Lorge, I. (1944) *The teacher's word book of 30 000 words*. New York: Bureau of Publications, Columbia University.

Thornton, A. and Raffin, M. (1978) Speech discrimination scores modelled as a binomial variable. *Journal of Speech and Hearing Research*, 21, 507–518.

Tillman, T. and Carhart, R. (1966) *An Expanded Test for Speech Discrimination Utilizing CNC Monosyllabic Words*. N.U. Auditory Test No. 6, USAF School of Aerospace.

Tillman, T. W., Carhart, R. and Wilber, L. (1963) *A test for speech discrimination composed of CNC monosyllabic words*. Northwestern University Auditory Test No 4. Technical Documentary Report No. SAM-TDR-62-135, USAF School of Aerospace Medicine, Brooks Air Force Base, Texas.

Tillman, T. W. and Gish, K. D. (1964) Comments on the effect of circumaural earphones on auditory thresholds. *Journal of the Acoustical Society of America*, 36, 969–970.

Tillman, T. W., Johnson, R. and Olsen, W. (1966) Earphones versus soundfield threshold sound pressure levels for spondee words. *Journal of the Acoustical Society of America*, 39, 125–133.

Tonnisson, W. (1976) Australian standardisation of CID everyday sentence test. *Proceedings of the 2nd National Conference of the Audiological Society of Australia*. Melbourne: ASA.

Tonisson, W. (1977) Australian Standardisation of C.I.D. Everyday Sentence Test, *Sydney: Annual Report 1976–77*, National Acoustic Laboratories.

Trammel, J., Farrar, C., Owens, S., Schepard, D., Thies, T. and Witlen, R. (1976) *Test of Auditory Comprehension*. North Hollywood: Foreworks.

Traynor, R. M., Smaldino, J. J., Kopra, L. L., Dunlop, R. J., Kopra, M., Abraham-son, J., Garstecki, D. C. and Rax, I. (1985) *High technology in aural rehabili-tation. A miniseminar*. Presented at the American Speech-Language-Hearing Association's Annual Convention in Washington, D.C.

Tyler, R. S. and Smith, P. A. (1983) Sentence identification in noise and hearing-handicap questionnaires. *Scandinavian Audiology*, 12, 285–292.

Tyler, R. S., Summerfield, Q., Wood, E. S. and Fernandes, M. A. (1982) Psychoa-coustic and phonetic temporal processing in normal and hearing-impaired lis-teners. *Journal of the Acoustical Society of America*, 72, 740–752.

Ulrich, J. H. (1957) An experimental study of the acquisition of information from three types of recorded television presentation. *Speech Monographs*, 2439–45.

Upfold, L. J. and Smither, M. F. (1981) Hearing aid fitting protocol. *British Journal of Audiology*, 15, 181–188.

Urbantschitsch, V. (1895) *Auditory training for deafmutism and for deafness acquired in later life*. Vienna: Urban and Schwarzenberg.

Utley, J. (1946) A test of lipreading ability. *Journal of Speech Disorders*, 11, 109–116.

Ventry, I. M. (1976) Pure tone-spondee threshold relationship in functional hearing loss: a hypothesis. *Journal of Speech and Hearing Disorders*, 41 , 16–22.

Ventry, I. M. (1979) Comment on Guidelines (Letter to Editor). *ASHA* 6, 639.

Ventry, I. M. (1976) Puretone-spondee threshold relationships in functional hearing loss. *Journal of Speech and Hearing Disorders*, 41, 16–22.

Ventry, I. M. and Weinstein, B. E. (1982) The hearing handicap inventory for the elderly: A new tool. *Ear and Hearing*, 3, 128.

Victoreen, J. A. (1973) *Basic principle of otometry*. Springfield, Ill.: Charles C. Thomas.

Voiers, W. D. (1977) *Diagnostic Evaluation of Speech Intelligibility* (in Hawley, 1977).

Walden, B. E. and Montgomery, A. A. (1975) Dimensions of consonant perception in normal and hearing impaired listeners. *Journal of Speech and Hearing Research*, 18, 444–455.

Walden, B. E. Erdman, S. A., Montgomery, A. A., Schwartz, D. H. and Prosek, R. A. (1981) Some effects of training on speech recognition by hearing impaired adults. *Journal of Speech and Hearing Research*, 24, 207–216.

Walden, B. E., Prosek, R. A., Montogomery, A. A., Scherr, C. K. and Jones, C. J. (1977) Effects of training on the visual recognition of consonants. *Journal of Speech and Hearing Research*, 20, 130–145.

Walker, G., Byrne, D. and Dillon, H. (1982) Learning effects with a closed set nonsense syllable test. *Australian Journal of Audiology*, 4, 27–31.

Wall, L. G., Davis, L. A. and Myers, D. K. (1984) Four spondee threshold pro-cedures: a comparison. *Ear and Hearing*, 5(3), 171–174.

Wang, M. D. and Bilger, R. C. (1973) Consonant confusions in noise: A study of perceptual features. *Journal of the Acoustical Society of America*, 54, 1248–1266.

Wang, W. S-Y. and Crawford, J. (1960) Frequency studies of English consonants. *Language and Speech*, 3, 131–139.

Watson, L. A. and Tolan, T. (1949) Hearing Tests and Hearing Instruments. Balti-more: Williams and Wilkins.

Watson, T. J. (1957) Speech audiometry in children. In Ewing, A. W. G. (Ed.) *Educational Guidance and the Deaf Child*. Manchester: Manchester University Press.

Watts, M. J. and Pegg, K. S. (1977) The rehabilitation of adults with acquired hearing loss. *British Journal of Audiology*, 11, 103–110.

Weber, S. and Redell, R. C. (1976) A sentence test for measuring speech discrimina-tion in children. *Audiology, Hearing and Education*, 2, 25–30.

Weinstein, B. E. (1984) A review of hearing handicap scales. *Audiology*, 9(7), 91–109.

Weinstein, B. E. and Ventry, I. M. (1982) The assessment of hearing handicap in the elderly. *Hearing Aid Journal*, 1(35), 17.

Weinstein, B. E. and Ventry, I. (1983a) The audiologic correlates of hearing handicap in the elderly. *Journal of Speech and Hearing Research*, 26, 148–151.

Weinstein, B. and Ventry, I. (1983b) Audiometric correlates of the hearing handicap inventory for the elderly. *Journal of Speech and Hearing Disorders*, 48, 379–384.

Weisenberger, J. M., Miller, J. D., Moog, J. S. and Geers, A. E. (1985) *Evaluation of the Siemens minifonator vibrotactile aid: testing with adults.* Presented at the American Speech-Language-Hearing Association's Annual Convention in Washington, D.C.

White, S. C. (1980) Chapter 7 in *Speech Protocols in Audiology*, Rupp, R. R. and Stockwell, K. G. (eds.), New York: Grune and Stratton.

Wilde, R. (1985) Personal Communication.

Wills, R. (1985) *A reverberation time survey in school classrooms used by hearing impaired children with hearing aids, and in a hospital free field audiology test room.* MSc. Project Report. Polytechnic of the South Bank, London.

Wilson, R. H. and Antablin, J. K. (1980) A picture identification task as an estimate of the word-recognition performance of non-verbal adults. *Journal of Speech and Hearing Disorders*, 45, 223–238.

Wilson, R. H. and Margolis, R. H. (1983) Measurements of auditory thresholds for speech stimuli. pp. 79–126 in *Principles of Speech Audiometry*, Konkle, D. F. and Rintelmann, W. F. (Eds) Perspectives in Audiology Series. Lyle, L. Lloyd (Series Ed.) Baltimore: University Park Press.

Wilson, R. H., Morgan, D. E. and Dirks, D. D. (1973) A proposed SRT procedure and its statistical precedent. *Journal of Speech and Hearing Disorders*, 38, 184–191.

Wilson, R. H., Stream, R. W. and Dirks, D. D. (1973) Spread-of-masking effects on pure tones and several speech stimuli. *Journal of Speech and Hearing Research*, 16, 385–396.

Woodward, M. F. and Barber, C. G. (1960) Phoneme perception in lip reading. *Journal of Speech and Hearing Research*, 3, 212–222.

Zwicker, E. and Feldtheller, R. (1967) *Das Ohr als Nachrichtenempfänger.* (The human ear as a receiver of information) 2nd edition. Stuttgart: S. Hirzel Verlag.

Zwislocki, J. J. (1953) Acoustic attenuation between the ears. *Journal of the Acoustical Society of America*, 25, 752.

Zwislocki, J. J. (1971) *An ear-like coupler for earphone calibration. Report LSC-S-9.* Institute for Sensory Research. Syracuse University, Syracuse, New York.

Index

Named Speech Audiometric Tests and Lipreading Tests are shown in bold in the index.

A Weighting Network 81
Acoustic coupler 92
  coupler sensitivity factor 93
Acoustic immittance 111
Acoustic impedance of human ear 92
Acoustic intensity 9
Acoustic leakage (earphones) 92, 94
Acoustic nerve 111
Acoustic neuromata 121,125
Acoustic phonetics 2, 14
Acoustic cues 14, 32
Adaptive tests 32, 262–3
  procedure 260
    for children 268
Affix system 21
Affricates 18, 19, 20
Age effect on performance 66, 67, 124,
    242, 261
  aided performance 136, 140
Allophonic variations 37, 43
Alveolar consonants 19, 22, 172, 192
Amplitude 3
Aperiodic sound 176
Aphasia 61
Approximant 19, 20, 23, 27
Arabic speech audiometry 283
Articulation 209
  gain function 209
  Index 209, 234, 260
  testing 156
Artificial ear 83, 92
  sentences 40, 158
Aspirant 23
  turbulence 22

Assimilation 28
Audiogram (pure tone) 24, 130
Audiometric configurations 119, 136
  test rooms 84
Audiometers 77
  calibration 77, 212
Auditory cortex lesions 122
Auditory function categories 111
Auditory Numbers Test (ANT) 161, 250,
    269
Auditory/aural rehabilitation
  definition 130
  and nonsense syllables 222
  and speech audiometry 231–234
  planning 220
Auditory sensitivity 110
  space 24, 28
  space-time 29, 32
Auditory transmission channel 35
Auditory training 148, 177
Auditory-visual presentation in
    noise 201–203
Audio visual tests 72, 172–173, 241
  testing 196–204
  and elderly 198–203
Australian Deafness Council 249
  English 249
Average speech level 104

Basilar membrane 24, 25
Best-fit curve 116
Bilabial consonants 19, 22, 172, 192
  stops 22
Bisyllabic test material (Norway) 238

Binaural listening   94, 101
    interaction   123
    fusion of speech   123
**Binnie, Montgomery and Jackson
    Lipreading Test**   182
Binomial distribution   49, 226, 227, 231,
    261
BKB Sentence lists for children   72, 143,
    146, 150, 153, 165, 180, 252
    picture related (BKB-PR)   165
Bone conduction   217, 225
Bone vibrators   92, 93
    freefield sensitivity   101
Boothroyd word lists/AB isophonemic
    word lists   72, 81, 113, 114, 116, 119,
    121, 144, 146, 148, 150, 151, 164, 170,
    222, 248, 250, 261
Brainstem disorders   112, 123
British Society of Audiology   ix
    speech audiogram format   31
British Standards (BS)   78

CAL-PBM lists   250, 251
CAL Audiology manual   256
Calibration
    of audiometers   77–78, 105, 166, 212,
    244
    equipment   78
    tones   79, 82, 105, 244, 281
    check tones   95, 96
    of recorded material   116, 105
    objective   91
California Consonant Test (CCT)   208,
    223, 232
Cantonese speech audiometry   280, 284
Carhart procedure for hearing aid
    evaluation   137
Carrier sentences   38
    phrases   215, 219, 228, 239
CCITT   95
Central auditory disorder   111–112, 207,
    220
    evaluation   122–124, 242
Central speech tests   124, 242
CHABA sentences   224, 232
Children
    aboriginal   248
    auditory test   269
    deaf-lipreading   181
        consonant perception   197
    hearing impaired   119, 149, 155–170,
    175, 212, 216, 219, 251

speech perception thresholds   252
    reading ability   273
    tests for   143, 150, 159, 174, 229–31,
    242, 266–278
    unilateral hearing loss   273
CID (Central Institute for the Deaf)
    lists   81
Everyday Sentence Lists   184, 224,
    252, 260
    W-1 spondees   208, 211
    W-2   211, 256
    W-22   112, 141, 156, 208, 220, 221,
    224, 227, 232, 235, 256
Clark PB Lists   250
Closed set tests   30, 70, 161, 223
CNC Word lists   220, 221
Coarticulation   44
Cochlea distortion   134, 137
    implants   32, 149, 233, 235, 241
Collinearity   66
COMMTRAM (Communication training
    programme for profoundly deafened
    adults)   265
Communication ability   207
Compact disc (video disc)   234, 238,
    239, 243
Computer controlled audiometry   87,
    234
Competing noise   64
    speech   125, 242
**Concrete Object Speech Test for
    Children**   267
Conductive hearing loss   111, 121, 207,
    220
    in children   268, 273
Confusion clusters   192
Connected discourse   211, 232
    Tracking test   148, 173, 233
Consonant   14, 18
    cluster   14
    contrast   16, 18, 173
    identiication test (**NAL lipreading
        test**)   187
    frequency of occurrence   44
    perception   197
Consonantal segments   14
Contextual information   110
Continuous speech tests   30, 158, 260
Cortical disorders   112, 123
Craig Lipreading Inventory   180
CUNY Nonsense Syllable test   251, 258
CVC monosyllables   45, 53, 60

Decibel scale   9
Decoding (of speech)   12–24
Dental   19
Detection   209
  threshold   209
Dichotic signals   123
Dialect   14, 21, 36, 43, 48
Differential diagnosis   109–125, 207, 220
Difficult to test patients   219
DIN standards   89–107
DIP Test   230
Diphthong   14, 18, 20, 23, 24, 26, 43
Directional microphones   149
Disability   68, 130–134, 219
  relationship with handicap   133
Discrimination   210
  function   30
  score   65
  curve   75, 101
  in quiet and noise with hearing
    aids   140
  function (aided)   147
Distortion (speech perception)   63–65,
  134
Distorted speech tests   242
Duration   7

Earphones   82
  Beyer DT48   92, 94, 97
  Telephonics TDH39/49   83, 212, 244
  free-field calibration   92, 94, 99
  test and calibration   106
Ear simulator   93
Effort   16
Electro acoustic transmission
    channel   35
Electro tactile devices   235
Elision   28
Encoding speech   12, 14
Equalising word levels   91
Equipment   97, 243
Error patterns   71, 198
Everyday speech   40

FAAF Test   30, 71, 73, 125, 143, 146,
  147, 148, 150, 152, 281
FADAST   73, 148, 150, 173
Familiarisation   215
Features (speech)   14
Film Test of Lipreading   182
Filter networks for speech
    audiometers   97

Filtering – low pass   203
Five Sound Test   162, 269
Foot (stress group)   13
Forced choice tests   30, 47, 60
Foreign listeners   48
Formant   16, 175
  nasal   20
  amplitude   20
  motion   23
Fourier analysis   4
Free field
  calibration   92–94
  sensitivity level   92, 93, 97
  sound pressure level of speech   99
  testing   83, 132, 162, 212, 259
Free sound field   105
Frequency Distorted Speech Test   242
Frequency discrimination   24, 25, 26, 110
Frequency selectivity   24
Frequency resolution   63, 110
Frequency response of hearing aids   137
  of speech audiometers   94, 105, 97
  and speech test performance   66
Frequency of occurrence effect   58
  of phonemes   192, 280
  of English sounds   221
Fricative   18, 19, 20, 25
  homorganic   20
  turbulence   22
  dental   23
  place   28
Frication   28
Fry Word Lists   113, 117, 121, 157, 260,
  280
Fry Kerridge Sentences   280
Functional hearing loss   242
Fundamental frequency   4, 5, 11
  (speech)   15, 203
Fundamental, missing   9, 10

Gap detection test   176
German DIN Standards   89–107
  word lists   89
    for children   90
  numerals   89
  monosyllabic nouns   89
  reference level for hearing loss   90
  sentences (German)   90, 95
Greek   248

Hagerman Test   241
Hair cell loss   24

Half peak level (HPL) 115, 127
  elevation (HPLE) 115, 117, 119
Half lists v whole lists 226, 239
Halo effect 36
Handicap 130, 133, 140, 149, 207, 240
  prediction of 131
  measurement of degree 241
Harmonic(s) 4, 5, 10, 11
  analysis 4
  distortion 106, 281
  series 5
Hearing aid users 66
  benefit 134, 135, 137, 139, 140
  evaluation 135, 241, 262
  and patient satisfaction 14
  paired comparisons 139
  quality judgements 138–9
  slope of frequency response 137
Homophones 59, 232
Historical developments (speech
  recognition tests) 155–157
Hindi speech audiometry 282, 284
Helen Lipreading Test 183, 187, 197,
  198, 203, 241
HRRC Rhyme Test 250
Hearing central 40
  tactics 203
  peripheral 40
Hearing Handicap Inventory for the
  Elderly (HHIE) 134, 233
  questionnaire 132
  scale (HHS) 134
**Hearing Impaired Test of Receptive
  Communication (HITORC)** 274
Hearing level for numerals 105
Hearing loss impairment 11, 26, 28, 39,
  66, 109, 130, 179
  conductive loss 31, 67, 118
  elderly 198–203
  high frequency 228
  NVIII origin 118
  sensorineural 24, 31, 63
  for speech 280
  vascular lesions 118
Hearing measurement scale 132, 134
Hearing performance inventory 233

Immediate Appreciation Test 40
Impulse sound level meter 91
Increment size 213
Institute of Sound and Vibration
  Research, Southampton 121

Instructions to patient 128
Intelligibility 210
  curves 48, 52, 53, 60
    shape of 39
  individual test words 103
  maximum 52
  reference curves 97
  sentences (German) 90
  testing (standardisation) 84
Intensity discrimination 63, 110
  gating 203
Interdentals 192
International Civil Aviation Organisation
  (ICAO) Standards 259
International Electrotechnical
  Commission (IEC) Standards 77,
  78, 88, 92, 93, 94, 282 *and Appendix,
  page 287*
International Standards Organisation
  (ISO) Standards 78, 84, 85, 93, 107
Intervocalic Consonant Test 173
Intonation 2, 13, 14, 27, 172, 174
  marker 13
  pattern, nucleus of 12
Interrupted Speech Test 242
Isophonemic lists 46
Iso-performance contours 67
Items (and lists) 38

Just Noticeable Difference (JND) 25

Kendall Toy (KT) Test 162, 167, 250,
  267

Label(ing) speech 174
Labiodental 19, 192
Laryngeal 19
  activity 18
  tone 24
Larynx 2, 20
Length 9, 12, 15, 16, 18
Level equalisation 262
  of calibration signal and test words 96
Leq and speech level 262
Lingala speech audiometry 284
Linguistics 1, 12
Linguistic complexity of speech 14
  hierarchy 12
  properties of stimuli 58
  unit 13
Lipreading 71, 148, 150, 177, 179–205
List(s) 38, 48, 68

recording preparation 81
Listening tests 94
Live voice testing 105, 116, 142, 150, 162, 164, 182, 185, 212, 225, 266, 267
Logatoms 40
Loudness 8, 12, 15
  minimum detectable 9
  of words 91
Loudspeaker 83
  output 106
  placement 149, 212, 240

Manchester Junior (MJ) Lists 163, 167
  **Picture (MP) Vocabulary
    Test** 163, 168
  Sentence (MS) Test 164, 169
  Speech Reading Test 183
Manner (of production) 14, 19, 20, 172
  contrasts 28
  decisions 24
  errors 71
  group 22
Masking (for speech audiometry) 77, 127, 216, 225, 229
  effective level 85, 116
  insert earphone 240
  level difference 123
  wideband 116
Maximum speech identification
  discrimination score 112, 116, 119, 131, 132, 134, 239
Mechanical coupler (artificial
  mastoid) 78, 92, 93
**Medical Research Council (MRC) Word
  Lists** 113, 114, 256, 280
Menieres 118, 122
Message to Competition Ratio
  (MCR) 141, 147
Meters (VU, PPM) 81
Microcomputer control of tests 176
Middle ear disorders/surgery 111
**Minimal Auditory Capabilities (MAC)
  Battery** 233, 252
**Monash Diagnostic Test of Lipreading
  Ability** 180
**Monosyllabic Adaptive Speech Test
  (MAST)** 268, 270
  Word Tests 158
    and Cortical Disorders 123
    for Children 160
**Monosyllable, Trochee, Spondee
  (MONSTER)** Test 251, 258

Most Comfortable Level (MCL) 136, 225, 227, 228, 256, 260
Multiple choice tests 30, 87, 159, 161, 223
**Multiple Choice Discrimination Test
  (MCDT)** 223
Music scales 12

Nasal(s) 14, 19, 20, 23, 25
  formant 21
Nasality 21, 232
National Acoustic Laboratories
  (NAL) 249
NAL Lipreading Test 185–196, 205–206, 265
  Paediatric Audiological Protocols
    Manual 255
  PBM Lists 257
  **Tests of Auditory Language Learning
    (NALTALLK)** 273
Noise–Cafeteria 69, 149
  Speech babble 69
    spectrum 77
  for speech in noise tests 69, 138, 149, 241
Non-rhotic 21
Non auditory variables 123
Non-organic hearing loss 111, 119
  and pure tone audiogram 120
  speech tests for 242
Nonsense Syllables 156, 157, 160, 197, 220, 222
  Test (NST) 157, 222, 232, 251
Normal auditory function 111, 112
  response curve 86
  sensitivity 64
  subjective calibration 252
  threshold for speech 282
**North Western University (NU)
  Children's Perception of Speech (NU-
    CHIPS) Test** 161, 230, 268
  NU 4 Test 222
  NU 6 Test 208, 220, 222, 232, 251, 263
Nucleus of intonation pattern 12
  a tone group 13, 15

Obstruent Consonants 175
Octaves 12
Open response tests 29, 59, 60
Optimal Discrimination Score
  (ODS) 115, 116, 122

Paediatric Audiology Word Lists   105
  Audiological Protocols Manual
    (NAL)   255
**Paediatric Speech Intelligibility Test
  (PSI)**   148, 230, 235
  Australian Version   267
PAL Auditory Test No 9   211
  No 14   211
  20 PB-50 Lists   156
  PB 50 Lists   47, 122, 208, 220, 221,
    227, 256
  PB 50 in Noise (PBN)   259
  PBK Lists for Children   229
Palato-alveolar   19
Patient groups   47
  Instructions   117, 128
PB$_{max}$ 112, 115, 122, 227, 256, 262
Peak level indicator   91, 96
Peceptual disabilities   123
  phonetics   221
Peripheral auditory system   110
Period   3
  discrimination   27
Periodic sounds identification   176
Periodicity   11, 22, 26
  clues   13
  of speech signals   15
Performance-Intensity (PI)
    function   224, 225, 227, 261
PEST Procedure   264
Phoneme   14, 37, 43
  combinations   59
  recognition   37, 232
  scoring   117
Phonemic balance   42, 46, 160, 221, 239
  inventory   43, 45
Phonemic category   12
Phonetics   1, 2
Phonetic inventory   43
Phonetically Balanced (PB) word
    lists   112
  Familiar List (PBF)   161
  Kindergarten 50s (PBK-50s) Test   161
  Monosyllable List   256
  Objects (PBO) Test for Children   266
  Picture (PBT) Test for Children   266
Phone   37, 43
Phono-acoustic space   37
Phonograph   156
Phonological contrast   12
Phrase   12, 13
Pitch   9, 12, 15, 24, 26

change   15, 27
detection   26
marker (motion)   15, 16, 26
perception   13, 24, 176
range   14
Place of articulation   18, 19, 20, 172, 175
  contrasts   22, 28
  cues   28
  decisions   24
  errors   71
  processing   26
PLOTT Test   250, 269
Pointing to Picture Test   30
  (Two Alternative)   72
Practice effects   193
Presbyacusis   61, 183
Presentation level   227
Pronunciation   116
Prosodics   1, 15, 172, 176
Prosodic shape   22, 26
Pseudohypoacusis   207, 216, 218
Psychiatric patients   216, 219
Psychoacoustics   8
  tests   110, 125
Psychometric function   60, 116, 208, 218
Psychophysical scaling   8, 12
Pure tone sensitivity and speech
    intelligibility   60, 65, 114, 118,
    120, 121, 130, 175, 211, 215, 216
  Threshold Best Two Average
    (BTA)   117–119

QUAH Lipreading Test   184, 187
Qualitative uses of speech
    audiometry   150

RASP Test   123
Reaction time to speech   87, 264
Received Pronunciation (RP)   44
Recognition   37, 209
  threshold   209
Recording level   82
  requirements and standardisation   281
Recorded speech material, sound
    pressure level   94
Recorded versus live voice
    presentation   212, 228
Recruitment   9, 67, 120, 228
Redundancies   39, 40, 143, 158
Redundancy-reduction for cortical
    tests   123
Reed Hearing Test   166

Reference level for hearing loss for
    speech (Germany) 90
  recordings 105
Rehabilitation 232
  programme 240
    use of NAL lipreading test 195
    audio-visual test results 203
Rehabilitation Services, Australia 248
Resonance 16
Response (appropriate) 36
  correct/incorrect versus Level 56
  criteria 213
  channel 35
  element 38
  forced/free 58
  probability 58
  set 110
  from patient 117
Retrocochlear disorders and speech
    discrimination 122, 216
Reverberation 149, 240
Rhyme Test 30, 220, 223
  Diagnostic (DRT) 30, 223
  HHRC 250, 251, 258
  Modified (MRHT) 152, 223, 232, 250,
    251, 258
RNID Hearing Test Cards 166, 170
Roll-over index 122
Running speech 68
  as competing signal 124
Rush Hughes PB-50 Lists 221

Scoring 38
Segment 13, 14, 15
Sensory disorders, differentiation of
    sensory and peripheral neural 120
Sentence (tests) 39, 68, 96, 104, 158,
    187, 223, 252, 259
Self assessment inventories 233
Self-reported speech disability 66, 69
Semitones 12
Semivowels 23
Sibilants 23, 25
Signal to noise ratio 64, 69, 183, 203
SIiN Test 70, 72
**Skamris Film Test of Lipreading
    Skills** 182
Social adequacy index 256
  hearing handicap index 134
Socio-economic group 67
Soft palate 22
Sonorance 232

**Sound Effects Recognition Test
    (SERT)** 162, 230
Sound carriers for hearing tests 104
  diffraction 92, 94
  field 212, 240
  level meter 78, 91, 95, 106, 116, 162,
    281
  pattern tests 174–177
  pressure level of speech 91, 96, 103,
    105, 213
  spectrum 174
Speaker 35
  selection 47, 186
  sex 14
Spectrogram 8
Spectrum 4, 6
  of speech 16, 24
Speech acoustic properties 24
  audiogram 30, 31
  audiometry – for communication
    ability 41
    for differential diagnosis 33, 41
    definition and theory 33, 53, 75,
    110, 207
    errors in responses 54
    equipment 75, 97
    general factors 36
    how to use speech in speech
      audiometry 28
    information flow 75, 76
    method for monosyllabic word
      lists 127
    statistics of scores 48
  audiometers 84, 91, 94
    bandwidth 100
    standardisation 91, 105, 287–294
    testing and calibration 106
  awareness threshold 210
  chain 2
  contrast 14, 32
  conversational 16
  decision 14
  Detection Threshold (SDT) 29, 81,
    159, 210, 216, 281
  discrimination score 207
    testing 110, 209
    and handicap 133
    identification functions 111
    with monosyllables 115, 116, 127
  in noise 68, 69
    adaptive tests 71
    test for aircrew 259

intelligibility   110
   and distortion   66
   measure of   63
   reference curves   98
level   58, 68
material   35
   selection of   39
   familiarity of   46
perception   14, 22, 24, 36
processing model   63
production   14
quality   9, 12, 14, 16
reception threshold   29, 52, 70,
   112–119, 131, 209, 215, 237, 244
recognition threshold   210, 211, 213,
   216, 218
signal level calibration   244
simulating noise (CCITT)   95, 105
sounds   8, 15, 22
synthesis   32, 174
test areas of use   35
   for civil aviation   259
   criteria for children   159
   conditions   149
   critical/minimal differences   144,
      151–153
   for mild to moderate losses   264
   sensitivity   142
   for severe to profound losses   265
   standardisation   47, 61, 104, 253
   reliability   144
   types   148
timbre   12
transmission Evaluation Procedures
   (STEPs)   264
transmission Index   234
volume   101
SPIN Test   32, 197, 224, 232, 265
   Australian version   251, 252
   for hearing aid fitting   258
Spondee (word lists)   112, 119, 208, 237
   threshold   209
Staggered Spondaic Word (SSW)
   Test   124, 234
Stapedial reflex   111
Step size   213
Stimulus element   38
Stop(s)   18, 19, 20, 22, 23, 25
Stress   2, 14, 16
   pattern   22
Stressed/unstressed syllables   13, 15,
   27
Subject instructions   70

with minimal English   115
   response   70
Subjective loudness   91
Suppression   63
Syllable   13–28
Syllabic rate   28
   rhythm   172, 174
Syntax   12, 13, 39
Synthetic sentences   124, 208, 220
   Sentence Identification (SSI) Test   124,
      141, 157, 208, 224
Synthesized speech   88
Synthetic speech tests   32

Tamil speech audiometry   284
Tape recorders   78, 95, 243
Temporal processing   25, 26
Temporal distortion   121
Temporal resolution   63, 66, 110
Terminology   110, 207–210
Test of Auditory Comprehension
   (TAC)   270
   duration   40, 48
   interval   237, 281
   items, selection of   41
   material   37
   rooms   84
      background SPL   85
   validity   33
   word spacing   95
Tester   70, 158, 160
Testing time   95
Threshold, ASHA guidelines for
   determining the threshold level of
   speech   113, 209
   definition   209
   for identifiication of speech
      material   112, 119
   free field versus earphone   84
Time Compressed Speech Test   242
TIP Test   219
Token Test   274
Tone group   15, 26, 27
Transition, rate of   14, 175

Uncomfortable Loudness Level
   (ULL)   159
Utah Vowel Imitation Test (U-VIT)   235
Utley Lipreading Test   181, 187
Utterance   12, 13, 15

Velar   19
Velum   22

Vibrotactile sensation 103
  stimulators 32, 197, 235
Videodisc 234
Vietnamese speech audiometry 248
Visemes 232, 233
Visemic categories 182, 185, 195
Visual cue 22, 23, 110
Vocal tract 16, 17, 19, 23
Voice, male/female differences 47
  Onset Time (VOT) 21, 22, 175
Voicing 18, 20, 22, 172, 232
Vowels 12, 18, 172
  contrasts 16, 173, 176
  frequency of occurrence 45
  perception 16, 176
  space 17
  quadrilateral 16–17
  quality 26

Vocoid 13
Volume Unit (VU) Meter 91, 212, 244

Waveform 2–4
Whisper 13, 23
Word boundaries 172
  confusion matrix 57
  familiarity 160
  frequency 46, 47
  test group interchange 104
    equivalence 89
  level measurement 79–82
  **Intelligibility By Picture Identification
    (WIPI) Test** 161, 230, 250
  recognition 58
    score (WRS) 210
  response pattern 54, 55